Improving health in Europe

Characteristics, effectiveness and implementation of different strategies

The European Observatory on Health Systems and Policies supports and promotes evidence-based health policy-making through comprehensive and rigorous analysis of health systems in Europe. It brings together a wide range of policy-makers, academics and practitioners to analyse trends in health reform, drawing on experience from across Europe to illuminate policy issues.

The Observatory is a partnership hosted by the WHO Regional Office for Europe, which includes other international organizations (the European Commission, the World Bank); national and regional governments (Austria, Belgium, Finland, Ireland, Norway, Slovenia, Spain, Sweden, Switzerland, the United Kingdom and the Veneto Region of Italy); other health system organizations (the French National Union of Health Insurance Funds (UNCAM), the Health Foundation); and academia (the London School of Economics and Political Science (LSE) and the London School of Hygiene & Tropical Medicine (LSHTM)). The Observatory has a secretariat in Brussels and it has hubs in London (at LSE and LSHTM) and at the Technical University of Berlin.

Improving healthcare quality in Europe

Characteristics, effectiveness and implementation of different strategies

Edited by:

Reinhard Busse
Niek Klazinga
Dimitra Panteli
Wilm Quentin

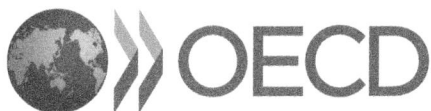

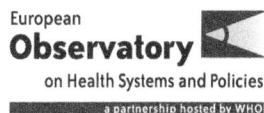

))OECD

European
Observatory
on Health Systems and Policies
a partnership hosted by WHO

Keywords:

QUALITY ASSURANCE, HEALTH CARE - methods
DELIVERY OF HEALTH CARE - standards
OUTCOME AND PROCESS ASSESSMENT (HEALTH CARE)
COST-BENEFIT ANALYSIS
HEALTH POLICY

ISBN 978 92 890 5175 0

OECD ISBN 978 92 648 0590 3

Printed in the United Kingdom

Table of contents

Part I

Chapter 1: An introduction to healthcare quality: defining and explaining its role in health systems   3

Reinhard Busse, Dimitra Panteli, Wilm Quentin

Chapter 2: Understanding healthcare quality strategies: a five-lens framework   19

Dimitra Panteli, Wilm Quentin, Reinhard Busse

Part III

Foreword

from the OECD

Policy-makers and care providers share with patients a key concern: ensuring that people using health services receive the best possible care, which is care that is safe, effective and responsive to their needs. Yet large variation in care outcomes persists both within and across countries. For example, avoidable hospital admissions for chronic conditions such as asthma and chronic obstructive pulmonary disease, indicators of quality of primary healthcare, vary by a factor of nearly 10 between the best and worst performing OECD countries. To take another example, thirty-day mortality after admission to hospital for acute myocardial infarction, an indicator of quality of acute care, varies by a factor of nearly three between Norway and Hungary.

These data signal that more should be done to improve quality, and that strategies to assure and improve quality care must remain at the core of healthcare policy in all OECD and EU countries. Luckily, policy-makers have an arsenal of strategies at their disposal. Many such policies are simple and cheap: think, for example, of basic hygiene policies, which are key to cutting the risk of resistant bacteria spreading in care settings. But policy-makers also must pay close attention to selecting the mix of strategies best fitting their unique conditions and goals. This can be tricky. Evidence about the effectiveness of specific strategies in specific settings is known, but making an informed choice across strategies that address the quality both of a specific healthcare service and of the system as a whole requires more careful consideration. Likewise, policy-makers need to carefully balance intrinsic providers' motivations for improving healthcare delivery with external accountability and transparency of performance, and encourage innovation without creating unnecessary administrative burdens.

Since 2003 the Organisation for Economic Co-operation and Development (OECD) has put quality of care on centre stage, helping countries to better benchmark Health Care Quality and Outcomes and improve quality and safety policies. This book supports this body of knowledge and adds to the fruitful collaboration between OECD and the European Observatory on Health Systems and Policies. It addresses the overall conceptual and measurement challenges and discusses a broad array of quality strategies across European countries. It serves both the policy-maker needing a quick overview of existing strategies and the manager, professional or healthcare user wanting to be informed about the scope and evidence behind specific strategies. It considers more recent strategies, such as the push for patient-centred care and value-based healthcare, alongside strategies such as accreditation, guidelines and audit and feed-back. Although European healthcare systems are the focus, the findings are of wider use to policy-makers seeking to raise quality standards worldwide.

Quality of healthcare services and systems does not come by itself but asks for an informed choice of strategies that work. This book will help to make these choices.

Francesca Colombo

Head Health Division
Organisation for Economic Co-operation and Development
Paris, June 2019

Foreword
from the European Observatory
on Health Systems and Policies

In discussions about universal health coverage, often the essential element of access to healthcare overshadows the understanding that better health can only be achieved if accessed services are also of high quality. The Sustainable Development Goals spell this out quite clearly: "Achieve universal health coverage, including financial risk protection, access to quality essential health-care services and access to safe, effective, quality and affordable essential medicines and vaccines for all" (Goal 3, Target 8). Indeed, ensuring that healthcare services are of good quality is an imperative for policy-makers at all levels and an important contributor to health system performance. As a knowledge-broker, the European Observatory on Health Systems and Policies is committed to transferring evidence into policy practice, by tailoring information for policy-makers in a timely and trustworthy manner (the "4T" principles). This is a particularly opportune time to set the focus of these activities on quality of healthcare.

Indeed, 2018 was a landmark year both for the Observatory and for the field of healthcare quality. The Observatory celebrated its 20th birthday – 20 years of generating evidence and tailoring it to the needs of policy-makers to enable better-informed health system decisions. At the same time important work on assuring and improving quality of care at different levels was published by leading organizations in the field, including WHO, alone (Handbook for national quality policy and strategy) and in collaboration with the OECD and the World Bank (Delivering quality health services: a global imperative for universal health coverage), as well as the National Academies of Sciences, Engineering and Medicine in the United States (Crossing the Global Quality Chasm: Improving Health Care Worldwide). The importance of patient safety, which is an essential component of good quality care and a stand-alone discipline, was reaffirmed at the Third Global Ministerial Summit on Patient Safety, held in Tokyo in April 2018. The summit focused on safety in the context of universal health coverage and culminated in the Tokyo Declaration on Patient Safety, which reiterates the global political commitment to the issue, as well as the necessity for collaboration between patients and practitioners in achieving safer care for all.

The year 2018 also marked the 10th anniversary of the Observatory's first comprehensive study on quality of care (Assuring the quality of health care in the European Union: a case for action, by Helena Legido-Quigley, Martin McKee, Ellen Nolte and Irene Glinos). The 2008 study is a well-cited resource, which provided important conceptual foundations and a mapping of quality-related initiatives in European countries. It highlighted the variability of practices among countries and the vast potential for improvement. It also helped the Observatory identify a significant unmet need for policy-makers: the availability of concentrated, comparable evidence that would help with prioritizing and/or aligning different quality initiatives to achieve separate but complementary goals within a comprehensive approach to quality improvement.

Over the years, and in line with health policy priorities, the Observatory has carried out work on individual strategies that contribute to quality of healthcare (for example on pharmaceutical regulation in 2004, 2016 and 2018; on human resources for health in 2006, 2011 and 2014; on health technology assessment in 2008; on audit and feedback in 2010; on clinical guidelines in 2013; and on public reporting in 2014). However, because "quality of care" is usually defined quite broadly, it is often unclear how the many organizations and movements aiming to improve it fit within a health system and how effective (and cost-effective) they can be. In a general effort to improve quality of care, should the focus be on more stringent regulations for health professionals, on a mandatory, rigorous accreditation of health provider organizations, or on financial incentives in the shape of pay-for-quality payment models? While the recent work on healthcare quality mentioned above provides vital resources to address such challenges, it does not answer these questions directly.

To bridge this gap, the Observatory worked together with the OECD to develop a conceptual framework for this study and to apply it for the collection, synthesis and presentation of evidence. This was motivated both by the experience of previous fruitful and successful collaboration between the two institutions (such as in the volume Paying for Performance in Health Care: Implications for health system performance and accountability, published in 2014) and by the OECD's vast expertise in developing healthcare quality indicators and comparing results across countries. The latter is reflected in the Health Care Quality Indicators (HCQI) project and the OECD's work on international health system performance comparisons.

Fuelled by the complementarity in roles and expertise of the Observatory and the OECD, this study breaks new ground in seven different ways:

i)   it provides conceptual clarity on the definition of quality of care and its link to (and distinction from) health system performance;

ii) it develops a comprehensive framework for categorizing and under-standing strategies aiming to assure or improve quality of care;

iii) it delineates an approach for evaluating different quality strategies based on available evidence regarding current (best) practice, effec-tiveness, cost-effectiveness and implementation;

iv) it fills an important gap by synthesizing and distilling existing knowl-edge on healthcare quality measurement;

v) it sheds light on the role of international and European governance and guidance for quality of healthcare;

vi) it presents – in a comprehensive yet accessible manner – the avail-able evidence on ten common quality strategies, including a culture of patient safety; and

vii) it clarifies the links between different strategies, paving the way for a coherent overall approach to improving healthcare quality.

The described approach fully embodies the principles underpinning the Observatory's work as a knowledge-broker. The Observatory was conceived at the first European Ministerial Conference on health systems in Ljubljana in 1996, as a response to the expressed need of Member States to systematically assess, compare and learn from health system developments and best practices across the European region. While this study focuses primarily on the European context, as a toolkit it can also be used by policy-makers outside Europe, reflect-ing the OECD's mission of promoting policies that will improve the economic and social well-being of people around the world.

Ensuring universal access to healthcare services of high quality is a global aspi-ration. This study joins its recent counterparts in arguing that the battle for healthcare quality is far from won, at any level. The European Observatory on Health Systems and Policies intends to continue its engagement in the field for years to come to aid policy-makers in understanding this dynamic field of knowledge and maintaining the necessary overview to navigate it.

Liisa-Maria Voipio-Pulkki

Chair, Steering Committee
European Observatory European Observatory on Health Systems and Policies

List of tables, figures and boxes

Tables

Figures

Boxes

List of abbreviations

ACGME	Accreditation Council on Graduate Medical Education (US)
AGREE	Appraisal of Guidelines, Research and Evaluation in Europe
AHRQ	Agency for Healthcare Research and Quality in the USA
AIRE	Appraisal of Indicators through Research and Evaluation
AMI	acute myocardial infarction
BSI	British Standards Institution
CABG	coronary artery bypass graft
CanMEDS	Canadian Medical Educational Directives for Specialists
CEN	Comité Européen de Normalisation (European Committee for Standardization)
CHF	congestive heart failure
CME	Continuing Medical Education
CPD	continuous professional development
CPMEC	Confederation of Postgraduate Medical Education Councils (Australia)
CPW	Clinical pathway
CQC	Care Quality Commission
DMP	disease management programme
DRG	Diagnosis-related group
EACCME	European Accreditation Council for Continuing Medical Education
ECAMSQ	European Council for Accreditation of Medical Specialist Qualifications
ECIBC	European Commission Initiative on Breast Cancer
EDAC	Evidence-based Design Assessment and Certification (US)
EDQM	European Directorate for the Quality of Medicines and HealthCare
EFN	European Federation of Nurses
EFQM	European Foundation for Quality Management
EMA	European Medicines Agency
EMR	electronic medical records
EPA	European Pathways Association

EPA	European Practice Assessment
EPAAC	European Partnership for Action against Cancer
EPSO	European Partnership of Supervisory Organisations
ESQH	European Society for Quality in Healthcare
EUDAMED	European Databank on Medical Devices
EuHPN	European Health Property Network
EUnetHTA	European network for Health Technology Assessment
EUNetPaS	European Network for Patient Safety
GMC	General Medical Council
GRADE	Grading of Recommendations Assessment, Development and Evaluation
HAC	hospital-acquired condition
HCPC	Health & Care Professions Council (UK)
HCQI	Health Care Quality Indicators project
HFA	Health for All
HSPA	health systems performance assessment
HSPSC	Hospital Survey on Patient Safety Culture
HTA	health technology assessment
ICD	International Classification of Diseases
INAHTA	International Network of Agencies for Health Technology Assessment
IOM	Institute of Medicine (US)
IQTIG	German Institute for Quality Assurance and Transparency in Health Care
ISO	International Organization for Standardization
ISQua	International Society for Quality in Healthcare
MAGIC	Making GRADE the Irresistible Choice
NASCE	Network of Accredited Clinical Skills Centres in Europe
NHS	National Health Service
NICE	National Institute for Health and Care Excellence
NKLM	National Competence Based Catalogue of Learning Objectives for Undergraduate Medical Education
NMC	Nursing and Midwifery Council (UK)
NQF	National Quality Forum (US)
N-RCT	Non-randomized controlled trials
OECD	Organisation for Economic Co-operation and Development
P4Q	Pay for Quality
PAS	Publicly Available Specification

PDCA	plan-do-check-act cycle
PDSA	plan-do-study-act cycle
PREM	patient-reported experience measures
PROM	patient-reported outcome measures
QALYs	quality-adjusted life-years
QIS	quality improvement systems
QM	quality management
QOF	Quality and Outcomes Framework
RCT	Randomized controlled trials
SAQ	Safety Attitudes Questionnaire
SDG	Sustainable Development Goals
SHI	Social health insurance
SimPatiE	Safety Improvement for Patients in Europe
SPR	single-occupancy patient rooms
UEMS	European Union of Medical Specialists

Author affiliations

Elke Berger, Research Fellow, Department of Health Care Management, Berlin University of Technology

Ian Brownwood, Coordinator Health Care Quality and Outcomes Health Division, Organisation for Economic Co-operation and Development

Reinhard Busse, Professor, Head of Department, Department of Health Care Management, Berlin University of Technology

Mirella Cacace, Professor of Health Care Systems and Health Policy, Catholic University of Applied Sciences Freiburg

Michael Cheng, Biomedical Engineer, Ottawa, Canada

Agnieszka Daval, Director Government and Public Affairs, Philips European Affairs Office

Robert Baatenburg de Jong, Professor and Chairman of the Department of Ear, Nose and Throat (ENT), Cancer Institute, Erasmus MC

Frederic Destrebecq, Executive Director, European Brain Council

Helene Eckhardt, Research Fellow, Department of Health Care Management, Berlin University of Technology

Jonathan Erskine, Executive Director, European Health Property Network, and Honorary Fellow, Durham University

Sara Evans Lacko, Associate Professorial Research Fellow, London School of Economics and Political Sciences, Personal Social Services Research Unit (PSSRU), UK

Signe Flottorp, Research Director, Division of Health Services, Norwegian Institute of Public Health, and Professor, Institute of Health and Society, University of Oslo, Norway

Pascal Garel, Chief Executive, European Hospital and Healthcare Federation (HOPE)

Max Geraedts, Professor, Institute for Health Services Research and Clinical Epidemiology, Department of Medicine, Philipps-Universität Marburg

Oliver Groene, Vice Chairman of the Board, OptiMedis AG, and Honorary Senior Lecturer, London School of Hygiene and Tropical Medicine, UK.

Noah Ivers, Family Physician, Chair in Implementation Science, Women's College Hospital, University of Toronto

Gro Jamtvedt, Dean and Professor, OsloMet – Oslo Metropolitan University, Faculty of Health Sciences

Leigh Kinsman, Joint Chair, professor of Evidence Based Nursing, School of Nursing and Midwifery, University of Newcastle and Mid North Coast Local Health District

Niek Klazinga, Head of the OECD Health Care Quality Indicator Programme, Organisation for Economic Co-operation and Development, and Professor of Social Medicine, Academic Medical Centre, University of Amsterdam

Oliver Komma, Outpatient Clinic Manager, MonorMED Outpatient Clinic

Anika Kreutzberg, Research Fellow, Department of Health Care Management, Berlin University of Technology

Finn Borlum Kristensen, Professor, Department of Public Health, University of Southern Denmark

Solvejg Kristensen, Programme Leader PRO-Psychiatry, Aalborg University Hospital – Psychiatry, Denmark

Helena Legido-Quigley, Associate Professor, Saw Swee Hock School of Public Health, National University of Singapore and London School of Hygiene and Tropical Medicine

Claudia Bettina Maier, Senior Research Fellow, Department of Health Care Management, Berlin University of Technology

Grant Mills, Senior Lecturer, The Bartlett School of Construction and Project Management, University College London

Camilla Palmhøj Nielsen, Research Director, DEFACTUM, Central Denmark Region

Günter Ollenschläger, Professor, Institute for Health Economics and Clinical Epidemiology (IGKE), University Hospital Cologne

Willy Palm, Senior Adviser, European Observatory on Health Systems and Policies

Dimitra Panteli, Senior Research Fellow, Department of Health Care Management, Berlin University of Technology

Veli-Matti Partanen, Researcher, Finnish Cancer Registry

Miek Peeters, Internal Market Affairs Officer, EFTA Surveillance Authority

Wilm Quentin, Senior Research Fellow, Department of Health Care Management, Berlin University of Technology

Christoph Reichebner, Research Assistant, Department of Health Care Management, Berlin University of Technology

Ulrich Ronellenfitsch, Assistant Professor of Surgery, Department of Visceral, Vascular and Endocrine Surgery, University Hospital Halle (Saale), Germany

Thomas Rotter, Associate Professor, Healthcare Quality Programmes, School of Nursing, Queen's University

Corinna Schaefer, PhD, Head of Department for Evidence-based Medicines and Guidelines, Medical Center for Quality in Health Care

Charles Shaw, Independent Consultant on Quality in Health Care

Peter C. Smith, Peter C. Smith, Professor Emeritus, Imperial College London and Professor, Centre for Health Economics, University of York.

Paulo Sousa, Professor, National School of Public Health, Universidade Nova de Lisboa

Cordula Wagner, Executive Director, Netherlands Institute of Health Services Research (NIVEL), and Professor of Patient Safety, VU University Medical Center Amsterdam

Acknowledgements

This volume is the result of a collaboration between the European Observatory on Health Systems and Policies and the Health Division of the Organisation for Economic Co-operation and Development (OECD). We are very grateful to all the authors for their hard work, patience and enthusiasm in this project. We wish to thank Marcial Velasco-Garrido, Jan-Arne Rottingen and Ellen Nolte for their conceptual support and engagement in the early stages of the project, as well as Friedrich Wittenbecher, Josep Figueras and Ewout van Ginneken for their support during different stages of the project.

We are particularly grateful to the reviewers of the volume for their helpful comments and suggestions: Thomas Custers, Damir Ivankovic, Basia Kutryba and Mike Rozijn.

Over the years, this project benefited from substantial technical support from staff at the Department of Health Care Management, Berlin University of Technology, including Judith Lukacs, Maximilien Hjortland and Christoph Reichebner.

The book incorporates input gathered at an initial authors' workshop in the summer of 2012, at a meeting with the European Commission's DG Santé in February 2013, at the Observatory's Steering Committee meeting in June 2016, at the European Public Health conference in Stockholm in November 2017, and at the Observatory Summer School in Venice in July 2018. We appreciate the contributions of those who participated in these events.

Finally, this book would not have appeared without the hard work of the production team led by Jonathan North, with the able assistance of Caroline White, Sarah Cook and Nick Gorman.

Part I

Chapter 1

An introduction to healthcare quality: defining and explaining its role in health systems

Reinhard Busse, Dimitra Panteli, Wilm Quentin

1.1 The relevance of quality in health policy

Quality of care is one of the most frequently quoted principles of health policy, and it is currently high up on the agenda of policy-makers at national, European and international levels (EC, 2016; OECD, 2017; WHO, 2018; WHO/OECD/World Bank, 2018). At the national level, addressing the issue of healthcare quality may be motivated by various reasons – ranging from a general commitment to high-quality healthcare provision as a public good or the renewed focus on patient outcomes in the context of popular value-based healthcare ideas to the identification of specific healthcare quality problems (*see* Box 1.1).

Box 1.1 *Reasons for (re)focusing on quality of care*

- Belief in and commitment to quality healthcare as a public good
- Growing awareness of gaps in safe, effective and person-centred care
- Increasing concerns about substantial practice variations in standards of healthcare delivery
- Renewed emphasis on improving patient outcomes in the context of currently popular value-based healthcare ideas
- Expectations from the public, media and civil society, with a growing public demand for transparency and accountability
- Drive towards universal health coverage and the understanding that improvements in access without appropriate attention to quality will not lead to the desired population health outcomes

---

- Growing recognition of the need to align the performance of public and private healthcare delivery in fragmented and mixed health markets
- Increasing understanding of the critical importance of trusted services for effective preparedness for outbreaks or other complex emergencies

Source: based on WHO, 2018, with modifications

At the European level, the European Council's Conclusions on the Common Values and Principles in European Union Health Systems highlight that "the overarching values of universality, access to good quality care, equity, and solidarity have been widely accepted in the work of the different EU institutions" (European Council, 2006). The European Commission (EC, 2014; EC, 2016) also recognizes quality as an important component of health system performance (i.e. the extent to which health systems meet their goals; we return to the link between quality and performance later in the chapter).

At the international level, quality is receiving increasing attention in the context of the Sustainable Development Goals (SDGs), as the SDGs include the imperative to "achieve universal health coverage, including financial risk protection, access to quality essential health-care services and access to safe, effective, quality and affordable essential medicines and vaccines for all". This is reflected in two World Health Organization (WHO) reports published in 2018, a handbook for national quality policies and strategies (WHO, 2018) and a guide aiming to facilitate the global understanding of quality as part of universal health coverage aspirations (WHO/OECD/World Bank, 2018).

A previous study on quality of care by the European Observatory on Health Systems and Policies (Legido-Quigley et al., 2008) noted that the literature on quality of care in health systems was already very extensive and difficult to systematize ten years ago – and this is even truer today. Research is available on a vast range of approaches or strategies for assuring or improving quality of care, often focusing on certain organizations (hospitals, health centres, practices) or particular areas of care (emergency care, maternal care, etc.) (Flodgren, Gonçalves & Pomey, 2016; Ivers et al., 2014; Houle et al., 2012; Gharaveis et al., 2018). This body of evidence has contributed to a better understanding of the effectiveness of particular interventions in particular settings for particular groups of patients. However, the available literature rarely addresses the question of the superiority of individual strategies and usually does not provide guidance to policy-makers on which strategy to implement in a particular setting.

In addition, despite the vast literature base and the universal acknowledgement of its importance in health systems, there is no common understanding of the term "quality of care", and there is disagreement about what it encompasses. The definition of quality often differs across contexts, disciplinary paradigms and levels of analysis. Yet, as prescribed by the seminal work of Avedis Donabedian (1980), assessing and improving quality predicates an understanding of what it entails. Therefore, the aim of this chapter is to provide clarity about the definition of quality and its relation to health system performance as well as introduce the level of analysis adopted in this book. The chapter concludes with a brief introduction to the aims and the structure of the book.

1.2 Definitions of healthcare quality

Early definitions of healthcare quality were shaped almost exclusively by health professionals and health service researchers. However, there has been increasing recognition that the preferences and views of patients, the public and other key players are highly relevant as well (Legido-Quigley et al., 2008). Table 1.1 summarizes some of the most influential definitions of healthcare quality from different contexts, starting with the definition of Donabedian (1980) and ending with the definition provided by WHO's handbook for national quality policy and strategy (WHO, 2018).

Table 1.1   *Selected definitions of quality, 1980–2018*

Donabedian (1980) In: *"Explorations in quality assessment and monitoring. The definition of quality and approaches to its assessment"*	Quality of care is the kind of care which is expected to maximize an inclusive measure of patient welfare, after one has taken account of the balance of expected gains and losses that attend the process of care in all its parts. *[More generally, quality in this work is "the ability to achieve desirable objectives using legitimate means".]*
Institute of Medicine, IOM (1990) In: *"Medicare: A Strategy for Quality Assurance"*	Quality of care is the degree to which health services for individuals and populations increase the likelihood of desired health outcomes and are consistent with current professional knowledge.
Council of Europe (1997) In: *"The development and implementation of quality improvement systems (QIS) in health care. Recommendation No. R (97) 17"*	Quality of care is the degree to which the treatment dispensed increases the patient's chances of achieving the desired results and diminishes the chances of undesirable results, having regard to the current state of knowledge.
European Commission (2010) In: *"Quality of Health care: policy actions at EU level. Reflection paper for the European Council"*	[Good quality care is] health care that is effective, safe and responds to the needs and preference of patients. *The Paper also notes that "Other dimensions of quality of care, such as efficiency, access and equity, are seen as being part of a wider debate and are being addressed in other fora."*
WHO (2018) In: *"Handbook for national quality policy and strategy"*	Quality health services across the world should be: • Effective: providing evidence-based health care services to those who need them. • Safe: avoiding harm to people for whom the care is intended. • People-centred: providing care that responds to individual preferences, needs and values. In order to realize the benefits of quality health care, health services must be timely [...], equitable [...], integrated [...], and efficient [...]

Donabedian defined quality in general terms as "the ability to achieve desirable objectives using legitimate means". This definition reflects the fact that the term "quality" is not specific to healthcare and is used by many different people in various sectors of society. People use the term quality when they describe a range of positive aspects of hospitals and doctors – but also when they speak about food or cars. In fact, the widespread use of the term quality explains part of the confusion around the concept of healthcare quality when policy-makers or researchers use the term for all kinds of positive or desirable attributes of health systems. However, Donabedian also provides a more specific definition of quality of care, stating that it is "care which is expected to maximize an inclusive measure of patient welfare, after one has taken account of the balance of expected gains and losses that attend the process of care in all its parts" (Donabedian, 1980).

Donabedian's definition is interesting because it specifies that quality of care is related to the process of care in all its parts and that the goal of high-quality care is to maximize patient welfare. Patient welfare certainly includes the health status of the patient (later specified as encompassing physical, physiological and psychological dimensions; *see also* Donabedian, Wheeler & Wyszewianski, 1982). However, the concept of patient welfare is also in line with an approach that considers what patients find important. Furthermore, Donabedian's definition recognizes the natural limits of quality and its improvement, by highlighting that gains and losses are expected in the process of care.

A decade later the Institute of Medicine (IOM) in the US defined quality of care as "the degree to which health services for individuals and populations increase the likelihood of desired health outcomes and are consistent with current professional knowledge" (*see* Table 1.1). At first glance, the IOM's definition's focus on "health outcomes" seems to be more restrictive than Donabedian's notion of "patient welfare". However, in their elaboration of the definition, the IOM specified that these "desired" health outcomes were expected to reflect patient satisfaction and well-being next to broad health status or quality-of-life measures. The IOM's definition has inspired the understanding of quality by many other organizations in the USA and internationally.

In contrast to other popular definitions of quality in healthcare around that time (including Donabedian's), which mainly referred to medical or patient care, the IOM's definition set the focus on health services in general (as "health care implies a broad set of services, including acute, chronic, preventive, restorative, and rehabilitative care, which are delivered in many different settings by many different health care providers") and on individuals and populations (rather than patients), thus strengthening the link of quality with prevention and health promotion. Finally, the concept of "current professional knowledge" both reinforced the movement for evidence-based care and highlighted that the concept of quality is dynamic and continuously evolving. In that sense, providers can only be assessed against the current state of knowledge as a service that is considered "good quality" at any given time may be regarded as "poor quality" twenty years later in light of newer insights and alternatives.

The definition of quality by the Council of Europe included in Table 1.1, published seven years after the IOM's definition as part of the Council's recommendations on quality improvement systems for EU Member States, is the first to explicitly include considerations about the aspect of patient safety. It argues that quality of care is not only "the degree to which the treatment dispensed increases the patient's chances of achieving the desired results", which basically repeats the IOM definition, but it goes on to specify that high-quality care also "diminishes the chances of undesirable results" (The Council of Europe, 1997). In the same document the Council of Europe also explicitly defines a range of dimensions of quality of care – but, surprisingly, does not include safety among them.

The final two definitions included in Table 1.1 are from the European Commission (2010) and from WHO (2018). In contrast to those discussed so far, both of these definitions describe quality by specifying three main dimensions or attributes: effectiveness, safety and responsiveness or patient-centredness. It is not by chance that both definitions are similar as they were both strongly influenced by the work of the OECD's Health Care Quality Indicators (HCQI) project (Arah et al., 2006; *see* below). These final two definitions are interesting also because they list a number of further attributes of healthcare and healthcare systems that are related to quality of care, including access, timeliness, equity and efficiency. However, they note that these other elements are either "part of a wider debate" (EC, 2010) or "necessary to realize the benefits of quality health care" (WHO, 2018), explicitly distinguishing core dimensions of quality from other attributes of good healthcare.

In fact, the dimensions of quality of care have been the focus of considerable debate over the past forty years. The next section focuses on this international discussion around the dimensions of quality of care.

1.3 Dimensions of healthcare quality

As mentioned earlier, Donabedian posited that assessing and improving quality of care presupposes an understanding of what it does and does not entail. Different definitions of quality often specify relatively long lists of various attributes that they recognize as part of quality. Table 1.2 provides an overview of the dimensions of quality mentioned by ten selected definitions (including those in Table 1.1).

The table shows that effectiveness, patient safety and responsiveness/patient-centredness seem to have become universally accepted as core dimensions of quality of care. However, many definitions – also beyond those shown in Table 1.2 – include attributes such as appropriateness, timeliness, efficiency, access and equity. This is confusing and often blurs the line between quality of care and overall health system performance. In an attempt to order these concepts, the table classifies its entries into core dimensions of quality, subdimensions that contribute to core dimensions of quality, and other dimensions of health system performance.

This distinction is based on the framework of the OECD HCQI project, which was first published in 2006 (Arah et al., 2006). The purpose of the framework was to guide the development of indicators for international comparisons of healthcare quality. The HCQI project selected the three dimensions of effectiveness, safety and patient-centredness as the core dimensions of healthcare quality, arguing that other attributes, such as appropriateness, continuity, timeliness and acceptability, could easily be accommodated within these three dimensions. For example, appropriateness could be mapped into effectiveness, whereas continuity and acceptability could be absorbed into patient-centredness. Accessibility, efficiency and equity were also considered to be important goals of health systems. However, the HCQI team argued – referring to the IOM (1990) definition – that only effectiveness, safety and responsiveness are attributes of healthcare that directly contribute to "increasing the likelihood of desired outcomes".

Some definitions included in Table 1.2 were developed for specific purposes and this is reflected in their content. As mentioned above, the Council of Europe (1997) definition was developed to guide the development of quality improvement systems. Therefore, it is not surprising that it includes the assessment of the process of care as an element of quality on top of accessibility, efficacy, effectiveness, efficiency and patient satisfaction.

In 2001 the IOM published "Crossing the Quality Chasm", an influential report which specified that healthcare should pursue six major aims: it should be safe, effective, patient-centred, timely, efficient and equitable. These six principles have been adopted by many organizations inside and outside the United States as the six dimensions of quality, despite the fact that the IOM itself clearly set them out as "performance expectations" ("a list of performance characteristics that, if addressed and improved, would lead to better achievement of that overarching purpose. To this end, the committee proposes six specific aims for improvement. Health care should be …"; IOM, 2001). For example, WHO (2006b) adapted these principles as quality dimensions in its guidance for making strategic choices in health systems, transforming the concept of timeliness into "accessibility" to include geographic availability and progressivity of health service provision. However, this contributed to the confusion and debate about quality versus other dimensions of performance.

The European Commission's Expert Panel on Effective Ways for Investing in Health Care also opted for a broad consideration of quality, including the dimensions of appropriateness, equity and efficiency in its recommendations for the future EU agenda on quality of care in 2014 (EC, 2014). Similarly, WHO (2016) used timeliness (as originally described by the IOM) instead of accessibility (as used by WHO in 2006b), and added integration in healthcare provision as a dimension of high-quality care, in line with the approach taken by the Health Care Council of Canada (Health Care Council of Canada, 2013). The understanding of integrated care as part of patient-centredness can also be found in the updated version of the HCQI framework published by the OECD in 2015 (Carinci et al., 2015).

This long and inconsistent list of different dimensions inevitably contributes to the confusion about the concept of quality of care. However, conceptual clarity about quality is crucial, as it will influence the types of healthcare policies and strategies that are adopted to improve it. Part of the confusion around the demarcation between quality of care and health system performance originates from insufficiently distinguishing between intermediate and final goals of health systems and between different levels at which quality can be addressed.

The next section aims to provide more clarity about the role of quality in health systems and health systems performance assessment by highlighting the difference between healthcare service quality and healthcare system quality. In so doing, the section sets the background for the way quality is understood in the remainder of the book.

1.4 The role of quality in health systems and health system performance assessment

Numerous frameworks have been developed over the past 20 years with the aim of facilitating a better understanding of health systems and enabling health system performance assessments (Papanicolas, 2013; Fekri, Macarayan & Klazinga, 2018). Most of these frameworks implicitly or explicitly include quality as an important health system goal but they differ in how they define quality and how they describe its contribution to overall health system goals. A particularly influential framework is the WHO (2006a) "building blocks" framework for health systems strengthening (*see* Fig. 1.1). The framework conceptualizes health systems in terms of building blocks, including service delivery, health workforce, information, medical products, financing and leadership/governance. In addition, the framework defines quality and safety as intermediate goals of health systems, together with access and coverage. Achievement of these intermediate goals will ultimately contribute to achieving overall health system goals of improved health, responsiveness, financial protection and improved efficiency.

Table 1.2 *Quality dimensions in ten selected definitions of quality, 1980–2018*

		Donabedian (1980)	IOM (1990)	Council of Europe (1997)	IOM (2001)	OECD (2006)	WHO (2006b)	EC (2010)	EC (2014)	WHO (2016)	WHO (2018)
Core dimensions of healthcare quality	Effectiveness	X	X	X	X	X	X	X	X	X	X
	Safety			X	X	X	X	X	X	X	X
	Responsiveness			X	Patient-centredness	X	Patient-centredness	X	Patient-centredness	Patient-centredness	Patient-centredness
	Acceptability						X				
	Appropriateness			X					X		
	Continuity										
Subdimensions (related to core dimensions)	Timeliness				X					X	X
	Satisfaction		X	X							
	Health improvement		X	X							
	Other	Patient Welfare		Assessment of care process				Patient's preferences		Integration	Integration
Other dimensions of health systems performance	Efficiency		X	X	X	X	X	X	X	X	X
	Access			X		X	X				
	Equity		X	X	X	X	X	X	X	X	X

Fig. 1.1   *Quality is an intermediate goal of health systems*

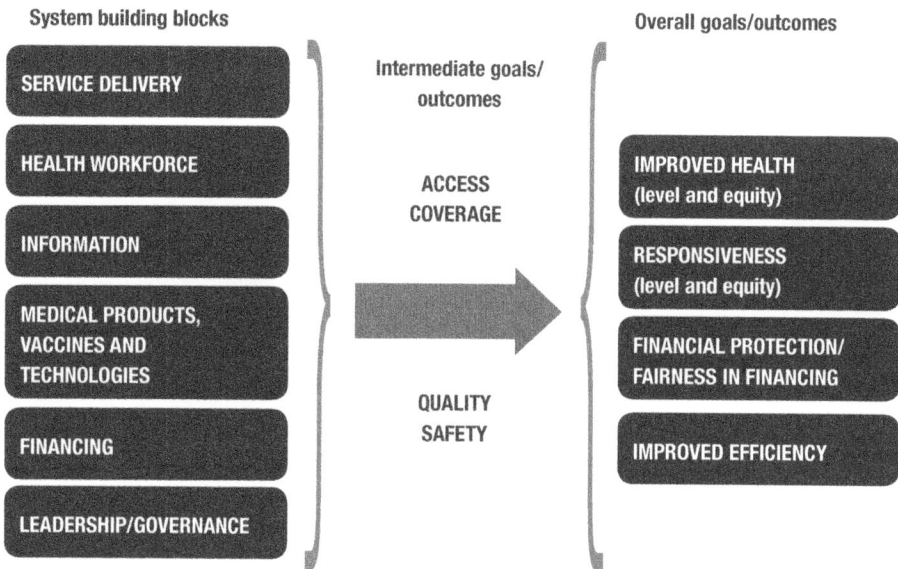

System building blocks   Overall goals/outcomes

SERVICE DELIVERY	Intermediate goals/ outcomes	
HEALTH WORKFORCE	ACCESS COVERAGE	IMPROVED HEALTH (level and equity)
INFORMATION		RESPONSIVENESS (level and equity)
MEDICAL PRODUCTS, VACCINES AND TECHNOLOGIES		FINANCIAL PROTECTION/ FAIRNESS IN FINANCING
FINANCING	QUALITY SAFETY	IMPROVED EFFICIENCY
LEADERSHIP/GOVERNANCE		

Source: WHO, 2006

It is worth noting that quality and safety are mentioned separately in the framework, while most of the definitions of quality discussed above include safety as a core dimension of quality. For more information about the relationship between quality and safety, *see also* Chapter 11.

As mentioned above, Donabedian defined quality in general terms as "the ability to achieve desirable objectives using legitimate means" (Donabedian, 1980). Combining Donabedian's general definition of quality with the WHO building blocks framework (Fig. 1.1), one could argue that a health system is "of high quality" when it achieves these (overall and intermediate) goals using legitimate means. In addition, Donabedian highlighted that it is important to distinguish between different levels when assessing healthcare quality (Donabedian, 1988). He distinguished between four levels at which quality can be assessed – individual practitioners, the care setting, the care received (and implemented) by the patient, and the care received by the community. Others have conceptualized different levels at which policy developments with regard to quality may take place: the health system (or "macro") level, the organizational ("meso") level and the clinical ("micro") level (Øvretveit, 2001).

While the exact definition of levels is not important, it is essential to recognize that the definition of quality changes depending on the level at which it is assessed. For simplicity purposes, we condense Donabedian's four tiers into two conceptually distinct levels (*see* Fig. 1.2). The first, narrower level is the level of health services, which may include preventive, acute, chronic and palliative care (Arah et al., 2006). At this level, there seems to be an emerging consensus that "quality of care is the degree to which health services for individuals and populations are effective, safe and people-centred" (WHO, 2018).

The second level is the level of the healthcare system as a whole. Healthcare systems are "of high quality" when they achieve the overall goals of improved health, responsiveness, financial protection and efficiency. Many of the definitions of healthcare quality included in Table 1.2 seem to be concerned with healthcare system quality as they include these attributes among stated quality dimensions. However, such a broad definition of healthcare quality can be problematic in the context of quality improvement: while it is undoubtedly important to address access and efficiency in health systems, confusion about the focus of quality improvement initiatives may distract attention away from those strategies that truly contribute to increasing effectiveness, safety and patient-centredness of care.

Fig. 1.2 *Two levels of healthcare quality*

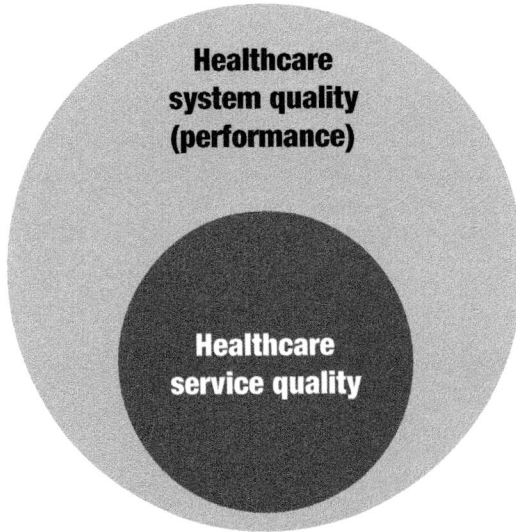

To avoid confusion and achieve conceptual clarity, we therefore propose reserving the use of the term "healthcare quality" for the first level, i.e. the healthcare services level. Concerning the second level, i.e. the health(care) system level, there seems to be an international trend towards using the term "health system performance" to describe the degree to which health systems achieve their overall and intermediate goals.

Frameworks to assess health system performance by the OECD (Carinci, 2015) and the European Commission (2014) include healthcare quality at the service level as a core dimension – besides other elements of performance such as accessibility, efficiency and population health. In other words, health system performance is a better term for health system "quality" (according to Donabedian's broad definition of the term), and healthcare service quality is one of its core components.

The relationship between quality and the achievement of final health system goals is aptly illustrated in another, relatively recent framework for health system performance comparisons (Fig. 1.3). The framework has condensed the four intermediate goals of the WHO building blocks model into only two: access (including coverage) and quality (including safety). It posits that population health outcomes and system responsiveness depend on the extent to which the entire population has access to care and the extent to which health services are of good quality (i.e. they are effective, safe and patient-centred). The resources, financial or otherwise, required to produce final health system goals determine efficiency in the system.

Fig. 1.3   *The link between health system performance and quality of healthcare services*

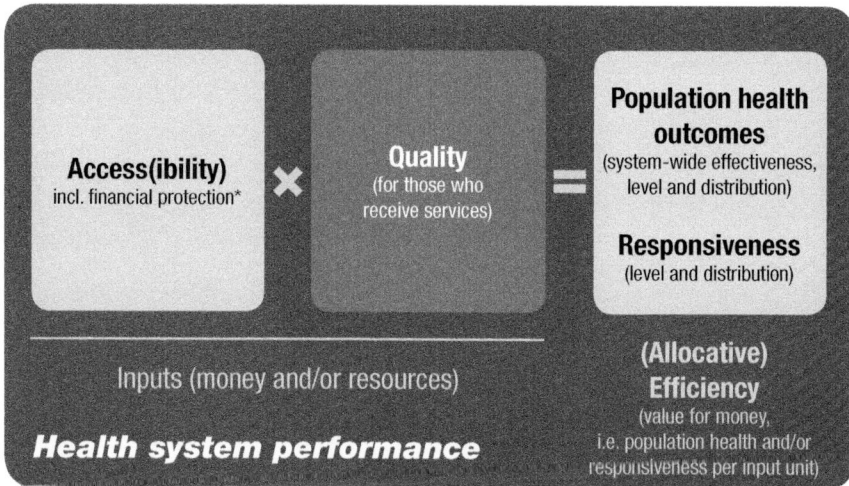

Access(ibility)
incl. financial protection*

×

Quality
(for those who receive services)

=

Population health outcomes
(system-wide effectiveness, level and distribution)

Responsiveness
(level and distribution)

Inputs (money and/or resources)

(Allocative) Efficiency
(value for money, i.e. population health and/or responsiveness per input unit)

Health system performance

Source: Busse, 2017.
Note: *Financial protection is both an enabling condition for access as well as a final outcome.

The framework highlights that health systems have to ensure both access to care *and* quality in order to achieve the final health system goals. However, it is important to distinguish conceptually between access and quality because very different strategies are needed to improve access (for example, improving financial protection, ensuring geographic availability of providers) than are needed to improve quality of care. This book focuses on quality and explores the potential of different strategies to improve it.

1.5 What are quality improvement strategies? Aims and structure of this book

As mentioned in the Preface, the purpose of the book is to provide a framework for understanding, measuring and ultimately improving the quality of healthcare through a variety of strategies. In general, a strategy can be viewed as an approach or plan that is designed or selected to achieve a desired outcome (for example, attain a goal or reach a solution to a problem). The 2018 WHO Handbook for National Quality Policy and Strategy differentiates between the two titular concepts by underlining that policy refers to an agreed ambition for the health system with an explicit statement of intention, i.e. a "course of action". Accordingly, it would usually mainly outline broad priorities to be addressed rather than the concrete steps to address them. The corresponding strategy, on the other hand, provides a clear roadmap for achieving these priorities (WHO, 2018). In this conceptualization, a number of tools, or interventions, can be used to implement the strategy and aid in the attainment of its milestones.

For the purpose of this book, we use the term "strategy" more narrowly and in a sectoral way to denote a mechanism of action geared towards achieving specific quality assurance or improvement goals by addressing specific targets within healthcare provision (for example, health professionals, provider organizations or health technologies). For example, we consider accreditation of healthcare providers and clinical practice guidelines as quality strategies, whereas the same concepts would be described as "quality interventions", "quality initiatives", "quality improvement tools" or "quality improvement activities" elsewhere.

Table 1.3 summarizes a range of selected quality strategies (or interventions) and clusters them into system level strategies, institutional/organizational strategies and patient/community level strategies. This categorization follows the one used by the OECD in its Country Quality Reviews and the recent report on the economics of patient safety (OECD, 2017; Slawomirksi, Auraaen & Klazinga, 2017). Table 1.3 also includes strategies listed in the 2018 WHO Handbook (WHO, 2018), as well as a few others. The strategies discussed in more detail in the second part of this book are marked in grey in the table.

As becomes evident in Table 1.3, the focus of this book is on system level and organizational/institutional level strategies. Its aim is to provide guidance to policy-makers who have to make choices about investing political and economic resources into the implementation or scale-up of different options from this vast number of different strategies. The book does not attempt to rank the best quality strategies to be implemented across countries, because different strategies will need to be prioritized depending on the motivation, the identified quality improvement needs and the existing structures or initiatives already in place. Instead, it hopes (1) to provide an overview of the experience with the

Table 1.3 *A selection of prominent quality strategies (marked in grey are the strategies discussed in Chapters 5 to 14 of this book)*

System level strategies	Organizational/institutional level strategies	Patient/community level interventions
Legal framework for quality assurance and improvement	Clinical quality governance systems	Formalized patient and community engagement and empowerment
Training and supervision of the workforce	Clinical decision support tools	Improving health literacy
Regulation and licensing of physicians and other health professionals	Clinical guidelines	Shared decision-making
Regulation and licensing of technologies (pharmaceuticals and devices)	Clinical pathways and protocols	Peer support and expert patient groups
Regulation and licensing of provider organizations/institutions	Clinical audit and feedback	Monitoring patient experience of care
External assessments: accreditation, certification and supervision of providers	Morbidity and mortality reviews	Patient self-management tools
Public reporting and comparative benchmarking	Collaborative and team-based improvement cycles	Self-management
Quality-based purchasing and contracting	Procedural/surgical checklists	
Pay-for-quality initiatives	Adverse event reporting	
Electronic Health Record (HER) systems	Human resource interventions	
Disease Management Programmes	Establishing a patient safety culture	

Source: authors' own compilation based on Slawomirksi, Auraaen & Klazinga, 2017, and WHO, 2018.

selected strategies to date in Europe and beyond, (2) to summarize the available evidence on their effectiveness and – where available – cost-effectiveness and the prerequisites for their implementation, and (3) to provide recommendations to policy-makers about how to select and actually implement different strategies.

The book is structured in three parts. Part I includes four chapters and deals with cross-cutting issues that are relevant for all quality strategies. Part II includes ten chapters each dealing with specific strategies. Part III focuses on overall conclusions for policy-makers.

The aim of Part I is to clarify concepts and frameworks that can help policy-makers to make sense of the different quality strategies explored in Part II. Chapter 2 introduces a comprehensive framework that enables a systematic analysis of the key characteristics of different quality strategies. Chapter 3 summarizes different approaches and data sources for measuring quality. Chapter 4 explores the role of international governance and guidance, in particular at EU level, to foster and support quality in European countries.

Part II, comprising Chapters 5 to 14, provides clearly structured and detailed information about ten of the quality strategies presented in Table 1.3 (those marked in grey). Each chapter in Part II follows roughly the same structure, explaining the rationale of the strategy, exploring its use in Europe and summarizing the available evidence about its effectiveness and cost-effectiveness. This is followed by a discussion of practical aspects related to the implementation of the strategy and conclusions for policy-makers. In addition, each chapter is accompanied by an abstract that follows the same structure as the chapter and summarizes the main points on one or two pages.

Finally, Part III concludes with the main findings from the previous parts of the book, summarizing the available evidence about quality strategies in Europe and providing recommendations for policy-makers.

References

Arah OA et al. (2006). A conceptual framework for the OECD Health Care Quality Indicators Project. *International Journal for Quality in Health Care*, 18(S1):5–13.

Busse R (2017). High Performing Health Systems: Conceptualizing, Defining, Measuring and Managing. Presentation at the "Value in Health Forum: Standards, Quality and Economics". Edmonton, 19 January 2017.

Carinci F et al. (2015). Towards actionable international comparisons of health system performance: expert revision of the OECD framework and quality indicators. *International Journal for Quality in Health Care*, 27(2):137–46.

Donabedian A (1980). The Definition of Quality and Approaches to Its Assessment. Vol 1. Explorations in Quality Assessment and Monitoring. Ann Arbor, Michigan, USA: Health Administration Press.

Donabedian A (1988). The quality of care. How can it be assessed? *Journal of the American Medical Association*, 260(12):1743–8.

Donabedian A, Wheeler JR, Wyszewianski L (1982). Quality, cost, and health: an integrative model. *Medical Care*, 20(10):975–92.

EC (2010). EU Actions on Patient Safety and Quality of Healthcare. European Commission, Healthcare Systems Unit. Madrid: European Commission.

EC (2014). Communication from the Commission – On effective, accessible and resilient health systems. European Commission. Brussels: European Commission.

EC (2016). So What? Strategies across Europe to assess quality of care. Report by the Expert Group on Health Systems Performance Assessment. European Commission (EC). Brussels: European Commission.

European Council (2006). Council Conclusions on Common values and principles in European Union Health Systems. *Official Journal of the European Union*, C146:1–2.

Fekri O, Macarayan ER, Klazinga N (2018). Health system performance assessment in the WHO European Region: which domains and indicators have been used by Member States for its measurement? Copenhagen: WHO Regional Office for Europe (Health Evidence Network (HEN) synthesis report 55).

Flodgren G, Gonçalves-Bradley DC, Pomey MP (2016). External inspection of compliance with standards for improved healthcare outcomes. Cochrane Database Syst Rev. 12: CD008992. doi: 10.1002/14651858.CD008992.pub3.

Gharaveis A et al. (2018). The Impact of Visibility on Teamwork, Collaborative Communication, and Security in Emergency Departments: An Exploratory Study. *HERD: Health Environments Research & Design Journal*, 11(4):37–49.

Health Council of Canada (2013). Better health, better care, better value for all: refocussing health care reform in Canada. Toronto, Health Care Council of Canada; 2013.

Houle SK et al. (2012). Does performance-based remuneration for individual health care practitioners affect patient care? A systematic review. *Annals of Internal Medicine*, 157(12):889–99.

IOM (1990). Medicare: A Strategy for Quality Assurance: Volume 1. Washington (DC), US: National Academies Press.

IOM (2001). Crossing the Quality Chasm: A New Health System for the 21st Century. Washington (DC), US: National Academies Press.

Ivers N et al. (2014). Growing literature, stagnant science? Systematic review, meta-regression and cumulative analysis of audit and feedback interventions in health care. *Journal of General Internal Medicine*, 29(11):1534–41.

Legido-Quigley H et al. (2008). Assuring the Quality of Health Care in the European Union: A case for action. Observatory Studies Series, 12. Copenhagen: WHO on behalf of the European Observatory on Health Systems and Policies.

OECD (2017). Caring for Quality in Health: Lessons learnt from 15 reviews of health care quality. OECD Reviews of Health Care Quality. Paris: OECD Publishing. Available at: http://dx.doi.org/10.1787/9789264267787-en, accessed 9 April 2019.

Øvretveit J (2001). Quality evaluation and indicator comparison in health care. *International Journal of Health Planning Management*, 16:229–41.

Papanicolas I (2013). International frameworks for health system comparison. In: Papanicolas I & Smith P (eds.): Health system performance comparison: An agenda for policy, information and research. European Observatory on Health Systems and Policies, Open University Press. New York.

Slawomirski L, Auraaen A, Klazinga N (2017). The economics of patient safety. Paris: Organisation for Economic Co-operation and Development.

The Council of Europe (1997). The development and implementation of quality improvement systems (QIS) in health care. Recommendation No. R (97) 17 and explanatory memorandum. Strasbourg: The Council of Europe.

WHO (2006a). Everybody's business: Strengthening health systems to improve health outcomes: WHO's framework for action. Geneva: World Health Organization.

WHO (2006b). Quality of care: a process for making strategic choices in health systems. Geneva: World Health Organization.

WHO (2016). WHO global strategy on people centred and integrated health services. Interim Report. Geneva: World Health Organization.

WHO (2018). Handbook for national quality policy and strategy – A practical approach for developing policy and strategy to improve quality of care. Geneva: World Health Organization.

WHO/OECD/World Bank (2018). Delivering quality health services: a global imperative for universal health coverage. Geneva: World Health Organization, Organisation for Economic Co-operation and Development, and The World Bank. Licence: CC BY-NC-SA 3.0 IGO.

Chapter 2

Understanding healthcare quality strategies: a five-lens framework

Dimitra Panteli, Wilm Quentin, Reinhard Busse

2.1 Introduction

The previous chapter defined healthcare quality as the degree to which health services for individuals and populations are effective, safe and people-centred. In doing so, it clarified the concept of healthcare quality and distinguished it from health system performance. It also explained how the term "quality strategy" is used in this book; however, it did not link the theoretical work behind understanding, measuring and improving healthcare quality to the characteristics of specific quality strategies (or "initiatives", or "activities" or "interventions", as they are called elsewhere; *see* Chapter 1).

Several conceptual frameworks exist that aim at characterizing different aspects of quality or explaining pathways for effecting change in healthcare. However, existing frameworks have traditionally focused on specific aspects of healthcare quality or on particular quality improvement strategies. For example, some frameworks have attempted to classify different types of indicator for measuring healthcare quality (for example, Donabedian, 1966), while other frameworks have contributed to a better understanding of the different steps needed to achieve quality improvements (for example, Juran & Godfrey, 1999). However, no single framework is available that enables a systematic comparison of the characteristics of the various (and varied) quality strategies mentioned in Chapter 1 and further discussed in Part II of this book.

To bridge this gap and facilitate a better understanding of the characteristics of these strategies, and of how they can contribute to assessing, assuring or improving quality of care, a comprehensive framework was developed for this book and is presented here. The framework draws on several existing concepts and approaches, or "lenses", for thinking about quality assessment and implementation of change, which are discussed in the following sections.

2.2 The first and second lens: three dimensions of quality and four functions of healthcare

The first two lenses of the five-lens framework developed for this book are based on the framework developed by the Organisation for Economic Co-Operation and Development (OECD) for the Health Care Quality Indicators (HCQI) project (*see* Fig. 2.1). The framework was first published in 2006 (Arah et al., 2006) and updated in 2015 (Carinci et al., 2015). The purpose of the OECD HCQI framework is to guide the efforts of the Organisation to develop healthcare quality indicators and compare results across countries, as part of a larger agenda focusing on international health systems performance comparisons.

Fig. 2.1 "zooms in" on the relevant part of the HCQI framework, which is conceptualized as a matrix with the dimensions of quality in columns and patients' healthcare needs in rows. The three dimensions of quality (effectiveness, safety and patient-centredness) have already been discussed in Chapter 1; they summarize the most important components of healthcare (service) quality. The four categories of patients' healthcare needs are based on the most important reasons for which people seek care, following the Institute of Medicine's influential work on quality (IOM, 2001):

- Staying healthy ('primary prevention' in Fig. 2.1): getting help to avoid illness and remain well

- Getting better: getting help to recover from an illness or injury

Fig. 2.1 *Framework of the OECD Health Care Quality Indicators project*

Healthcare needs	Quality dimension		
	Effectiveness	Safety	Responsiveness/patient-centredness
1. Primary prevention			
2. Getting better			
3. Living with illness or disability/ chronic care			Individual patient experiences / Integrated care
4. Coping with end of life			

Source: Carinci et al., 2015

- Living with illness or disability: getting help with managing an ongoing, chronic condition or dealing with a disability that affects function

- Coping with the end of life: getting help to deal with a terminal illness

The logic behind the inclusion of these needs categories into the quality framework is that patients seek different types of care depending on their needs. For example, in order to stay healthy, patients seek preventive care, and in order to get better, they seek acute care. Similarly, chronic care corresponds to patients' needs of living with illness or disability, and palliative care corresponds to the need for coping with end of life. Indicators and quality strategies have to be planned differently for different types of services, depending on patients' needs and the corresponding necessary healthcare. For example, inpatient mortality is frequently used as an indicator of quality for acute care (for example, mortality of patients admitted because of acute myocardial infarction), but it cannot serve as a quality indicator for palliative care, for obvious reasons.

As mentioned above, the OECD HCQI project has used this framework to define its scope and develop indicators for the different fields in the matrix. One of the updates included in the 2015 version of the framework (shown in Fig. 2.1) was that the dimension of patient-centredness was split into the two areas of "individual patient experiences" and "integrated care". This was meant to facilitate the creation of related indicators and reflects the international acknowledgement of the importance of integrated care (*see also* Chapter 1 for a reflection on how the proposed dimensions of healthcare quality have evolved over time). Also, in the 2015 version, the initial wording of "staying healthy" was changed to "primary prevention" to provide a clearer distinction from "living with illness and disability – chronic care", as many patients living with a managed chronic condition may consider themselves as seeking care to stay healthy (Carinci et al., 2015).

Drawing from the conceptualization behind the OECD HCQI project, the first lens of the framework developed for this book consists of the three dimensions of quality, i.e. effectiveness, safety and responsiveness. The second lens encompasses the four functions of care that correspond to the categories of patients' healthcare needs described above, i.e. primary prevention, acute care, chronic care and palliative care.

2.3 The third lens: three major activities of quality strategies

The most influential framework used to conceptualize approaches for the improvement of quality – not only in healthcare but in many industries – is the plan-do-check-act (PDCA) cycle, also known as the plan-do-study-act (PDSA) cycle (Reed & Card, 2016). The PDCA cycle is a four-step model for implementing change that has been applied by many healthcare institutions and public health programmes. It also provides the theoretical underpinning for several of the quality strategies presented in Part II of the book, for example, audit and feedback, and external assessment strategies (*see* Chapters 10 and 8).

The method of quality management behind the PDCA cycle originated in industrial design, specifically Walter Shewhart and Edward Deming's description of iterative processes for catalysing change. The PDCA cycle guides users through a prescribed four-stage learning approach to introduce, evaluate and progressively adapt changes aimed at improvement (Taylor et al., 2014). Fig. 2.2 presents the four stages of the PDCA cycle as originally described by Deming.

Fig. 2.2   *The Plan-Do-Check-Act (PDCA) cycle*

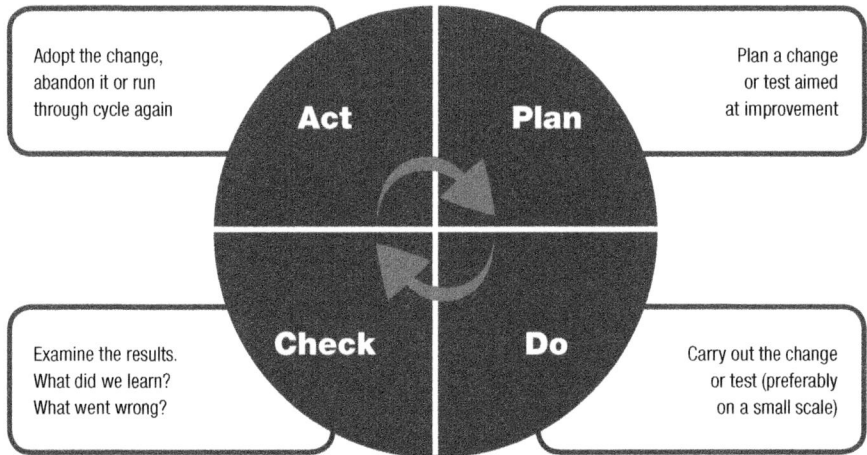

Act — Adopt the change, abandon it or run through cycle again

Plan — Plan a change or test aimed at improvement

Check — Examine the results. What did we learn? What went wrong?

Do — Carry out the change or test (preferably on a small scale)

Source: based on Taylor et al., 2014

Other quality improvement scholars have developed similar and somewhat related concepts. For example, the Juran trilogy defines three cyclical stages of managerial processes that are often used in discussions around healthcare improvement (Juran & Godfrey, 1999), including (1) quality planning, (2) quality control, and (3) quality improvement. On the one hand, the trilogy draws attention to the fact that these are three separable domains or activities that can be addressed by particular quality interventions (WHO, 2018a). On the other hand, the cyclical conceptualization of the trilogy highlights that all three elements are necessary and complementary if improvements are to be assured.

Similar to the Juran trilogy, WHO defined three generic domains – or areas of focus – of quality strategies that are useful when thinking about approaches addressing different target groups, such as professionals or providers (WHO, 2008): (1) legislation and regulation, (2) monitoring and measurement, (3) assuring and improving the quality of healthcare services (as 3a) and healthcare systems (as 3b). The idea behind specifying these domains was to guide national governments in their assessment of existing approaches and identification of necessary interventions to improve national quality strategies. A focus on these three cornerstones of quality improvement has proven useful for the analysis of national quality strategies (see, for instance, WHO, 2018b).

Based on these considerations, the third lens of the framework developed for this book builds on these concepts and defines three major activities (or areas of focus) of different quality strategies: (1) setting standards, (2) monitoring, and (3) assuring improvements (*see* Fig. 2.3). Some of the strategies presented in Part II of the book provide the basis for defining standards (for example, clinical guidelines, see Chapter 9), while others focus on monitoring (for example, accreditation and certification, *see* Chapter 8) and/or on assuring improvements (for example, public reporting, *see* Chapter 13), while yet others address more than one element. Focusing on the characteristic feature of each strategy in this respect is useful as it can help clarify why it should contribute to improved quality of care.

Fig. 2.3   *Three major activities of different quality strategies (with examples covered in this book)*

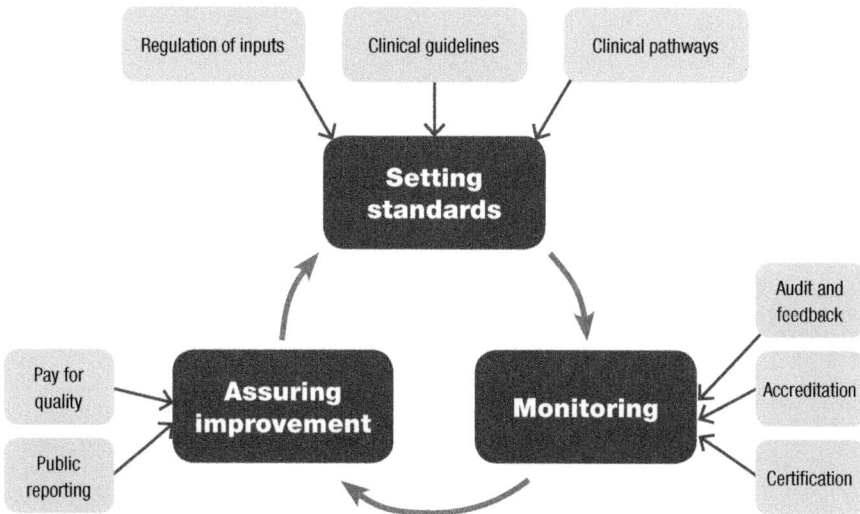

Source: authors' own compilation, inspired by WHO, 2018b

However, following the idea of the PDCA cycle, these three activities are conceptualized in the five-lens framework as a cyclical process (*see* Fig. 2.3). This means that all three activities are necessary in order to achieve change. For example, setting standards does not lead to change by itself if these standards are not monitored – and in order to achieve improvements of quality, actors will have to take the necessary actions to implement change.

2.4 The fourth lens: Donabedian's distinction between structure, process and outcome

Donabedian's approach to describing and evaluating the quality of care has been widely accepted and is possibly one of the very few points of consensus in the field (Ayanian & Markel, 2016). In his landmark 1966 article "Evaluating the quality of medical care", Donabedian built on the concept of "input–process–output" used in industrial manufacturing to propose the triad of structure, process and outcome for the evaluation of the quality of healthcare (*see* Fig. 2.4).

He defined "structure" (or input) as the attributes of the setting in which care occurs. This includes all the resources needed for the provision of healthcare, such as material resources (facilities, capital, equipment, drugs, etc.), intellectual resources (medical knowledge, information systems) and human resources (healthcare professionals). "Process" denotes the components of care delivered, encompassing the use of resources in terms of what is done in giving and receiving care, divided into patient-related processes (prescription patterns, intervention rates, referral rates, etc.) and organizational aspects (supply with drugs, management of waiting lists, payment of healthcare staff, collection of funds, etc.). Finally, "outcome" describes the effects of healthcare on the health status of patients and populations. Donabedian distinguishes between final outcomes, such as mortality, morbidity, disability or quality of life, and intermediate outcomes, for instance, blood pressure, body weight, personal well-being, functional ability, coping ability and improved knowledge (Donabedian 1988).

Fig. 2.4 also visualizes Donabedian's position that "good structure increases the likelihood of good process, and good process increases the likelihood of good

Fig. 2.4   *Donabedian's Structure-Process-Outcome (SPO) framework for Quality Assessment*

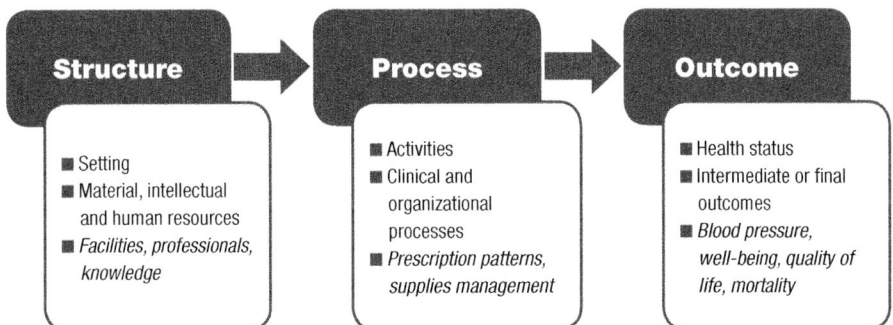

Source: authors' own compilation based on Donabedian, 1988

outcome" (Donabedian, 1988). For example, the availability of the right mix of qualified professionals at a hospital increases the likelihood that a heart surgery will be performed following current professional standards, and this in turn increases the likelihood of patient survival.

Accordingly, the fourth lens of the framework adopts Donabedian's distinction between structures, processes and outcomes. Again, this distinction is useful because several strategies presented in Part II of this book focus more on one of these elements than on the others. For example, regulation of professionals focuses on the quality of inputs, while clinical guidelines focus on the quality of care processes. Ultimately, the goal of all improvement strategies is better outcomes; the primary mechanism for achieving this goal, however, will vary.

2.5 The fifth and final lens: five targets of quality strategies

The final lens in the five-lens framework distinguishes between five different units of focus (or "targets", from this point forward) of different strategies (WHO, 2008). Quality strategies can address individual health professionals (for example, physicians or nurses), health technologies (for example, medicines, medical devices), and provider organizations (for example, hospitals or primary care centres). Furthermore, quality strategies can aim at patients or at payers in the health system (WHO, 2008). Table 2.1 provides examples of different strategies targeted at health professionals, health technologies, healthcare provider organizations, patients and payers (*see also* WHO, 2018a). The distinction between

Table 2.1 *Targets of various quality strategies*

Potential targets	Possible strategies
Health professionals	Regulation and licensing, certification/revalidation, training and continuous medical education, establishing a patient-safety culture, clinical guidelines, clinical pathways, clinical audit and feedback, explicit description of professional competencies, quality-measurement, peer-review, setting norms and standards for professional misconduct, medical workforce planning, task-substitution, introduction of new professions, pay-for-quality (P4Q).
Medical products and technologies	Regulation and licensing of technologies (pharmaceuticals and devices), regulation and monitoring of risks, health technology assessment and an overall national innovation strategy.
Healthcare provider organizations	Regulation and licensing, quality indicators, external assessments: accreditation, certification and supervision of providers, electronic health records, risk-management, adverse event reporting, nationally standardized databases, quality improvement and safety programmes, accreditation of integrated delivery systems, organizational innovation, pay-for-quality (P4Q).
Patients	Legislation on patient rights, patient/community participation, systematic measurement of patient experiences, public reporting and comparative benchmarking.
Payers	Valuing quality in monetary terms, production of quality information, pay-for-quality (P4Q) initiatives and the issuing of national quality reports.

Source: adapted from WHO, 2008 and WHO, 2018a

targets of strategies is important because the level of decision-making, regulatory mechanisms and relevant stakeholders to involve in planning, implementation and monitoring varies depending on the target.

2.6 Putting it together: the five-lens framework of healthcare quality strategies

Fig. 2.5 presents the five-lens framework, which integrates the different concepts and approaches presented so far. The framework does not assume a hierarchical order of the different lenses: rather, these are meant as five complementary conceptual perspectives; using them in combination can provide a more complete and more actionable picture of different quality strategies.

To reiterate, the five lenses include – moving from innermost to outermost:

1. The three core dimensions of quality: safety, effectiveness and patient-centredness.

2. The four functions of health care: primary prevention, acute care, chronic care and palliative care.

3. The three main activities of quality strategies: setting standards, monitoring and assuring improvements.

4. Donabedian's triad: structures, processes and outcomes.

5. The five main targets of quality strategies: health professionals, health technologies, provider organizations, patients and payers.

The five lenses of the framework draw attention to the characteristics of different quality strategies and guide the discussion of their potential contribution to healthcare quality in each chapter of Part II of the book. The conceptualization of the framework in terms of concentric cyclic arrows indicates that different strategies combine different features on each lens. However, in general, strategies do not fall unambiguously into one category per lens of the framework – and there are also areas of overlap between different strategies. As such, the framework does not aim to classify quality strategies to a unique taxonomic position; it rather hopes to describe their characteristics in a manner that enables a better understanding of their contribution to quality assurance and/or improvement and their use in different European countries.

For example, using the framework, audit and feedback (*see* Chapter 10) can be characterized as a strategy that usually focuses on effectiveness and safety in various settings (prevention, acute care, chronic care and palliative care), by monitoring (and assuring improvements) of care processes (for example, adherence to guidelines) of health professionals. By contrast, pay-for-quality (P4Q) as a quality strategy (*see* Chapter 14) can be characterized as usually focusing on effectiveness and safety in preventive, acute or chronic care by providing incentives to assure improvements in structures, processes or outcomes of provider organizations or professionals.

Fig. 2.5   *Comprehensive framework for describing and classifying quality strategies*

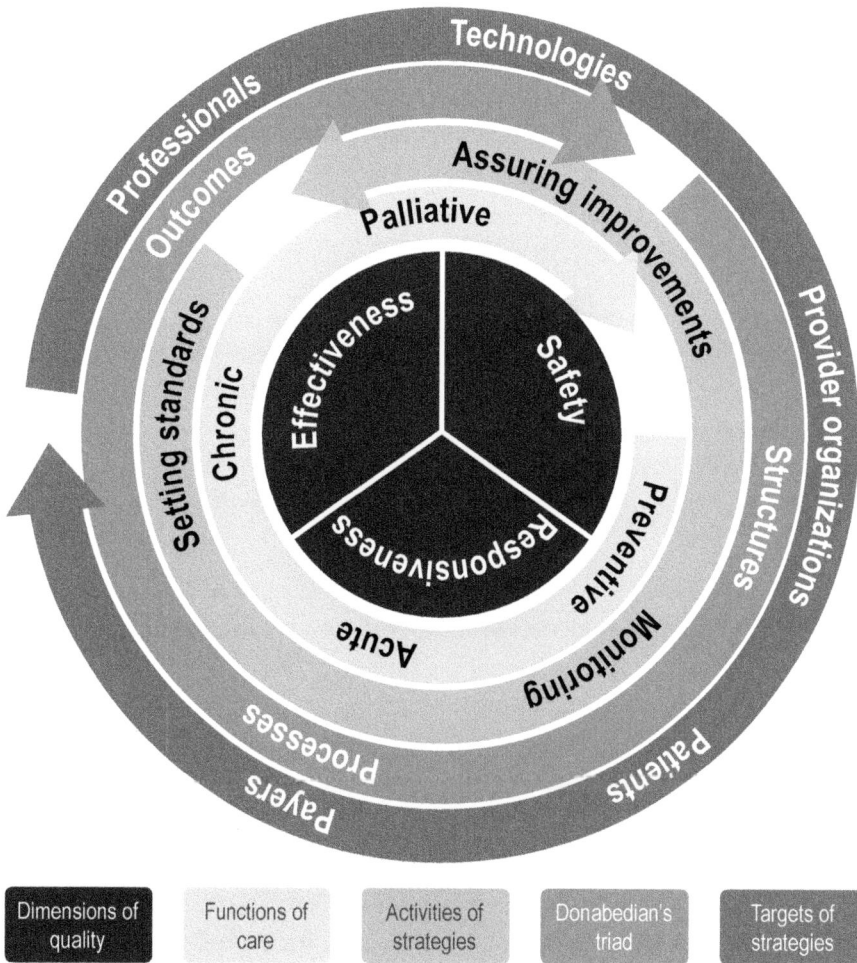

Source: authors' compilation

2.7 Quality strategies discussed in this book

As mentioned in Chapter 1, numerous strategies have emerged over the years claiming to contribute to assuring or improving quality of care. For instance, the OECD lists 42 strategies for patient safety alone (Slawomirksi, Auraaen

& Klazinga, 2017), and Table 1.3 at the end of Chapter 1 includes 28 quality strategies; neither of those lists is exhaustive. Given the multiplicity of different quality strategies and the various levels on which they can be implemented, policy-makers often struggle to make sense of them and to judge their relative effectiveness and cost-effectiveness for the purposes of prioritization.

Any book on quality strategies is inevitably selective, as it is impossible to provide an exhaustive overview and discussion. The strategies discussed in detail in the second part of this book were selected based on the experience of the European Observatory on Health Systems and Policies and comprise those most frequently discussed by policy-makers in Europe. However, this does not mean that other not are less important or should not be considered for implementation. In particular, the book includes only one strategy explicitly targeting patients, i.e. public reporting (*see* Chapter 13). Other strategies, such as systematic measurement of patient experience or strategies to support patient participation could potentially have an important impact on increasing patient-centredness of healthcare service provision. Similarly, the book does not place much emphasis on digital innovations, such as electronic health records or clinical decision support systems to improve effectiveness and safety of care, despite their potential impact on changing service provision. Nevertheless, among the included strategies there is at least one corresponding to each element of the five-lens framework, i.e. there is at least one strategy concerned with payers (or providers or professionals, etc.), one strategy concerned with structures (or processes or outcomes), and so on.

Many different categorizations of quality strategies are possible along the five lenses of the framework described above. For the sake of simplicity, Table 2.2 categorizes the strategies discussed in the second part of the book into three groups using lenses three and four of the five-lens framework: (1) strategies that set standards for health system structures and inputs, (2) strategies that focus on steering and monitoring health system processes, and (3) strategies that leverage processes and outcomes with the aim of assuring improvements.

Table 2.2 also shows the common structure largely followed by all chapters in Part II of the book. First, chapters describe the characteristic features of the quality strategy at hand, i.e. what are its target(s) (professionals, technologies, provider organizations, patients or payers; lens five of the framework described above) and main activity (setting standards, monitoring or assuring improvements; lens three). In addition, each chapter describes the underlying rationale of why the strategy should contribute to healthcare quality by explaining how it may affect safety, effectiveness and/or patient-centredness (lens 1) of care through changes of structures, processes and/or outcomes (lens 4). Secondly, the chapters provide an overview of what is being done in European countries in respect to the specific quality strategy, considering – among other things – whether the strategy

Table 2.2 *Overview of chapter structure and topics addressed in Part 2 of the book*

Chapter structure	Settings standards for Health System Structures and Inputs	Steering and Monitoring Quality of Health System Processes	Leveraging Processes and Outcomes of Care to assure improvements
1. *What are the characteristics of the strategy?* 2. *What is being done in European countries?* 3. *What do we know about the strategy's (cost-)effectiveness?* 4. *How can the strategy be implemented?* 5. *Conclusions: lessons for policy-makers*	• Regulation of Health Professionals • Regulation of health technologies: Health Technology Assessment • Regulation of Healthcare Facilities • External institutional strategies: accreditation, certification, supervision	• Clinical Guidelines • Audit and Feedback • Patient Safety Strategies • Clinical Pathways	• Public Reporting • Financial Incentives

is mostly applied in preventive care, acute care, chronic care or palliative care (lens 2). They then summarize the available evidence with regard to the strategy's effectiveness and cost-effectiveness, often building on existing systematic reviews or reviews of reviews. They follow up by addressing questions of implementation, for example, what institutional and organizational requirements are necessary to implement the strategy. Finally, each chapter provides conclusions for policy-makers bringing together the available evidence and highlighting the relationship of the strategy to other strategies.

2.8 Concluding remarks

This chapter described the development of a comprehensive five-lens framework that brings together influential concepts and approaches for understanding, assuring and improving quality of care. The framework facilitates a better grasp of the key characteristics of individual quality strategies and guides the discussion about their potential contribution to high-quality healthcare in Part II of the book. This discussion of quality strategies hopes to contribute to greater conceptual clarity about their key characteristics and to enable policy-makers to develop national strategic plans on the basis of the best available evidence.

References

Arah OA et al. (2006). A conceptual framework for the OECD Health Care Quality Indicators Project. *International Journal for Quality in Health Care*, 18(S1):5–13.

Ayanian ZJ, Markel H (2016). Donabedian's Lasting Framework for Health Care Quality. *The New England Journal of Medicine*, 375:205–7.

Carinci F et al. (2015). Towards actionable international comparisons of health system performance: expert revision of the OECD framework and quality indicators. *International Journal for Quality in Health Care*, 27(2):137–46.

Donabedian A (1966). Evaluating the quality of medical care. *Milbank Quarterly*, 691–729.

Donabedian A (1988). The quality of care. How can it be assessed? *Journal of the American Medical Association*, 260(12):1743–8.

IOM (2001). Envisioning the National Health Care Quality Report. Washington (DC), US: National Academies Press.

Juran JM, Godfrey A (1999). Juran's Quality Handbook. New York: McGraw-Hill.

Reed JE, Card AJ (2016). The problem with Plan-Do-Study-Act cycles. *BMJ Quality & Safety*, 25:147–52.

Slawomirski L, Auraaen A, Klazinga N (2017). The economics of patient safety. Paris: Organisation for Economic Co-operation and Development.

Taylor MJ et al. (2014). Systematic review of the application of the plan-do-study-act method to improve quality in healthcare. *BMJ Quality & Safety*, 23(4):290–8.

WHO (2008). Guidance on developing quality and safety strategies with a health system approach. Copenhagen: World Health Organization (Regional Office for Europe).

WHO (2018a). Handbook for national quality policy and strategy – A practical approach for developing policy and strategy to improve quality of care. Geneva: World Health Organization.

WHO (2018b). Quality of care review in Kyrgyzstan. Copenhagen: World Health Organization (Regional Office for Europe).

Chapter 3

Measuring healthcare quality

Wilm Quentin, Veli-Matti Partanen, Ian Brownwood, Niek Klazinga

3.1 Introduction

The field of quality measurement in healthcare has developed considerably in the past few decades and has attracted growing interest among researchers, policy-makers and the general public (Papanicolas & Smith, 2013; EC, 2016; OECD, 2019). Researchers and policy-makers are increasingly seeking to develop more systematic ways of measuring and benchmarking quality of care of different providers. Quality of care is now systematically reported as part of overall health system performance reports in many countries, including Australia, Belgium, Canada, Italy, Mexico, Spain, the Netherlands, and most Nordic countries. At the same time, international efforts in comparing and benchmarking quality of care across countries are mounting. The Organisation for Economic Co-operation and Development (OECD) and the EU Commission have both expanded their efforts at assessing and comparing healthcare quality internationally (Carinci et al., 2015; EC, 2016). Furthermore, a growing focus on value-based healthcare (Porter, 2010) has sparked renewed interest in the standardization of measurement of outcomes (ICHOM, 2019), and notably the measurement of patient-reported outcomes has gained momentum (OECD, 2019).

The increasing interest in quality measurement has been accompanied and supported by the growing ability to measure and analyse quality of care, driven, amongst others, by significant changes in information technology and associated advances in measurement methodology. National policy-makers recognize that without measurement it is difficult to assure high quality of service provision in a country, as it is impossible to identify good and bad providers or good and bad practitioners without reliable information about quality of care. Measuring quality of care is important for a range of different stakeholders within healthcare systems, and it builds the basis for numerous quality assurance and improvement strategies discussed in Part II of this book. In particular, accreditation and certification (*see* Chapter 8), audit and feedback (*see* Chapter 10), public reporting (*see* Chapter 13) and pay for quality (*see* Chapter 14) rely heavily on the availability of reliable information about the quality of care provided by different providers and/or professionals. Common to all strategies in Part II is that without robust measurement of quality, it is impossible to determine the extent to which new regulations or quality improvement interventions actually work and improve quality as expected, or if there are also adverse effects related to these changes.

This chapter presents different approaches, frameworks and data sources used in quality measurement as well as methodological challenges, such as risk-adjustment, that need to be considered when making inferences about quality measures. In line with the focus of this book (*see* Chapter 1), the chapter focuses on measuring quality of healthcare services, i.e. on the quality dimensions of effectiveness, patient safety and patient-centredness. Other dimensions of health system performance, such as accessibility and efficiency, are not covered in this chapter as they are the focus of other volumes about health system performance assessment (*see*, for example, Smith et al., 2009; Papanicolas & Smith, 2013; Cylus, Papanicolas & Smith, 2016). The chapter also provides examples of quality measurement systems in place in different countries. An overview of the history of quality measurement (with a focus on the United States) is given in Marjoua & Bozic (2012). Overviews of measurement challenges related to international comparisons are provided by Forde, Morgan & Klazinga (2013) and Papanicolas & Smith (2013).

3.2 How can quality be measured? From a concept of quality to quality indicators

Most quality measurement initiatives are concerned with the development and assessment of quality indicators (Lawrence & Olesen, 1997; Mainz, 2003; EC, 2016). Therefore, it is useful to step back and reflect on the idea of an indicator more generally. In the social sciences, an indicator is defined as "a quantitative measure that provides information about a variable that is difficult to measure directly" (Calhoun, 2002). Obviously, quality of care is difficult to measure directly because it is a theoretical concept that can encompass different aspects depending on the exact definition and the context of measurement.

Chapter 1 has defined quality of care as "the degree to which health services for individuals and populations are effective, safe and people-centred". However, the chapter also highlighted that there is considerable confusion about the concept of quality because different institutions and people often mean different things when using it. To a certain degree, this is inevitable and even desirable because quality of care does mean different things in different contexts. However, this context dependency also makes clarity about the exact conceptualization of quality in a particular setting particularly important, before measurement can be initiated.

In line with the definition of quality in this book, quality indicators are defined as quantitative measures that provide information about the effectiveness, safety and/ or people-centredness of care. Of course, numerous other definitions of quality indicators are possible (Mainz, 2003; Lawrence & Olesen, 1997). In addition, some institutions, such as the National Quality Forum (NQF) in the USA, use the term *quality measure* instead of *quality indicator*. Other institutions, such as the NHS Indicator Methodology and Assurance Service and the German Institute for Quality Assurance and Transparency in Health Care (IQTIG), define further attributes of quality indicators (IQTIG, 2018; NHS Digital, 2019a). According to these definitions, quality indicators should provide:

1. a quality goal, i.e. a clear statement about the intended goal or objective, for example, inpatient mortality of patients admitted with pneumonia should be as low as possible;

2. a measurement concept, i.e. a specified method for data collection and calculation of the indicator, for example, the proportion of inpatients with a primary diagnosis of pneumonia who died during the inpatient stay; and

3. an appraisal concept, i.e. a description of how a measure is expected to be used to judge quality, for example, if inpatient mortality is below 10%, this is considered to be good quality.

Often the terms *measures* and *indicators* are used interchangeably. However, it makes sense to reserve the term quality *indicator* for *measures* that are accompanied by an appraisal concept (IQTIG, 2018). This is because measures without an appraisal concept are unable to indicate whether measured values represent good or bad quality of care. For example, the readmission rate is a measure for the number of readmissions. However, it becomes a quality indicator if a threshold is defined that indicates "higher than normal" readmissions, which could, in turn, indicate poor quality of care. Another term that is frequently used interchangeably with *quality indicator*, in particular in the USA, is *quality metric*. However, a *quality metric* also does not necessarily define an appraisal concept, which could potentially distinguish it from an indicator. At the same time, the term *quality metric* is sometimes used more broadly for an entire system that aims to evaluate quality of care using a range of indicators.

Operationalizing the theoretical concept of quality by translating it into a set of quality indicators requires a clear understanding of the purpose and context of measurement. Chapter 2 has introduced a five-lens framework for describing and classifying quality strategies. Several of these lenses are also useful for better understanding the different aspects and contexts that need to be taken into account when measuring healthcare quality. First, it is clear that different indicators are needed to assess the three dimensions of quality, i.e. effectiveness, safety and/or patient-centredness, because they relate to very different concepts, such as patient health, medical errors and patient satisfaction.

Secondly, quality measurement has to differ depending on the concerned function of the healthcare system, i.e. depending on whether one is aiming to measure quality in preventive, acute, chronic or palliative care. For example, changes in health outcomes due to preventive care will often be measurable only after a long time has elapsed, while they will be visible more quickly in the area of acute care. Thirdly, quality measurement will vary depending on the target of the quality measurement initiative, i.e. payers, provider organizations, professionals, technologies and/or patients. For example, in some contexts it might be useful to assess the quality of care received by all patients covered by different payer organizations (for example, different health insurers or regions) but more frequently quality measurement will focus on care provided by different provider organizations. In international comparisons, entire countries will constitute another level or target of measurement.

In addition, operationalizing quality for measurement will always require a focus on a limited set of quality aspects for a particular group of patients. For example, quality measurement may focus on patients with hip fracture treated in hospitals and define aspects of care that are related to effectiveness (for example, surgery performed within 24 hours of admission), safety (for example, anticoagulation to prevent thromboembolism), and/or patient-centredness of care (for example, patient was offered choice of spinal or general anaesthesia) (Voeten et al., 2018). However, again, the choice of indicators – and also potentially of different appraisal concepts for indicators used for the same quality aspects – will depend on the exact purpose of measurement.

3.3 Different purposes of quality measurement and users of quality information

It is useful to distinguish between two main purposes of quality measurement: The first purpose is to use quality measurement in quality assurance systems as a *summative mechanism* for external accountability and verification. The second purpose is to use quality measurement as a *formative mechanism* for quality improvement. Depending on the purpose, quality measurement systems face different challenges with regard to indicators, data sources and the level of precision required.

Table 3.1 highlights the differences between quality assurance and quality improvement (Freeman, 2002; Gardner, Olney & Dickinson, 2018). Measurement for quality assurance and accountability is focused on identifying and overcoming problems with quality of care and assuring a sufficient level of quality across providers. Quality assurance is the focus of many external assessment strategies (*see* also Chapter 8), and providers of insufficient quality may ultimately lose their licence and be prohibited from providing care. Assuring accountability is one of the main purposes of public reporting initiatives (*see* Chapter 13), and measured quality of care may contribute to trust in healthcare services and allow patients to choose higher-quality providers.

Quality measurement for quality assurance and accountability makes summative judgements about the quality of care provided. The idea is that "real" differences will be detected as a result of the measurement initiative. Therefore, a high level of precision is necessary and advanced statistical techniques may need to be employed to make sure that detected differences between providers are "real" and attributable to provider performance. Otherwise, measurement will encounter significant justified resistance from providers because its potential consequences, such as losing the licence or losing patients to other providers, would be unfair. Appraisal concepts of indicators for quality assurance will usually focus on assuring a minimum quality of care and identifying poor-quality providers. However, if the purpose is to incentivize high quality of care through pay for quality initiatives, the appraisal concept will likely focus on identifying providers delivering excellent quality of care.

By contrast, measurement for quality improvement is change oriented and quality information is used at the local level to promote continuous efforts of providers to improve their performance. Indicators have to be actionable and hence are often more process oriented. When used for quality improvement, quality measurement does not necessarily need to be perfect because it is only informative. Other sources of data and local information are considered as well in order to provide context for measured quality of care. The results of quality measurement are only used to start discussions about quality differences and to motivate change in provider behaviour, for example, in audit and feedback initiatives (*see* Chapter 10). Freeman (2002) sums up the described differences between quality improvement and quality assurance as follows: "Quality improvement models use indicators to develop discussion further, assurance models use them to foreclose it."

Different stakeholders in healthcare systems pursue different objectives and as a result they have different information needs (Smith et al., 2009; EC, 2016). For example, governments and regulators are usually focused on quality assurance and accountability. They use related information mostly to assure that the quality

Table 3.1 *The purpose of quality measurement: quality assurance versus quality improvement.*

	Quality Assurance and Accountability	Quality Improvement
Focus	Avoiding quality problems Verification and assurance Measurement oriented	Learning to promote continuous improvement Change oriented
Rationale	Provide external accountability and renew legitimacy	Promote change and improvement in care quality
Locus of power and control	External managerial power	Internal professional authority
Culture	Comparisons in order to take summative judgements on care quality League tables Blame and shame	Comparisons in order to learn from differences and encourage improvement Informal benchmarking to promote discussion and change
Precision required	High precision Use of statistics to identify "real" differences	Lower precision
Epistemology	Empirical Statistical validity and reliability important	Interpretative Use of other data sources and local information to provide context
Examples	External assessment Pay for quality Public reporting	Internal audit and feedback Continuous quality improvement

Source: authors' compilation based on Freeman, 2002 and Gardner, Olney & Dickinson, 2018

of care provided to patients is of a sufficient level to avoid harm – although they are clearly also interested in assuring a certain level of effectiveness. By contrast, providers and professionals are more interested in using quality information to enable quality improvement by identifying areas where they deviate from scientific standards or benchmarks, which point to possibilities for improvement (*see* Chapter 10). Finally, patients and citizens may demand quality information in order to be assured that adequate health services will be available in case of need and to be able to choose providers of good-quality care (*see* Chapter 13). The stakeholders and their purposes of quality measurement have, of course, an important influence on the selection of indicators and data needs (*see* below).

While the distinction between quality assurance and quality improvement is useful, the difference is not always clear-cut. First, from a societal perspective, quality assurance aims at stamping out poor-quality care and thus contributes to improving average quality of care. Secondly, proponents of several of the strategies that are included under quality assurance in Table 3.1, such as external assessment (*see also* Chapter 8) or public reporting (*see also* Chapter 13), in fact claim that these strategies do contribute to improving quality of care and assuring public trust in healthcare services. In fact, as pointed out in the relevant chapters, the rationale of external assessment and public reporting is that these strategies will lead to changes within organizations that will ultimately contribute to improving quality of care. Clearly, there also need to be incentives and/or motivations for change, i.e. while internal quality improvement processes often rely on professionalism, external accountability mechanisms seek to motivate through external incentives and disincentives – but this is beyond the scope of this chapter.

3.4 Types of quality indicators

There are many options for classifying different types of quality indicators (Mainz, 2003). One option is to distinguish between rate-based indicators and simple count-based indicators, usually used for rare "sentinel" events. Rate-based indicators are the more common form of indicators. They are expressed as proportions or rates with clearly defined numerators and denominators, for example, the proportion of hip fracture patients who receive antibiotic prophylaxis before surgery. Count-based indicators are often used for operationalizing the safety dimension of quality and they identify individual events that are intrinsically undesirable. Examples include "never events", such as a foreign body left in during surgery or surgery on the wrong side of the body. If the measurement purpose is quality improvement, each individual event would trigger further analysis and investigation to avoid similar problems in the future.

Another option is to distinguish between generic and disease-specific indicators. Generic indicators measure aspects of care that are relevant to all patients. One example of a generic indicator is the proportion of patients who waited more than six hours in the emergency department. Disease-specific indicators are relevant only for patients with a particular diagnosis, such as the proportion of patients with lung cancer who are alive 30 days after surgery.

Yet other options relate to the different lenses of the framework presented in Chapter 2. Indicators can be classified depending on the dimension of quality that they assess, i.e. effectiveness, patient safety and/or patient-centredness (the first lens); and with regard to the assessed function of healthcare, i.e. prevention, acute, chronic and/or palliative care (the second lens). Furthermore, it is possible to distinguish between patient-based indicators and event-based indicators. Patient-based indicators are indicators that are developed based on data that are linked across settings, allowing the identification of the pathway of care provided to individual patients. Event-based indicators are related to a specific event, for example, a hospital admission.

However, the most frequently used framework for distinguishing between different types of quality indicators is Donabedian's classification of structure, process and outcome indicators (Donabedian, 1980). Donabedian's triad builds the fourth lens of the framework presented in Chapter 2. The idea is that the

Table 3.2 *Examples of structure, process and outcome quality indicators for different dimensions of quality*

Dimension of quality	Donabedian's triad		
	Structure	Process	Outcome
Effectiveness	Availability of staff and equipment Training expenditure for staff	Aspirin at arrival for patients with acute myocardial infarction HPV vaccination for female adolescents Beta blockers after a myocardial infarction	Hospital readmission rate Heart surgery mortality rate Rate of preventable hospital admissions Activities of daily living Patient-reported outcome measures (PROMs)
Patient safety	Availability of safe medicines Volume of surgeries performed	Safe surgery checklist use Staff compliance with hand hygiene guidelines False-positive rates of cancer screening tests	Complications of diagnosis or treatment Incidence of hospital-acquired infections (HAI) Foreign body left in during procedure
Patient-centredness	Patient rights Availability of patient information	Regular doctor spending enough time with patients during consultation Patient-reported experience measures (PREMs)	Activities of daily living Patient satisfaction Willingness to recommend the hospital Patient-reported outcome measures (PROMs)

Source: authors' compilation, based on Lighter, 2015

structures where health care is provided have an effect on the processes of care, which in turn will influence patient health outcomes. Table 3.2 provides some examples of structure, process and outcome indicators related to the different dimensions of quality.

In general, structural quality indicators are used to assess the setting of care, such as the adequacy of facilities and equipment, staffing ratios, qualifications of medical staff and administrative structures. Structural indicators related to effectiveness include the availability of staff with an appropriate skill mix, while the availability of safe medicines and the volume of surgeries performed are considered to be more related to patient safety. Structural indicators for patient-centredness can include the organizational implementation of a patients' rights charter or the availability of patient information. Although institutional structures are certainly important for providing high-quality care, it is often difficult to establish a clear link between structures and clinical processes or outcomes, which reduces, to a certain extent, the relevance of structural measures.

Process indicators are used to assess whether actions indicating high-quality care are undertaken during service provision. Ideally, process indicators are built on reliable scientific evidence that compliance with these indicators is related to better outcomes of care. Sometimes process indicators are developed on the basis of clinical guidelines (*see also* Chapter 9) or some other golden standard. For example, a process indicator of effective care for AMI patients may assess if patients are given aspirin on arrival. A process indicator of safety in surgery may assess if a safety checklist is used during surgery, and process indicators for patient-centredness may analyse patient-reported experience measures (PREMs). Process measures account for the majority of most quality measurement frameworks (Cheng et al., 2014; Fujita, Moles & Chen, 2018; NQF, 2019a).

Finally, outcome indicators provide information about whether healthcare services help people stay alive and healthy. Outcome indicators are usually concrete and highly relevant to patients. For example, outcome indicators of effective ambulatory care include hospitalization rates for preventable conditions. Indicators of effective inpatient care for patients with acute myocardial infarction often include mortality rates within 30 days after admission, preferably calculated as a patient-based indicator (i.e. capturing deaths in any setting outside the hospital) and not as an event-based indicator (i.e. capturing death only within the hospital). Outcome indicators of patient safety may include complications of treatment, such as hospital acquired infections or foreign bodies left in during surgery. Outcome indicators of patient-centredness may assess patient satisfaction or patients' willingness to recommend the hospital. Outcome indicators are increasingly used in quality measurement programmes, in particular in the USA, because they are of greater interest to patients and payers (Baker & Chassin, 2017).

3.5 Advantages and disadvantages of different types of indicators

Different types of indicators have their various strengths and weaknesses:

- Generic indicators have the advantage that they assess aspects of healthcare quality that are relevant to all patients. Therefore, generic indicators are potentially meaningful for a greater audience of patients, payers and policy-makers.

- Disease-specific indicators are better able to capture different aspects of healthcare quality that are relevant for improving patient care. In fact, most aspects of healthcare quality are disease-specific because effectiveness, safety and patient-centredness mean different things for different groups of diseases. For example, prescribing aspirin at discharge is an indicator of providing effective care for patients after acute myocardial infarction. However, if older patients are prescribed aspirin for extended periods of time without receiving gastro-protective medicines, this is an indicator of safety problems in primary care (NHS BSA, 2019).

Likewise, structure, process and outcome indicators each have their comparative strengths and weaknesses. These are summarized in Table 3.3. The strength of structural measures is that they are easily available, reportable and verifiable because structures are stable and easy to observe. However, the main weakness is that the link between structures and clinical processes or outcomes is often indirect and dependent on the actions of healthcare providers.

Process indicators are also measured relatively easily, and interpretation is often straightforward because there is often no need for risk-adjustment. In addition, poor performance on process indicators can be directly attributed to the actions of providers, thus giving clear indication for improvement, for example, by better adherence to clinical guidelines (Rubin, Pronovost & Diette, 2001). However, healthcare is complex and process indicators usually focus only on very specific procedures for a specific group of patients. Therefore, hundreds of indicators are needed to enable a comprehensive analysis of the quality of care provided by a professional or an institution. Relying only on a small set of process indicators carries the risk of distorting service provision towards a focus on measured areas of care while disregarding other (potentially more) important tasks that are harder to monitor.

Outcome indicators place the focus of quality assessments on the actual goals of service provision. Outcome indicators are often more meaningful to patients and policy-makers. The use of outcome indicators may also encourage innovations in service provision if these lead to better outcomes than following established processes of care. However, attributing health outcomes to the services provided by individual organizations or professionals is often difficult because outcomes are influenced by many factors outside the control of a provider (Lilford et al., 2004). In addition, outcomes may require a long time before they manifest themselves, which makes outcome measures more difficult to use for quality measurement (Donabedian, 1980). Furthermore, poor performance on outcome indicators does not necessarily provide direct indication for action as the outcomes may be related to a range of actions of different individuals who worked in a particular setting at a prior point in time.

3.6 Aggregating information in composite indicators

Given the complexity of healthcare provision and the wide range of relevant quality aspects, many quality measurement systems produce a large number of quality indicators. However, the availability of numerous different indicators may make it difficult for patients to select the best providers for their needs and for policy-makers to know whether overall quality of healthcare provision is improving. In addition, purchasers may struggle with identifying good-quality providers if they do not have a metric for aggregating conflicting results from

Table 3.3 *Strengths and weaknesses of different types of indicators*

	Structure indicators	Process indicators	Outcome indicators
STRENGTHS	**Easily available.** Many structural factors are evident and easily reportable **Stable.** Structural factors are relatively stable and often easy to observe	**Easily available.** Utilization of health technologies is often easily measured **Easily interpreted.** Compliance with process indicators can often be interpreted as good quality without the need for case-mix adjustment or inter-unit comparisons **Attribution.** Processes are directly dependent on actions of providers **Smaller sample size needed.** Significant quality deficiencies can be detected more easily **Unobtrusive.** Care processes can frequently be assessed unobtrusively from stored data **Indicators for action.** Failures identified provide clear guidance on what must be remedied	**Focus.** Directs attention towards the patient and helps nurture a "whole system" perspective **Goals.** Represent the goals of care more clearly **Meaningful.** More meaningful to patients and policy-makers **Innovation.** Encourages providers to experiment with new modes of delivery **Far-sighted.** Encourages providers to adopt long-term strategies (for example, health promotion) that may realize long-term benefits **Resistant to manipulation.** Less open to manipulation but providers may engage in risk-selection or upcoding to influence risk-adjustment
WEAKNESSES	**Link to quality is very weak.** Can only indicate potential capacity for providing quality care **Subject to response bias.** Over-reporting of resources or idealizing organizational aspects (for example, having a quality management system in place)	**Salience.** Processes of care may have little meaning to patients unless the link to outcomes can be explained **Specificity.** Processes indicators are highly specific to single diseases or procedures and numerous indicators may be required to represent quality of care provided **Ossification.** May stifle innovation and the development of new modes of care **Obsolescence.** Usefulness may dissipate as technology and modes of care change **Adverse behaviour.** Can be manipulated relatively easily and may give rise to gaming and other adverse behaviours	**Measurement definition.** Relatively easy to measure some outcome aspects validly and reliably (for example, death) but others are notoriously difficult (for example, wound infection) **Attribution.** May be influenced by many factors outside the control of a healthcare organization **Sample size.** Requires large sample size to detect a statistically significant effect **Timing.** May take a long time to observe **Interpretation.** Difficult to interpret if the processes that produced them are complex or occurred distant from the observed outcome **Ambiguity.** Good outcomes can often be achieved despite poor processes of care (and vice versa)

Source: authors' compilation based on Freeman, 2002 and Davies, 2005

different indicators. As a result, some users of quality information might base their decisions on only a few selected indicators that they understand, although these may not be the most important ones, and the information provided by many other relevant indicators will be lost (Goddard & Jacobs, 2009).

In response to these problems, many quality measurement initiatives have developed methods for combining different indicators into composite indicators or composite scores (Shwartz, Restuccia & Rosen, 2015). The use of composite indicators allows the aggregation of different aspects of quality into one measure to give a clearer picture of the overall quality of healthcare providers. The advantage is that the indicator summarizes information from a potentially wide range of individual indicators, thus providing a comprehensive assessment of quality. Composite indicators can serve many purposes: patients can select providers based on composite scores; hospital managers can use composite indicators to benchmark their hospitals against others, policy-makers can use composite indicators to assess progress over time, and researchers can use composite indicators for further analyses, for example, to identify factors associated with good quality of care. Table 3.4 summarizes some of the advantages and disadvantages of composite indicators.

The main disadvantages of composite indicators include that there are different (valid) options for aggregating individual indicators into composite indicators and that the methodological choices made during indicator construction will influence the measured performance. In addition, composite indicators may lead to simplistic conclusions and disguise serious failings in some dimensions. Furthermore, because of the influence of methodological choices on results, the selection of constituting indicators and weights could become the subject of political dispute. Finally, composite indicators do not allow the identification of specific problem areas and thus they need to be used in conjunction with individual quality indicators in order to enable quality improvement.

There are at least three important methodological choices that have to be made to construct a composite indicator. First, individual indicators have to be chosen to be combined in the composite indicator. Of course, the selection of indicators and the quality of chosen indicators will be decisive for the reliability of the overall composite indicator. Secondly, individual indicators have to be transformed into a common scale to enable aggregation. There are many methods available for this rescaling of the results, including ranking, normalizing (for example, using z-scores), calculating the proportion of the range of scores, and grouping scores into categories (for example, 5 stars) (Shwartz, Restuccia & Rosen, 2015). All of these methods have their comparative advantages and disadvantages and there is no consensus about which one should be used for the construction of composite indicators.

Table 3.4 *Advantages and disadvantages of composite indicators*

Advantages	Disadvantages
• Condense complex, multidimensional aspects of quality into a single indicator.	• Performance on indicator depends on methodological choices made to construct the composite.
• Easier to interpret than a battery of many separate indicators.	• May send misleading messages if poorly constructed or misinterpreted.
• Enable assessments of progress of providers or countries over time.	• May invite simplistic conclusions.
• Reduce the number of indicators without dropping the underlying information base.	• May be misused, if the composite construction process is not transparent and/or lacks sound statistical or conceptual principles.
• Place issues of provider or country performance and progress at the centre of the policy arena.	• The selection of indicators and weights could be the subject of political dispute.
• Facilitate communication with general public and promote accountability.	• May disguise serious failings in some dimensions and increase the difficulty of identifying remedial action, if the construction process is not transparent.
• Help to construct/underpin narratives for lay and literate audiences.	• May lead to inappropriate decisions if dimensions of performance that are difficult to measure are ignored.
• Enable users to compare complex dimensions effectively.	

Source: based on OECD, 2008

Thirdly, weights have to be attached to the individual indicators, which signal the relative importance of the different components of the composite indicator. Potentially, the ranking of providers can change dramatically depending on the weights given to individual indicators (Goddard & Jacobs, 2009). Again, several options exist. The most straightforward way is to use equal weights for every indicator but this is unlikely to reflect the relative importance of individual measures. Another option is to base the weights on expert judgement or preferences of the target audience. Further options include opportunity-based weighting, also called denominator-based weights because more weight is given to indicators for more prevalent conditions (for example, higher weights for diabetes-related indicators than for acromegaly-related indicators), and numerator-based weights which give more weight to indicators covering a larger number of events (for example, higher weight on medication interaction than on wrong-side surgery). Finally, yet another option is to use an all-or-none approach at the patient level, where a score of one is given only if all requirements for an individual patient have been met (for example, all five recommended pre-operative processes were performed).

Again, there is no clear guidance on how best to construct a composite indicator. However, what is important is that indicator construction is transparent and that methodological choices and rationales are clearly explained to facilitate understanding. Furthermore, different choices will provide different incentives for improvement and these need to be considered during composite construction.

3.7 Selection of indicators

A wide range of existing indicators is available that can form the basis for the development of new quality measurement initiatives. For example, the National Quality Forum (NQF) in the USA provides an online database with more than a thousand quality indicators that can be searched by type of indicator (structure, process, outcome), by clinical area (for example, dental, cancer or eye care), by target of measurement (for example, provider, payer, population), and by endorsement status (i.e. whether they meet the NQF's measure evaluation criteria) (NQF, 2019a). The OECD Health Care Quality Indicator Project provides a list of 55 quality indicators for cross-country analyses of the quality of primary care, acute care and mental care, as well as patient safety and patient experiences (OECD HCQI, 2016). The Australian Commission on Safety and Quality in Health Care has developed a broad set of indicators for hospitals, primary care, patient safety and patient experience, among others (ACSQHC, 2019).

The English Quality and Outcomes Framework (QOF) includes 77 indicators for evaluating the quality of primary care (NHS Employers, 2018), and these indicators have inspired several other countries to develop their own quality indicators for primary care. The NHS also publishes indicators for the assessment of medication safety (NHS BSA, 2019). In addition, several recent reviews have summarized available quality indicators for different areas of care, for example, palliative care (Pfaff & Markaki, 2017), mental health (Parameswaran, Spaeth-Rublee & Alan Pincus, 2015), primary care for patients with serious mental illnesses (Kronenberg et al., 2017), cardiovascular care (Campbell et al., 2008), and for responsible use of medicines (Fujita, Moles & Chen, 2018). Different chapters in this book will refer to indicators as part of specific quality strategies such as public reporting (*see* Chapter 13).

In fact, there is a plethora of indicators that can potentially be used for measurement for the various purposes described previously (*see* section above: Different purposes of quality measurement and users of quality information). However, because data collection and analysis may consume considerable resources, and because quality measurement may have unintended consequences, initiatives have to carefully select (or newly develop) indicators based on the identified quality problem, the interested stakeholders and the purpose of measurement (Evans et al., 2009).

Quality measurement that aims to monitor and/or address problems related to specific diseases, for example, cardiovascular or gastrointestinal diseases, or particular groups of patients, for example, geriatric patients or paediatric patients, will likely require disease-specific indicators. By contrast, quality measurement aiming to address problems related to the organization of care (for example, waiting times in emergency departments), to specific providers (for example, falls during inpatient stays), or professionals (for example, insufficiently qualified personnel) will likely require generic indicators. Quality problems related to the effectiveness of care are likely to require rate-based disease-specific indicators, while safety problems are more likely to be addressed through (often generic) sentinel event indicators. Problems with regard to patient-centredness will likely require indicators based on patient surveys and expressed as rates.

The interested stakeholders and the purpose of measurement should determine the desired level of detail and the focus of measurement on structures, processes or outcomes. This is illustrated in Table 3.5, which summarizes the information needs of different stakeholders in relation to their different purposes. For example, governments responsible for assuring overall quality and accountability of healthcare service provision will require relatively few aggregated composite indicators, mostly of health outcomes, to monitor overall system level performance and to assure value for money. By contrast, provider organizations and professionals, which are mostly interested in quality improvement, are likely to demand a high number of disease-specific process indicators, which allows identification of areas for quality improvement.

Another issue that needs to be considered when choosing quality indicators is the question of finding the right balance between coverage and practicality. Relying on only a few indicators causes some aspects of care quality to be neglected and

Table 3.5 *Information needs of health system stakeholders with regard to quality of care*

Stakeholder	Purpose	Information needs
Governments	Quality assurance and accountability	Few aggregated composite generic indicators with a focus on outcomes
Regulators	Quality assurance	Moderate number of aggregated composite indicators for structures, processes and outcomes
Purchasers and payers	Quality assurance	Few aggregated composite generic indicators
	Quality improvement	A large number of disease-specific indicators for structures, processes and outcomes
Provider organizations	Quality improvement	High number of disease-specific indicators, focus on processes
Professionals	Quality improvement	High number of disease-specific indicators, focus on processes
Patients	Quality assurance and accountability	Disease-specific aggregated information on outcomes, processes and structures – with option to disaggregate
Citizens	Quality assurance and accountability	Aggregated generic information on outcomes, structures and processes

Source: authors' compilation

potentially to distract attention away from non-measured areas. It may also be necessary to have more than one indicator for one quality aspect, for example, mortality, readmissions and a PREM. However, maintaining too many indicators will be expensive and impractical to use. Finally, the quality of quality indicators should be a determining factor in selecting indicators for measurement.

3.8 Quality of quality indicators

There are numerous guidelines and criteria available for evaluating the quality of quality indicators. In 2006 the OECD Health Care Quality Indicators Project published a list of criteria for the selection of quality indicators (Kelley & Hurst, 2006). A relatively widely used tool for the evaluation of quality indicators has been developed at the University of Amsterdam, the Appraisal of Indicators through Research and Evaluation (AIRE) instrument (de Koning, Burgers & Klazinga, 2007). The NQF in the USA has published its measure evaluation criteria, which form the basis for evaluations of the eligibility of quality indicators for endorsement (NQF, 2019b). In Germany yet another tool for the assessment of quality indicators – the QUALIFY instrument – was developed by the Federal Office for Quality Assurance (BQS) in 2007, and the Institute for Quality Assurance and Transparency in Health Care (IQTIG) defined a similar set of criteria in 2018 (IQTIG, 2018).

In general, the criteria defined by the different tools are quite similar but each tool adds certain aspects to the list. Box 3.1 summarizes the criteria defined by the various tools grouped along the dimensions of relevance, scientific soundness, feasibility and meaningfulness. The relevance of an indicator can be determined based on its effect on health or health expenditures, the importance that it has for the relevant stakeholders, the potential for improvement (for example, as determined by available evidence about practice variation), and the clarity of the purpose and the healthcare context for which the indicator was developed. The latter point is important because many of the following criteria are dependent on the specific purpose.

For example, the desired level for the criteria of validity, sensitivity and specificity will differ depending on whether the purpose is external quality assurance or internal quality improvement. Similarly, if the purpose is to assure a minimum level of quality across all providers, the appraisal concept has to focus on minimum acceptable requirements, while it will have to distinguish between good and very good performers if the aim is to reward high-quality providers through a pay for quality approach (*see* Chapter 14).

Important aspects that need to be considered with regard to feasibility of measurement include whether previous experience exists with the use of the measure, whether the necessary information is available or can be collected in the required timeframe, whether the costs of measurement are acceptable, and whether the data will allow meaningful analyses for relevant subgroups of the population (for example, by socioeconomic status). Furthermore, the meaningfulness of the indicator is an important criterion, i.e. whether the indicator allows useful comparisons, whether the results are user-friendly for the target audience, and whether the distinction between high and low quality is meaningful for the target audience.

Box 3.1   *Criteria for indicators*

Relevance

- *Impact of disease or risk on health and health expenditures.* What is the impact on health and on health expenditure associated with each disease, risk or patient group?
- *Importance.* Are relevant stakeholders concerned about the quality problem and have they endorsed the indicator?
- *Potential for improvement.* Does evidence exist that there is less-than-optimal performance, for example, variation across providers?
- *Clarity of purpose and context.* Are the purpose of the indicator and the organizational and healthcare contexts clearly described?

Scientific soundness

- *Validity.* Does the indicator measure what it is intended to measure? The indicator should make sense logically and clinically (face validity); it should correlate well with other indicators of the same aspects of the quality of care (construct validity) and should capture meaningful (i.e. evidence-based) aspects of the quality of care (content validity).
- *Sensitivity and specificity.* Does the indicator detect only a few false positives and false negatives?
- *Reliability.* Does the measure provide stable results across various populations and circumstances?
- *Explicitness of the evidence base.* Is scientific evidence available to support the measure (for example, systematic reviews, guidelines, etc.)?
- *Adequacy of the appraisal concept.* Are reference values fit for purpose, and do they allow identification of good and bad providers?

Feasibility

- *Previous experience.* Is the measure in use in pilot programmes or in other countries?
- *Availability of required data across the system.* Can information needed for the measure be collected in the scale and timeframe required?
- *Cost or burden of measurement.* How much will it cost to collect the data needed for the measure?

continued
overleaf   >

- *Capacity of data and measure to support subgroup analyses.* Can the measure be used to compare different groups of the population (for example, by socioeconomic status to assess disparities)?

Meaningfulness

- *Comparability:* does the indicator permit meaningful comparisons across providers, regions, and/or countries?
- *User-friendliness:* is the indicator easily understood and does it relate to things that are important for the target audience?
- *Discriminatory power:* does the indicator distinguish clearly between good and bad performers?

Sources: Hurtado, Swift & Corrigan, 2001; Mainz, 2003; Kelley & Hurst, 2006; de Koning, Burgers & Klazinga, 2007; Evans et al., 2009; Lüngen & Rath, 2011; IQTIG, 2018; NQF, 2019b

3.9 Data sources for measuring quality

Many different kinds of data are available that can potentially be used for quality measurement. The most often used data sources are administrative data, medical records of providers and data stored in different – often disease-specific – registers, such as cancer registers. In addition, surveys of patients or healthcare personnel can be useful to gain additional insights into particular dimensions of quality. Finally, other approaches, such as direct observation of a physician's activities by a qualified colleague, are useful under specific conditions (for example, in a research context) but usually not possible for continuous measurement of quality.

There are many challenges with regard to the quality of the available data. These challenges can be categorized into four key aspects: (1) completeness, (2) comprehensiveness, (3) validity and (4) timeliness. Completeness means that the data properly include all patients with no missing cases. Comprehensiveness refers to whether the data contain all relevant variables needed for analysis, such as diagnosis codes, results of laboratory tests or procedures performed. Validity means that the data accurately reflect reality and are free of bias and errors. Finally, timeliness means that the data are available for use without considerable delay.

Data sources differ in their attributes and have different strengths and weaknesses, which are presented below and summarized in Table 3.6. The availability of data for research and quality measurement purposes differs substantially between countries. Some countries have more restrictive data privacy protection legislation in place, and also the possibility of linking different databases using unique personal identifiers is not available in all countries (Oderkirk, 2013; Mainz, Hess & Johnsen, 2019). Healthcare providers may also use patient data only for internal quality improvement purposes and prohibit transfer of data to external bodies. Nevertheless, with the increasing diffusion of IT technology in the form of electronic health records, administrative databases and clinical registries, opportunities of data linkage are increasing, potentially creating new and better options for quality measurement.

3.9.1 Administrative data

Administrative data are not primarily generated for quality or research purposes but by definition for administrative and management purposes (for example, billing data, routine documentation) and have the advantage of being readily available and easily accessible in electronic form. Healthcare providers, in particular hospitals, are usually mandated to maintain administrative records, which are used

Table 3.6 *Strengths and weaknesses of different data sources*

Data Source	Strengths	Weaknesses	Indications
Administrative	• Readily available at a national level and in electronic format • Allows comparison and analysis through standardized classifications and codes • High data quality given it is used for administrative purposes, such as billing	• Lacks much of the clinical information recorded in the medical record • Coding can be systematically affected by use for funding purposes • Generally not trusted by clinicians as much as clinical data systems • Relies on sound documentation and clinical coding	• National and international comparisons where standardization of coding is critical • Process and outcome indicators where few clinical data are required • Linking to other data sets, including mortality data
Medical Record	• Principal source of clinical information at patient level • Provides information on medical, nursing and allied healthcare • Enables opportunities for longitudinal data, at least within the facility • Electronic systems facilitate data access and coverage of patient care	• Paper-based systems require significant effort to retrieve and aggregate data • Relies on sound documentation • Paper-based systems lack linkage across facilities • Electronic systems require significant investment to capture comprehensive clinical data	• Facilitate quality improvement within care facilities • Use in research studies and ad hoc audits • Electronic records facilitate routine monitoring and greater aggregation within and across services over time
Registry	• Allows purposeful collection of high-quality data through strong planning and governance • High level of trust in data quality by clinicians • Readily accessible electronically and can draw on data sources from across facilities and settings	• Requires significant investment in establishment and maintenance • Can be isolated from ongoing clinical practice due to time lags and governance • Often specific in focus and requires linkage to obtain a broader clinical view	• National and international comparisons where coverage and standardization are critical • Indicators where specific clinical data are routinely required • Used in preference to administrative data for specific conditions or dimensions of quality

continued overleaf >

Data Source	Strengths	Weaknesses	Indications
Survey	• Allows greater scope to collect qualitative information • Can be designed for specific purposes and ad hoc studies • Does not necessarily require all members of a population to provide data • Allows greater depth of insights into specific areas, depending on methods	• Requires careful survey design to ensure validity of the data and avoid misleading conclusions • Often fraught with issues regarding representativeness, due to selection bias, non-response bias and sample size • Can be burdensome for respondents, particularly if the survey is repeated • Cohort follow can be problematic for longitudinal data	• Enables information not captured by other data sources, including patient and staff reported data
Direct observation	• Does not necessarily rely on patient, clinician or other staff documentation or reporting • Can be independent and systematically carried out across a facility and system • Provides a basis for collecting data when routine and other data systems are not viable • Allows direct verification of observable events and situations • Can incorporate documentations and subject reported information	• Requires significant investment in training inspectors and coordinating and carrying out inspections • Risk of significant inter-rater variability • Not generally feasible for information to be collected frequently • Not all quality issues can be obtained through observation, requiring access to documentation or other data sources	• Enables information not captured by other data sources, including patient and staff reported data. • Amenable to certain measures dependent on observation, and often not well documented or reported including pressure ulcers, restraint and other safety events

Sources: Steinwachs & Hughes, 2008; Iezzoni, 2009; Busse, 2012

in many countries for quality measurement purposes. In addition, governments usually have registers of births and deaths that are potentially relevant for quality measurement but which are often not used by existing measurement systems.

Administrative discharge data from hospitals usually include a patient identifier, demographic information, primary and secondary diagnoses coded using the International Classification of Diseases (ICD), coded information about medical and surgical procedures, dates of services provided, provider identifiers and many other bits of information (Iezzoni, 2009).

However, more detailed clinical information on severity of disease (for example, available from lab test results) or information about functional impairment or quality of life are not available in administrative data. The strength of administrative data is that they are comprehensive and complete with few problems of missing data. The most important problem of administrative data is that they are generated by healthcare providers, usually for payment purposes. This means that coding may be influenced by the incentives of the payment system, and – once used for purposes of quality measurement – also by incentives attached to the measured quality of care.

3.9.2 Medical record data

Medical records contain the most in-depth clinical information and document the patient's condition or problem, tests and treatments received and follow-up care. The completeness of medical record data varies greatly between and within countries and healthcare providers. Especially in primary care where the GP is familiar with the patient, proper documentation is often lacking. Also, if the patient changes provider during the treatment process and each provider keeps their own medical records, the different records would need to be combined to get a complete picture of the process (Steinwachs & Hughes, 2008).

Abstracting information from medical records can be expensive and time-consuming since medical records are rarely standardized. Another important aspect is to make sure that the information from medical records is gathered in a systematic way to avoid information bias. This can be done by defining clinical variables explicitly, writing detailed abstraction guidelines and training staff to maintain data quality. Medical record review is used mostly in internal quality improvement initiatives and research studies.

With the growth of electronic medical and electronic health records, the use of this data for more systematic quality measurement will likely increase in the future. The potential benefits of using electronic records are considerable as this may allow real-time routine analysis of the most detailed clinical information available, including information from imaging tests, prescriptions and pathology systems (Kannan et al., 2017). However, it will be necessary to address persisting challenges with regard to accuracy, completeness and comparability of the data collected in electronic records to enable reliable measurement of quality of care on the basis of this data (Chan et al., 2010).

3.9.3 Disease-specific registries

There are many disease-specific registries containing data that can be used for healthcare quality measurement purposes. Cancer registries exist in most developed countries and, while their main purpose is to register cancer cases and provide information on cancer incidence in their catchment area, the data can also be used for monitoring and evaluation of screening programmes and estimating cancer survival by follow-up of cancer patients (Bray & Parkin, 2009). In Scandinavian countries significant efforts have gone into standardizing cancer registries to enable cross-country comparability. Nevertheless, numerous differences persist with regard to registration routines and classification systems, which are important when comparing time trends in the Nordic countries (Pukkala et al., 2018).

In some countries there is a large number of clinical registries that are used for quality measurement. For example, in Sweden there are over a hundred clinical quality registries, which work on a voluntary basis as all patients must be informed and have the right to opt-out. These registries are mainly for specific diseases and they include disease-specific data, such as severity of disease at diagnosis, diagnostics and treatment, laboratory tests, patient-reported outcome measures, and other relevant factors such as body mass index, smoking status or medication. Most of the clinical registries focus on specialized care and are based on reporting from hospitals or specialized day care centres (Emilsson et al., 2015).

With increasing diffusion of electronic health records, it is possible to generate and feed disease-specific population registries based on electronic abstraction (Kannan et al., 2017). Potentially, this may significantly reduce the costs of data collection for registries. Furthermore, linking of data from different registries with other administrative data sources can increasingly be used to generate datasets that enable more profound analyses.

3.9.4 Survey data

Survey data are another widely used source of quality information. Surveys are the only option for gaining information about patient experiences with healthcare services and thus are an important source of information about patient-centredness of care. Substantial progress has been made over recent years to improve standardization of both patient-reported experience measures (PREMs) and patient-reported outcome measures (PROMs) in order to facilitate international comparability (Fujisawa & Klazinga, 2017).

Surveys of patient experiences capture the patients' views on health service delivery (for example, communication with nurses and doctors, staff responsiveness, discharge and care coordination). Most OECD countries have developed at least one national survey measuring PREMs over the past decade or so (Fujisawa & Klazinga, 2017), and efforts are under way to further increase cooperation and collaboration to facilitate comparability (OECD, 2017).

Surveys of patient-reported outcomes capture the patient's perspective on their health status (for example, symptoms, functioning, mental health). PROMs surveys can use generic tools (for example, the SF-36 or EQ-5D) or disease-specific tools, which are usually more sensitive to change (Fitzpatrick, 2009). The NHS in the United Kingdom requires all providers to report PROMs for two elective procedures: hip replacement and knee replacement. Both generic (EQ-5D and EQ VAS) and disease-specific (Oxford Hip Score, Oxford Knee Score and Aberdeen Varicose Vein Questionnaire) instruments are used (NHS Digital, 2019b).

Finally, several countries also use surveys of patient satisfaction in order to monitor provider performance. However, satisfaction is difficult to compare internationally because it is influenced by patients' expectations about how they will be treated, which vary widely across countries and also within countries (Busse, 2012).

3.9.5 Direct observation

Direct observation is sometimes used for research purposes or as part of peer-review processes. Direct observation allows the study of clinical processes, such as the adherence to clinical guidelines and the availability of basic structures. Observation is normally considered to be too resource-intensive for continuous quality measurement. However, site visits and peer-reviews are often added to routine monitoring of secondary (administrative) data to investigate providers with unexplained variation in quality and to better understand the context where these data are produced.

3.10 Attribution and risk-adjustment

Two further conceptual and methodological considerations are essential when embarking on quality measurement or making use of quality data, in particular with regard to outcome indicators. Both are related to the question of responsibility for differences in measured quality of care or, in other words, related to the question of attributing causality to responsible agents (Terris & Aron, 2009). Ideally, quality measurement is based on indicators that have been purposefully developed to reflect the quality of care provided by individuals, teams, provider organizations (for example, hospitals) or other units of analysis (for example, networks, regions, countries) (*see also* above, Quality of quality indicators). However, many existing quality indicators do not reflect only the quality of care provided by the target of measurement but also a host of factors that are outside the direct control of an individual provider or provider organization.

For example, surgeon-specific mortality data for patients undergoing coronary artery bypass graft (CABG) have been publicly reported in England and several states of the USA for many years (Radford et al., 2015; Romano et al., 2011). Yet debate continues whether results actually reflect the individual surgeon's quality of care or rather the quality of the wider hospital team (for example, including anaesthesia, intensive care unit quality) or the organization and management of the hospital (for example, the organization of resuscitation teams within hospitals) (Westaby et al., 2015). Nevertheless, with data released at the level of the surgeon, responsibility is publicly attributed to the individual and not to the organization.

Other examples where attributing causality and responsibility is difficult include outcome indicators defined using time periods (for example, 30-day mortality after hospitalization for ischemic stroke) because patients may be transferred between different providers and because measured quality will depend on care received after discharge. Similarly, attribution can be problematic for patients with chronic conditions, for example, attributing causality for hospitalizations of patients with heart failure – a quality indicator in the USA – is difficult because these patients may see numerous providers, such as one (or more) primary care physician(s) and specialists, for example, nephrologists and/or cardiologists.

What these examples illustrate is that attribution of quality differences to providers is difficult. However, it is important to accurately attribute causality because it is unfair to hold individuals or organizations accountable for factors outside their control. In addition, if responsibility is attributed incorrectly, quality improvement measures will be in vain, as they will miss the appropriate target. Therefore, when developing quality indicators, it is important that a causal pathway can be established between the agents under assessment and the outcome proposed as a quality measure. Furthermore, possible confounders, such as the influence of other providers or higher levels of the healthcare system on the outcome of interest, should be carefully explored in collaboration with relevant stakeholders (Terris & Aron, 2009).

Of course, many important confounders outside the control of providers have not yet been mentioned as the most important confounders are patient-level clinical factors and patient preferences. Prevalence of these factors may differ across patient populations and influence the outcomes of care. For example, severely ill patients or patients with multiple coexisting conditions are at risk of having worse outcomes than healthy individuals despite receiving high-quality care. Therefore, providers treating sicker patients are at risk of performing poorly on measured quality of care, in particular when measured through outcome indicators.

Risk-adjustment (sometimes called case-mix adjustment) aims to control for these differences (risk-factors) that would otherwise lead to biased results. Almost all outcome indicators require risk-adjustment to adjust for patient-level risk factors that are outside the control of providers. In addition, healthcare processes may be influenced by patients' attitudes and perceptions, which should be taken into account for risk-adjustment of process indicators if relevant. Ideally, risk-adjustment assures that measured differences in the quality of care are not biased by differences in the underlying patient populations treated by different providers or in different regions.

An overview of potential patient (risk-) factors that may influence outcomes of care is presented in Table 3.7. Demographic characteristics (for example, age), clinical (for example, co-morbidities) and socioeconomic factors, health-related behaviours (for example, alcohol use, nutrition) and attitudes may potentially have an effect on outcomes of care. By controlling for these factors, risk-adjustment methods will produce estimates that are better comparable across individuals, provider organizations or other units of analysis.

The field of risk-adjustment is developing rapidly and increasingly sophisticated methods are available for ensuring fair comparisons across providers, especially for conditions involving surgery, risk of death and post-operative complications (Iezzoni, 2009). Presentation of specific risk-adjustment methods is beyond the scope of this chapter but some general methods include direct and indirect standardization, multiple regression analysis and other statistical techniques. The selection of potential confounding factors needs to be done carefully, taking into account the ultimate purpose and use of the quality indicator that needs adjustment.

In fact, the choice of risk-adjustment factors is not a purely technical exercise but relies on assumptions that are often not clearly spelled out. For example, in several countries the hospital readmission rate is used as a quality indicator in pay for quality programmes (Kristensen, Bech & Quentin, 2015). If it is believed that age influences readmission rates in a way hospitals cannot affect, age should be included in the risk-adjustment formula. However, if it is thought that hospitals can influence elderly patients' readmission rates by special discharge programmes for the elderly, age may not be considered a "risk" but rather an indicator for the hospitals to use for identifying patients with special needs. The same arguments apply also for socioeconomic status. On the one hand, there are good reasons to adjust for socioeconomic variables because patients living in poorer neighbourhoods tend to have higher readmission rates. On the other hand, including socioeconomic variables in a risk-adjustment formula would implicitly mean that it was acceptable for hospitals located in poorer areas to have more readmissions.

The assumptions and methodological choices made when selecting variables for risk-adjustment may have a powerful effect on risk-adjusted measured quality of care. Some critics (for example, Lilford et al., 2004) have argued that comparative outcome data should not be used externally to make judgements about quality of hospital care. More recent criticism of risk-adjustment methods has suggested

Table 3.7 *Potential patient risk-factors*

Demographic characteristics	Socioeconomic factors	Attitudes and perceptions
• age	• educational attainment	• cultural beliefs and behaviours
• sex/gender	• health literacy	• religious beliefs and behaviours, spirituality
• race and ethnicity	• language(s)	
	• employment and occupation	• overall health status and quality of life
	• economic resources	
	• family characteristics and household composition	• preferences, values and expectations for healthcare services
	• housing and neighbourhood characteristics	
	• health insurance coverage	

Clinical factors	Health-related behaviours and activities
• acute physiological stability	• tobacco use
• principal diagnosis	• alcohol, illicit drug use
• severity of principal diagnosis	• sexual practices ('safe sex')
• extent and severity of co-morbidities	• diet and nutrition
• physical functioning	• physical activity, exercise
• vision, hearing, speech functioning	• obesity and overweight
• cognitive functioning	
• mental illness, emotional health	

Source: Iezzoni, 2009

that risk-adjustment methods of current quality measurement systems could be evaluated by assigning ranks similar to those used to rate the quality of evidence (Braithwaite, 2018). Accordingly, A-level risk-adjustment would adjust for all known causes of negative consequences that are beyond the control of clinicians yet influence outcomes. C-level risk-adjustment would fail to control for several important factors that cause negative consequences, while B-level risk-adjustment would be somewhere in between.

3.11 Conclusion

This chapter has introduced some basic concepts and methods for the measurement of healthcare quality and presented a number of related challenges. Many different stakeholders have varying needs for information on healthcare quality and the development of quality measurement systems should always take into account the purpose of measurement and the needs of different stakeholders. Quality measurement is important for quality assurance and accountability to make sure that providers are delivering good-quality care but they are also vital for quality improvement programmes to ensure that these interventions lead to increases in care quality.

The development and use of quality measures should always be fit-for-purpose. For example, outcome-based quality indicators, such as those used by the OECD, are useful for international comparisons or national agenda-setting but providers such as hospitals or health centres may need more specific indicators related to processes of care in order to enable quality improvement. The Donabedian framework of structure, process and outcome indicators provides a comprehensive, easily understandable model for classifying different types of indicator, and it has guided indicator development of most existing quality measurement systems.

Quality indicators should be of high quality and should be carefully chosen and implemented in cooperation with providers and clinicians. The increasing availability of clinical data in the form of electronic health records is multiplying possibilities for quality measurement on the basis of more detailed indicators. In addition, risk-adjustment is important to avoid high-quality providers being incorrectly and unfairly identified as providing poor quality of care – and vice versa, to avoid that poor providers appear to be providing good quality of care. Again, the increasing availability of data from electronic medical records may expand the options for better risk-adjustment.

However, most quality measurement initiatives will continue to focus – for reasons of practicality and data availability – only on a limited set of quality indicators. This means that one of the fundamental risks of quality measurement will continue to be important: quality measurement will always direct attention to those areas that are covered by quality indicators, potentially at the expense of other important aspects of quality that are more difficult to assess through quality measurement.

Nevertheless, without quality information policy-makers lack the knowledge base to steer health systems, patients can only rely on personal experiences or those of friends for choosing healthcare providers, and healthcare providers have no way of knowing whether their quality improvement programmes have worked as expected.

Quality information is a tool and it can do serious damage if used inappropriately. Seven basic principles of using quality indicators are summarized in Box 3.2. It is critical to be aware of the limitations of quality measurement and to be cautious of using quality information for quality strategies that provide powerful incentives to providers, such as public reporting (*see* Chapter 13) or P4Q schemes (*see* Chapter 14), as these may lead to potential unintended consequences such as gaming or patient selection.

Box 3.2 *Seven principles to take into account when using quality indicators*

Principle 1: Indicators have to be fit-for-purpose

The choice of quality indicators should proceed from a clear definition of its intended purpose. Indicators designed with an external focus (i.e. oversight, accountability, identifying outliers, patient choice) will require different characteristics from those designed with an internal focus (i.e. quality improvement). For external use the quality measures should be sensitive to identify quality problems, and they should be capable of showing meaningful differences between providers. For internal use more specific quality measures are necessary to monitor progress over time and to provide signals that offer clear and actionable management responses.

Principle 2: Quality of measurement depends on quality of data and indicators

The reliability of quality measures relates to the quality of the data on which they are based and the robustness of the method used to construct them. Reliability can be a concern where quality indicators are derived from databases that are only indirectly linked to the primary process of care delivery and data recording, for example, administrative billing data.

Principle 3: Quality measurement has limits

Quality of care has different dimensions (effectiveness, safety, patient-centredness) and one specific healthcare provider (for example, a hospital or GP practice) provides care via various processes involving many different professionals and technologies. Conclusions about all different quality aspects and all underlying services made on the basis of only a few indicators are likely to miss important non-measured aspects of care. Organizational context and local knowledge of confounding circumstances must be taken into account when interpreting even well-constructed indicators.

Principle 4: Outcome measures require risk-adjustment

Despite much progress, the validity of outcome measures is often debatable. Collecting information on outcomes like mortality and complications is useful but often it is hard to determine whether differences found are actually the result of differences in quality of care. For example, without risk-adjustment for complications and co-morbidities, differences in mortality found between hospitals may not be due to differences in the quality of care provided. One hospital may deal only with straightforward, uncomplicated patients whereas others (such as specialist centres) may treat the most complicated cases.

Principle 5: Composite indicators improve simplicity but may be misleading

Attempts have been made to construct composite indicators that summarize a broader suite of underlying measures. Although this approach has certain attractions – notably simplicity – the results can be misleading. Weaknesses of the underlying indicators are often disguised and the weighting between the various constituent indicators is often not based on empirical information or not reported at all. Thus, the summary "score" may suggest a clear result (for example, that one provider is better than another) but if underlying data and methods are weak, users may come to incorrect conclusions.

Principle 6: A league table raises interest but is not always fair

The same methodological limitations that apply to compound indicators also apply to league tables. Weaknesses in the underlying components may be masked, weighting is not necessarily user-based and ranking suggests real differences in the units being measured, i.e. hospitals, countries, etc. Additionally, without the presence of properly calculated confidence estimates, rank orders that imply absolute differences in quality may in fact be nothing more significant than chance. League tables, especially those published through official channels, should therefore be handled with care.

Principle 7: Be aware of gaming and unintended consequences

Overall reporting of information on quality of care can lead to performance improvement. Nevertheless, reporting on certain aspects of care can lead to adverse effects such as gaming or outright cheating. For example, reporting on hospital mortality rates has in the past led hospital professionals to try to improve their rates by promoting that patients die elsewhere. Furthermore, if indicators focus on major diseases like diabetes and chronic heart failure, this may lessen interest in diseases that are less prominent in reporting and rewarding systems. Additionally, reporting on negative outcomes (safety, complications) should be balanced by reporting on positive outcomes (improved functioning, survival) – doing so will help to promote a balanced culture of risk control and risk taking in healthcare.

Source: based on OECD, 2010

References

ACSQHC (2019). Indicators of Safety and Quality. Australian Commission on Safety and Quality in Health Care (ACSQHC): https://www.safetyandquality.gov.au/our-work/indicators/#Patientreported, accessed 21 March 2019.

Baker DW, Chassin MR (2017). Holding Providers Accountable for Health Care Outcomes. *Annals of Internal Medicine*, 167(6):418–23.

Braithwaite RS (2018). Risk Adjustment for Quality Measures Is Neither Binary nor Mandatory. *Journal of the American Medical Association*, 319(20):2077–8.

Bray F, Parkin DM (2009). Evaluation of data quality in the cancer registry: Principles and methods. Part I: Comparability, validity and timeliness. *European Journal of Cancer*, 45(5):747–55.

Busse R (2012). Being responsive to citizens' expectations: the role of health services in responsiveness and satisfaction. In: McKee M, Figueras J (eds.) Health Systems: Health, wealth and societal well-being. Maidenhead: Open University Press/McGraw-Hill.

Calhoun C (2002). Oxford dictionary of social sciences. New York: Oxford University Press.

Campbell SM et al. (2008). Quality indicators for the prevention and management of cardiovascular disease in primary care in nine European countries. *European Journal of Cardiovascular Prevention & Rehabilitation*, 15(5):509–15.

Carinci F et al. (2015). Towards actionable international comparisons of health system performance: expert revision of the OECD framework and quality indicators. *International Journal for Quality in Health Care*, 27(2):137–46.

Chan KS et al. (2010). Electronic health records and the reliability and validity of quality measures: a review of the literature. *Medical Care Research and Review*, 67(5):503–27.

Cheng EM et al. (2014). Quality measurement: here to stay. *Neurology Clinical Practice*, 4(5):441–6.

Cylus J, Papanicolas I, Smith P (2016). Health system efficiency: how to make measurement matter for policy and management. Copenhagen: WHO, on behalf of the European Observatory on Health Systems and Policies.

Davies H (2005). Measuring and reporting the quality of health care: issues and evidence from the international research literature. NHS Quality Improvement Scotland.

Donabedian A (1980). The Definition of Quality and Approaches to Its Assessment. Vol 1. Explorations in Quality Assessment and Monitoring. Ann Arbor, Michigan, USA: Health Administration Press.

EC (2016). So What? Strategies across Europe to assess quality of care. Report by the Expert Group on Health Systems Performance Assessment. European Commission (EC). Brussels: European Commission.

Emilsson L et al. (2015). Review of 103 Swedish Healthcare Quality Registries. *Journal of Internal Medicine*, 277(1):94–136

Evans SM et al. (2009). Prioritizing quality indicator development across the healthcare system: identifying what to measure. *Internal Medicine Journal*, 39(10):648–54.

Fitzpatrick R (2009). Patient-reported outcome measures and performance measurement. In: Smith P et al. (eds.) Performance Measurement for Health System Improvement: Experiences, Challenges and Prospects. Cambridge: Cambridge University Press.

Forde I, Morgan D, Klazinga N (2013). Resolving the challenges in the international comparison of health systems: the must do's and the trade-offs. *Health Policy*, 112(1–2):4–8.

Freeman T (2002). Using performance indicators to improve health care quality in the public sector: a review of the literature. *Health Services Management Research*, 15:126–37.

Fujisawa R, Klazinga N (2017). Measuring patient experiences (PREMS): Progress made by the OECD and its member countries between 2006 and 2016. Paris: Organisation for Economic Co-operation and Development (OECD).

Fujita K, Moles RJ, Chen TF (2018). Quality indicators for responsible use of medicines: a systematic review. *BMJ Open*, 8:e020437.

Gardner K, Olney S, Dickinson H (2018). Getting smarter with data: understanding tensions in the use of data in assurance and improvement-oriented performance management systems to improve their implementation. *Health Research Policy and Systems*, 16(125).

Goddard M, Jacobs R (2009). Using composite indicators to measure performance in health care. In: Smith P et al. (eds.) Performance Measurement for Health System Improvement: Experiences, Challenges and Prospects. Cambridge: Cambridge University Press.

Hurtado MP, Swift EK, Corrigan JM (2001). Envisioning the National Health Care Quality Report. Washington, DC: National Academy Press.

ICHOM (2019). Standard Sets. International Consortium for Health Outcomes Measurement (ICHOM): https://www.ichom.org/standard-sets/, accessed 8 February 2019.

Iezzoni L (2009). Risk adjustment for performance measurement. In: Smith P et al. (eds.) Performance Measurement for Health System Improvement: Experiences, Challenges and Prospects. Cambridge: Cambridge University Press.

IQTIG (2018). Methodische Grundlagen V1.1.s. Entwurf für das Stellungnahmeverfahren. Institut für Qualitätssicherung und Transparenz im Gesundheitswesen (IQTIG). Available at: https://iqtig.org/das-iqtig/grundlagen/methodische-grundlagen/, accessed 18 March 2019.

Kannan V et al. (2017). Rapid Development of Specialty Population Registries and Quality Measures from Electronic Health Record Data. *Methods of information in medicine*, 56(99):e74–e83.

Kelley E, Hurst J (2006). Health Care Quality Indicators Project: Conceptual framework paper. Paris: Organization for Economic Co-operation and Development (OECD). Available at: https://www.oecd.org/els/health-systems/36262363.pdf, accessed on 22/03/2019.

De Koning J, Burgers J, Klazinga N (2007). Appraisal of indicators through research and evaluation (AIRE). Available at: https://www.zorginzicht.nl/kennisbank/PublishingImages/Paginas/AIRE-instrument/AIRE%20Instrument%202.0.pdf, accessed 21 March 2019.

Kristensen SR, Bech M, Quentin W (2015). A roadmap for comparing readmission policies with application to Denmark, England and the United States. *Health Policy*, 119(3):264–73.

Kronenberg C et al. (2017). Identifying primary care quality indicators for people with serious mental illness: a systematic review. *British Journal of General Practice*, 67(661):e519–e530.

Lawrence M, Olesen F (1997). Indicators of Quality in Health Care. *European Journal of General Practice*, 3(3):103–8.

Lighter D (2015). How (and why) do quality improvement professionals measure performance? *International Journal of Pediatrics and Adolescent Medicine*, 2(1):7–11.

Lilford R et al. (2004). Use and misuse of process and outcome data in managing performance of acute medical care: avoiding institutional stigma. *Lancet*, 363(9424):1147–54.

Lohr KN (1990). Medicare: A Strategy for Quality Assurance. Washington (DC), US: National Academies Press.

Lüngen M, Rath T (2011). Analyse und Evaluierung des QUALIFY Instruments zur Bewertung von Qualitätsindikatoren anhand eines strukturierten qualitativen Interviews. *Zeitschrift für Evidenz, Fortbildung und Qualität im Gesundheitswesen*, 105(1):38–43.

Mainz J (2003). Defining and classifying indicators for quality improvement. *International Journal for Quality in Health Care*, 15(6):523–30.

Mainz J, Hess MH, Johnsen SP (2019). Perspectives on Quality: the Danish unique personal identifier and the Danish Civil Registration System as a tool for research and quality improvement. *International Journal for Quality in Health Care* (efirst): https://doi.org/10.1093/intqhc/mzz008.

Marjoua Y, Bozic K (2012) Brief history of quality movement in US healthcare. *Current reviews in musculoskeletal medicine*, 5(4):265–73.

NHS BSA (2019). Medication Safety – Indicators Specification. NHS Business Services Authority (NHS BSA). Available at: https://www.nhsbsa.nhs.uk/sites/default/files/2019-02/Medication%20Safety%20-%20Indicators%20Specification.pdf, accessed 21 March 2019.

NHS Digital (2019a). Indicator Methodology and Assurance Service. NHS Digital, Leeds. Available at: https://digital.nhs.uk/services/indicator-methodology-and-assurance-service, accessed 18 March 2019.

NHS Digital (2019b). Patient Reported Outcome Measures (PROMs). NHS Digital, Leeds. Available at: https://digital.nhs.uk/data-and-information/data-tools-and-services/data-services/patient-reported-outcome-measures-proms, accessed 22 March 2019.

NHS Employers (2018). 2018/19 General Medical Services (GMS) contract Quality and Outcomes Framework (QOF). Available at: https://www.nhsemployers.org/-/media/Employers/Documents/Primary-care-contracts/QOF/2018-19/2018-19-QOF-guidance-for-stakeholders.pdf, accessed 21 March 2019.

NQF (2019a). Quality Positioning System. National Quality Forum (NQF). Available at: http://www.qualityforum.org/QPS/QPSTool.aspx, accessed 19 March 2019.

NQF (2019b). Measure evaluation criteria. National Quality Forum (NQF). Available at: http://www.qualityforum.org/measuring_performance/submitting_standards/measure_evaluation_criteria.aspx, accessed 19 March 2019.

Oderkirk J (2013). International comparisons of health system performance among OECD countries: opportunities and data privacy protection challenges. *Health Policy*, 112(1–2):9–18

OECD (2008). Handbook on Constructing Composite Indicators: Methodology and user guide. Organisation for Economic Co-operation and Development (OECD). Available at: https://www.oecd.org/sdd/42495745.pdf, accessed 22 March 2019.

OECD (2010). Improving Value in Health Care: Measuring Quality. Organisation for Economic Co-operation and Development. Available at: https://www.oecd-ilibrary.org/

docserver/9789264094819-en.pdf?expires=1545066637&id=id&accname=ocid56023174 a&checksum=1B31D6EB98B6160BF8A5265774A54D61, accessed 17 December 2018.

OECD (2017). Recommendations to OECD Ministers of Health from the High Level Reflection Group on the future of health statistics. Strengthening the international comparison of health system performance through patient-reported indicators. Paris: Organisation for Economic Co-operation and Development.

OECD (2019). Patient-Reported Indicators Survey (PaRIS). Paris: Organisation for Economic Co-operation and Development. Available at: http://www.oecd.org/health/paris.htm, accessed 8 February 2019.

OECD HCQI (2016). Definitions for Health Care Quality Indicators 2016–2017. HCQI Data Collection. Organisation for Economic Co-operation and Development Health Care Quality Indicators Project. Available at: http://www.oecd.org/els/health-systems/Definitions-of-Health-Care-Quality-Indicators.pdf, accessed 21 March 2019.

Papanicolas I, Smith P (2013). Health system performance comparison: an agenda for policy, information and research. WHO, on behalf of the European Observatory. Open University Press, Maidenhead.

Parameswaran SG, Spaeth-Rublee B, Alan Pincus H (2015). Measuring the Quality of Mental Health Care: Consensus Perspectives from Selected Industrialized Countries. *Administration and Policy in Mental Health*, 42:288–95.

Pfaff K, Markaki A (2017). Compassionate collaborative care: an integrative review of quality indicators in end-of-life care. *BMC Palliative Care*, 16:65.

Porter M (2010). What is value in health care? *New England Journal of Medicine*, 363(26):2477–81.

Pukkala E et al. (2018). Nordic Cancer Registries – an overview of their procedures and data comparability. *Acta Oncologica*, 57(4):440–55.

Radford PD et al. (2015). Publication of surgeon specific outcome data: a review of implementation, controversies and the potential impact on surgical training. *International Journal of Surgery*, 13:211–16.

Romano PS et al. (2011). Impact of public reporting of coronary artery bypass graft surgery performance data on market share, mortality, and patient selection. *Medical Care*, 49(12):1118–25.

Rubin HR, Pronovost P, Diette G (2001). The advantages and disadvantages of process-based measures of health care quality. *International Journal for Quality in Health Care*, 13(6):469–74.

Shwartz M, Restuccia JD, Rosen AK (2015). Composite Measures of Health Care Provider Performance: A Description of Approaches. *Milbank Quarterly*, 93(4):788–825.

Smith P et al. (2009). Introduction. In: Smith P et al. (eds.) Performance Measurement for Health System Improvement: Experiences, Challenges and Prospects. Cambridge: Cambridge University Press.

Steinwachs DM, Hughes RG (2008). Health Services Research: Scope and Significance. Patient Safety and Quality: An Evidence-Based Handbook for Nurses. Rockville (MD): Agency for Healthcare Research and Quality (US).

Terris DD, Aron DC (2009). Attribution and causality in health-care performance measurement. In: Smith P et al. (eds.) Performance Measurement for Health System Improvement: Experiences, Challenges and Prospects. Cambridge: Cambridge University Press.

Voeten SC et al. (2018). Quality indicators for hip fracture care, a systematic review. *Osteoporosis International*, 29(9):1963–85.

Westaby S et al. (2015). Surgeon-specific mortality data disguise wider failings in delivery of safe surgical services. *European Journal of Cardiothoracic Surgery*, 47(2):341–5.

Chapter 4

International and EU governance and guidance for national healthcare quality strategies

Willy Palm, Miek Peeters, Pascal Garel, Agnieszka Daval, Charles Shaw

4.1 Introduction

This chapter deals with international frameworks and guidance to foster and support quality strategies in European countries. As will be demonstrated in the chapter, the legal status and binding nature of various international governance and guidance instruments differ substantially. While some are meant to support national quality initiatives in healthcare, others have a more direct effect on determining quality and safety of healthcare goods and services. This is definitely the case for measures taken at EU level to ensure free movement of goods, persons and services.

One of the questions addressed in this chapter is how the international community can contribute to national policies related to quality of care. Four different ways can be distinguished, which – taken together – can be considered as defining the four main elements of an integrated international governance framework for quality in healthcare (Fig. 4.1):

- raising political awareness of the relevance of healthcare quality and creating a common vision on how to improve it;

- implementing this vision into actual policy frameworks by sharing experience and practice between countries;

- developing and providing standards and models (voluntary or mandatory) that can be transposed into national policy; and

- measuring, assessing and comparing quality by developing better information and better indicators and methodologies as well as dissemination strategies.

Fig. 4.1   *An integrated international governance framework for quality in healthcare*

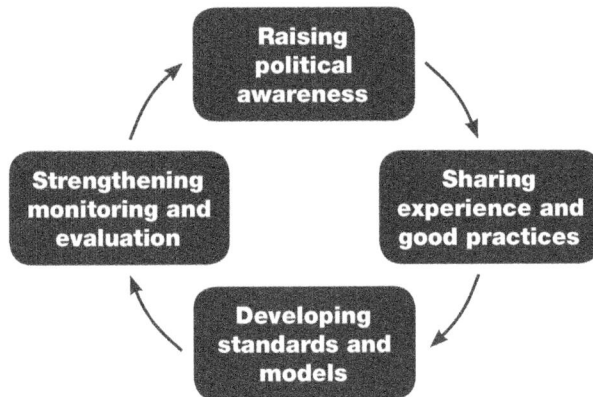

Based on this framework, the international dimension to healthcare quality will be explored in the first section. As different international organizations – both public and private – determine the international context in which Member States develop their quality policies, it will explore the interests of these organizations in addressing quality and analyse their influence on quality of healthcare in countries.

The following section will specifically focus on how quality in healthcare is addressed through EU policy. Traditionally, the emphasis has been mainly on the dimension of standardization (harmonization) as a way to ensuring free movement of goods, citizens and services and creating an internal market (also in healthcare). Promoting healthcare quality was thus not the prime motivation, and this is why other elements included in the framework (*see* Fig. 4.1) have gained relevance more recently in order to achieve a more integrated approach. At the same time, as a supranational institution the EU has considerable leverage on Member States to influence their national quality regulation and policies.

4.2 The international dimension to quality in healthcare

This section will briefly describe how different international organizations engaged in putting quality in healthcare on the political agenda and supporting countries in developing specific policies in this area. It is not always easy or possible to clearly disentangle the various dimensions of the quality governance framework. This section is not meant to provide a comprehensive analysis of what all international organizations do in all areas of the quality governance framework. Instead, it will provide some examples of the kind of support they are providing, and illustrate the complementary elements that can be observed in their approaches.

Raising political awareness and creating a common vision

Quality became an issue at international level only more recently. For a long time it was presumed that all care was of good quality, and the skills and practices of doctors and medical professionals were not called into question. It was only when national and international studies and projects started to demonstrate the huge heterogeneity in medical practice often associated with variations in health outcomes, as well as the high number of adverse events and medical errors, that it moved up the political agenda (Committee on Quality of Health Care in America, 1999).

Because quality was implicitly assumed to be an inherent attribute of healthcare, reference to quality is sometimes missing in earlier policy documents. For example, the Charter of fundamental rights of the EU includes a right to healthcare without explicit reference to quality (Charter of fundamental rights of the European Union, 2000: Article 35). Also the Council of Europe's Social Charter (1961) refers to the right of medical assistance (Article 13) without mentioning quality.

It is only the more recent Convention on Human Rights and Biomedicine (1997) that contains an obligation for Member States to provide "equitable access to health care of appropriate quality" (Article 3). Also, the EU Council's statement on the overarching values and principles underpinning health systems in the EU prescribes that access to good-quality care is one of the fundamental values besides universality, equity and solidarity (Council of the European Union, 2006). In addition, quality and safety are mentioned explicitly as common operating principles of health systems in the EU (*see* Box 4.1). In fact, all operating principles refer to some extent to quality: care that is based on ethics and evidence, patient involvement, redress, and privacy and confidentiality (Nys & Goffin, 2011).

Box 4.1 *Excerpt from the Council Conclusions on Common values and principles in European Union Health Systems (2006)*

— Quality:

All EU health systems strive to provide good quality care. This is achieved in particular through the obligation to continuous training of healthcare staff based on clearly defined national standards and ensuring that staff have access to advice about best practice in quality, stimulating innovation and spreading good practice, developing systems to ensure good clinical governance, and through monitoring quality in the health system. An important part of this agenda also relates to the principle

> *of safety. . . . Patients can expect each EU health system to secure a systematic approach to ensuring patient safety, including the monitoring of risk factors and adequate training for health professionals, and protection against misleading advertising of health products and treatments.*
>
> *— Safety:*
>
> *Patients can expect each EU health system to secure a systematic approach to ensuring patient safety, including the monitoring of risk factors and adequate training for health professionals, and protection against misleading advertising of health products and treatments.*

The active promotion of quality as an important lever for healthcare reform started in 1977 when the World Health Organization (WHO) launched its Health for All (HFA) strategy. The idea of quality assurance – comprising both external quality assessment and internal quality control – was considered an effective way for ensuring at the same time equal access to care, quality of life and user satisfaction as well as cost-effective use of resources. In target 31 of the HFA strategy, WHO Member States were urged to build effective mechanisms for ensuring quality of patient care, to provide structures and processes for ensuring continuous improvement in the quality of healthcare and appropriate development and use of new technologies. Under the revised HFA strategy for the 21st century that was adopted by the World Health Assembly in 1998, WHO Regional Office for Europe also emphasized continuous quality improvement as one of the core targets of its so-called Health21 framework for improving the health of Europeans (*see* Table 4.1).

Political statements and targets eventually led to the emergence of an international quality movement. In fact, the International Society for Quality in Healthcare (ISQua) was established in 1985 out of a WHO working group on training and quality assurance.[1] Other international organizations have followed, each one taking a specific focus or complementary function. The European Society for Quality in Healthcare (ESQH) since 1998 also actively promoted the improvement of quality in healthcare in Europe.

4.2.1 Sharing experiences and good practices to support national action

International organizations also actively promote the exchange of experience between countries. While some countries have developed over time quite comprehensive and integrated frameworks for assuring quality of healthcare, other countries still lack legislation in this field and initiatives are fragmented and

---

1   http://www.isqua.org/who-we-are/30th-anniversary/timeline-1985---2015.

Table 4.1   *WHO targets for ensuring quality in healthcare*

Health for all	Target 31, Ensuring quality of care
	By 1990, all Member States should have built effective mechanisms for ensuring quality of patient care within their health care systems.
	This could be achieved by establishing methods and procedures for systematically monitoring the quality of care given to patients and making assessment and regulation a permanent component of health professionals' regular activities; and providing all health personnel with training in quality assurance.
Health21	**Target 16, Managing for quality of care, focuses on outcomes as the ultimate measure of quality**
	By the year 2010, Member States should ensure that the clinical management of the health sector, from population-based health programmes to individual patient care at the clinical level, is oriented towards health outcomes.
	16.1 The effectiveness of major public health strategies should be assessed in terms of health outcomes, and decisions regarding alternative strategies for dealing with individual health problems should increasingly be taken by comparing health outcomes and their cost-effectiveness.
	16.2 All countries should have a nationwide mechanism for continuous monitoring and development of the quality of care for at least ten major health conditions, including measurement of health impact, cost-effectiveness and patient satisfaction.
	16.3 Health outcomes in at least five of the above health conditions should show a significant improvement, and surveys should show an increase in patients' satisfaction with the quality of services received and heightened respect for their rights.

subject to voluntary agreements (Legido-Quigley et al., 2013). This wide diversity indeed offers opportunities for mutual learning and sharing best practices.

In the first place, the international community helped in providing the conceptual framework for quality policies in healthcare, defining what quality is (*see also* Chapter 1), identifying its different dimensions, exploring its operational translation and developing tools and indicators for measurement and assessment. International organizations contributed significantly in helping governments to translate political awareness into concrete policy action, as well as by mapping the various approaches taken by individual countries in designing quality improvement strategies and organizing quality structures.

The work of WHO is the most evident example of these international efforts to support national actors with guidance on the definition and implementation of quality strategies. Next to its political advocacy role, WHO stimulated the international exchange by commissioning studies to document national quality structures and processes (for example, Shaw & Kalo, 2002). In addition, it developed models for national quality strategies, built comparative condition-specific databases (including stroke, diabetes and renal disease), created collaborative centres and training programmes in "quality of care development (QCD)". It also supported the development of common indicators in several areas of healthcare and of benchmarking tools to support quality work (for example, diabetes care and hospital infections). Other WHO activities have included the commissioning of monographs on specific technical issues in quality, with an emphasis on the integration of standards, measurement and improvement as a global, cyclical and continuing activity (Shaw & Kalo, 2002).

Later, WHO also developed similar activities to facilitate and support the development of patient safety policies and practices across all WHO Member States. In 2004 the WHO Global Alliance for Patient Safety was launched, following a resolution that urged countries to establish and strengthen science-based systems, necessary for improving patients' safety and the quality of healthcare, including the monitoring of drugs, medical equipment and technology (WHO, 2002).

4.2.2 Developing standards and models

Often the exchange of experience and practice leads to developing common approaches, models and standards. The Council of Europe is a good example of an international actor that has supported countries with the development of common standards and recommendations to foster quality in healthcare. Also, the European Union is an important source of standardization in various areas of the health sector through internal market regulation. This will be addressed in more detail in the next section.

As a promotor of human rights, democracy and the rule of law, the Council of Europe's activities in the area of healthcare quality are based on the Right to Protection of Health that is enshrined in the European Social Charter (Article 11). Through legally non-binding recommendations, the Council promotes quality-related policies in various fields (*see* Table 4.2). Two particularly important recommendations with regard to quality are recommendation No. R(97)17 on the development and implementation of quality improvement systems (QIS) (The Council of Europe, 1997), and recommendation Rec(2001)13 on evidence-based clinical practice guidelines (Committee of Ministers, 2001). In the first one, Member States are urged to develop and implement quality improvement systems (QIS), systems for continuously assuring and improving the quality of healthcare at all levels, following guidelines defined by a special committee of experts. The second one proposes a coherent and comprehensive national policy framework for the production, appraisal, updating and active dissemination of evidence-based clinical practice guidelines in order to improve the quality and effectiveness of healthcare. The text also calls for promoting international networking between organizations, research institutions, clearinghouses and other agencies that are producing evidence-based health information.

The Council's standard-setting work has been particularly important in the field of pharmaceuticals. Already in 1965 the Convention on the Elaboration

Table 4.2   *Some examples of Council of Europe recommendations with regards to quality in healthcare**

Blood	Recommendation No. R(95)15 on the preparation, use and quality assurance of blood components.
Cancer control	Recommendation No. R(89)13 of the Committee of Ministers to Member States on the organization of multidisciplinary care for cancer patients
	Recommendation No. R(80)6 of the Committee of Ministers to Member States concerning cancer control
Disabilities	Recommendation Rec(2006)5 of the Committee of Ministers to Member States on the Council of Europe Action Plan to promote the rights and full participation of people with disabilities in society: improving the quality of life of people with disabilities in Europe, 2006–2015
Health Policy, Development and Promotion	Recommendation Rec(2001)13 on developing a methodology for drawing up guidelines on best medical practices
	Recommendation No. R(97)17 of the Committee of Ministers to Member States on the development and implementation of quality improvement systems (QIS) in healthcare
Health services	Recommendation Rec(2006)7 of the Committee of Ministers to Member States on management of patient safety and prevention of adverse events in healthcare
	Recommendation Rec(99)21 of the Committee of Ministers to Member States on criteria for the management of waiting lists and waiting times in healthcare
	Recommendation Rec(84)20 on the prevention of hospital infections
Mental disorder	Recommendation Rec(2004)10 of the Committee of Ministers to Member States concerning the protection of human rights and dignity of persons with mental disorder
Palliative care	Recommendation Rec(2003)24 of the Committee of Ministers to Member States on the organization of palliative care
Patients' role	Recommendation Rec(2000)5 of the Committee of Ministers to Member States on the development of structures for citizen and patient participation in the decision-making process affecting healthcare
	Recommendation Rec(80)4 concerning the patient as an active participant in his own treatment
Transplantation	Recommendation Rec(2005)11 of the Committee of Ministers to Member States on the role and training of professionals responsible for organ donation (transplant "donor co-ordinators")
Vulnerable groups	Recommendation R(98)11 of the Committee of Ministers to Member States on the organization of healthcare services for the chronically ill

* Based on http://www.coe.int/t/dg3/health/recommendations_en.asp

of a European Pharmacopoeia was adopted to set compulsory standards for the production and quality control of medicines. The European Directorate for the Quality of Medicines and HealthCare (EDQM),[2] an institution of the Council of Europe, publishes and updates the European Pharmacopoeia. Also the more recent "Medicrime Convention" (2011) of the Council of Europe is a binding international instrument of criminal law to fight against the production and distribution of counterfeit medicines and similar crimes involving threats to public health (Alarcón-Jiménez, 2015).

---

2   https://www.edqm.eu/

Besides supporting the development of quality policies at country level, international action has also targeted the level of individual healthcare providers by setting standards for assessing their competence and the quality of the services they provide. The European Foundation for Quality Management (EFQM) framework for self-assessment or the European Practice Assessment (EPA) in primary care can be mentioned here as examples (Legido-Quigley et al., 2013). Also, the European Union of Medical Specialists (UEMS), representing national associations of medical specialists in the European Union and in associated countries, created in 2010 the European Council for Accreditation of Medical Specialist Qualifications (ECAMSQ). This model aims to assess the competence of individual medical specialists across Europe based on the core curricula developed by the Specialist Sections of the UEMS. For hospitals, several organizations, such as the Joint Commission International (JCI), Accreditation Canada International, Veritas (DNV GL), are providing global models for accreditation and certification (*see* Chapter 8).

The increasing international focus and work on quality is also acquiring a more economic dimension. With the growing internationalization in healthcare, the variations in quality standards are increasingly seen as an obstacle to international mobility and trade relations. International standardization and accreditation were considered ways to overcome these differences. The International Organization for Standardization (ISO) provides an industry-based model with a global network of national standards bodies through which different institutions can be assessed according to common standards (*see* Chapter 8). While there are only specific standards for medical diagnostic laboratories, other healthcare facilities can be assessed according to the ISO 9000 series, which combines a set of five standards on quality management and assurance that were originally used for the manufacturing industry.

At European level, the European Committee for Standardization (CEN) is officially recognized by the European Union and the European Free Trade Association as the competent body for developing and publishing European standards. Standards published by CEN are developed on a voluntary basis and drafted by experts in the field with more or less involvement of various stakeholders (industry, trade federations, public authorities, academia, civil society). However, this application of industry-based standardization in healthcare has been heavily criticized, especially when it moves into assessing specific medical treatments. Recently, the increased involvement of the CEN in standardizing particular healthcare services (*see* Table 4.3) and in launching a CEN Healthcare Services Focus Group (2016) encountered heavy opposition from various European stakeholder organizations in healthcare. Whereas the definition of uniform safety standards and specifications for medical products and devices is widely accepted as a way to ensure their trade and use across countries, voluntary

Table 4.3 *CEN Technical Committees on healthcare*

Committee	Subject	Standard reference
CEN/TC 394	Healthcare provision by chiropractors	EN 16224:2012
CEN/TC 403	Aesthetic surgery services	EN 16372:2014
CEN/TC 414	Osteopathic healthcare provision	EN 16686
CEN/TC 362	Health services – Quality management systems – Guide for the use of EN ISO 9004:2000 in health services for performance improvement	CEN/TR 15592:2007
	Quality management systems – EN ISO 9001:2015 for healthcare	EN 15224:2016
CEN/WS 068	Quality criteria for health checks	CWA 16642:2013
CEN/TC 449	Quality of care for elderly people in ordinary and residential care facilities	Under drafting
CEN/TC 450	Minimum requirements of patient involvement in person-centred care	Under drafting

Note: Three other standards exist: Medical laboratories – Requirements for quality and competence (EN ISO 15189), Services offered by hearing aid professionals (EN 15927), Early care services for babies born with cleft lip and/or palate (CEN/TR 16824), Services of medical doctors with additional qualification in Homoeopathy (MDQH) – Requirements for healthcare provision by Medical Doctors with additional qualification in Homoeopathy (EN 16872).

and market-driven international standardization in healthcare provision is more controversial, especially when being "conducted by a private body which is neither scientifically suited nor carries sufficient legitimacy to intervene in national competences" (European Hospital and Healthcare Federation et al., 2016).

A more widely acceptable and adapted avenue is the international support and coordination to develop clinical guidelines as one of the many tools available to healthcare professionals to improve the quality of healthcare (*see* Chapter 9; Legido-Quigley et al., 2013). The AGREE (Appraisal of Guidelines, Research and Evaluation in Europe) collaboration that was established in 1998 is a good example (Cluzeau et al., 2003). Its work culminated in the publication of the now validated and widely used AGREE tool, which identified six quality domains and 23 specific items, covering the key elements of the clinical guideline development process. Obviously, also the work of the international Cochrane collaboration has been vital to improving the quality of healthcare through the production and dissemination of systematic reviews on the effects of healthcare interventions (Council of Europe, 1997).

However, to increase the effectiveness of external assessment of health services, the three sources of standardization (research, regulation and accreditation) and their respective interested parties need to work together rather than competing with one another (Shaw. 2015). The European Commission's strategic vision for European standards recommends that "A systematic approach to research, innovation and standardisation should be adopted at European and national level" and proposes that Regulation (EC) 765/2008, which provides a legal framework for the EU-wide provision of accreditation services for the marketing of goods, should extend to services (EC, 2011). In 2013 the Joint Research Centre of the European Commission, together with the European standards organizations, launched an initiative, "Putting Science into Standards", to bring the scientific and standardization communities closer together (European Commission Joint Research Centre, 2013). It is in that context that a pilot project was launched to develop a voluntary European Quality Assurance Scheme for Breast Cancer Services (BCS), as part of the European Commission's Initiative on Breast Cancer (ECIBC, 2014). This project demonstrates the challenges of applying concepts of "certification" to healthcare, and of transposing standards for diagnostic services (ISO 15189) into clinical services in Europe.

4.2.3 Strengthening monitoring and evaluation and international comparison

A final essential component in an integrated approach to quality governance is the aspect of surveillance and assessment, which presupposes robust health information systems and includes tools and methods for measuring quality and for comparing performance between countries as well as between individual providers. It also covers compliance with international norms, standards and regulations (World Health Organization, 1998).

The Organisation for Economic Co-operation and Development (OECD) has played an important role in complementing and coordinating efforts of national and other international bodies in measuring and comparing the quality of health service provision in different countries. Following on from a ministerial conference held in Ottawa in 2001 which discussed good practices in measuring key components of health systems performance, the OECD launched its Health Care Quality Indicators Project. An expert group developed a conceptual framework and a set of quality indicators for assessing the impact of particular factors on the quality of health services (*see* Chapter 2). It developed specific indicators for measuring quality in specific disease areas (cancer, cardiovascular diseases), as well as for measuring patient safety and patient experience. Based on the data gathered, since 2012 the OECD has published country reviews on quality as well as international comparisons in the Health at a Glance series. Based on these quality reviews a report published in 2017 drew lessons to inform national policy-makers (OECD, 2017). The report calls for greater transparency; more specifically it recommends the development of better measures of patient outcomes, especially those reported by patients themselves. This is also why the OECD, with the support of the EU's Public Health Programme, is developing and testing new indicators on patient-reported experience measures (PREMs) and patient-reported outcome measures (PROMs).

4.3 The EU's approach to quality

This section will look in more detail at how quality of healthcare is addressed within the context of the European Union. On the one hand, the EU can enact regulations that are binding for Member States. On the other hand, quality in healthcare was initially addressed only indirectly as a precautionary measure accompanying the process of economic integration in the health sector. This is the reason why many of these measures focus mostly on safety – and less on other dimensions of quality.

Even if quality is among the values and principles that are commonly shared among EU Member States, the EU's scope for developing a common policy in this field is limited. Formally, all aspects that touch upon the definition of health policy and the organization and delivery of health services and medical care are of national competence (Article 168.5, Treaty on the Functioning of the EU (TFEU)). However, within the context of internal market rules that underpin the EU integration process, public health plays an increasingly important role. Since free movement of people, services or goods may endanger public health, countries have always been allowed to implement restrictions (Articles 36, 45.3, 52 and 62 TFEU). In addition, various health crises in the past – such as the Thalidomide crisis in the 1960s, the blood scandals in the 1980s, the food safety crises in the 1990s and more recently the problems with silicone-filled breast implants – have demonstrated the need to secure public health for proper functioning of the internal market.

In fact, since then the Maastricht Treaty securing public health has been explicitly enshrined in primary EU law: "A high level of human health protection shall be ensured in the definition and implementation of all Union policies and activities" (Article 168.1 TFEU). To achieve this, a shared competence between the Union and the Member States was instituted to address common safety concerns in public health matters for aspects defined in the Treaty (Article 4.2(k) TFEU). The EU was also entrusted with direct legislative power to set standards of quality and safety in two specific areas: (1) organs and substances of human origin, blood and blood derivatives and (2) medicinal products and devices for medical use (Article 168.4 (a) and (c) respectively). The development of common standards is justified by the fact that it facilitates free movement as it would systematically remove unjustified restrictions at national level.

In addition to this, the public health article of the Treaty (Article 168 TFEU) provides a mandate for the EU to support, coordinate or complement national policies on quality and safety, and to stimulate cooperation between countries. In particular, the Commission is encouraged to promote coordination of Member States' programmes and policies aimed at the establishment of guidelines and indicators, the organization of exchange of best practice, and the preparation of the necessary elements for periodic monitoring and evaluation (Article 168.2 para 2). The tools for developing this are commonly referred to as "soft law" (*see also* Greer & Vanhercke, 2010). They include instruments such as Recommendations, Communications, the Open Method of Coordination, high-level reflection processes or working parties, action programmes, Joint Actions, etc. (*see also* Greer et al., 2014).

These two different approaches will be further elaborated in the next sections. First, we will explore how quality and safety are secured through EU provisions and policies that are meant to ensure free movement and establish an internal market. Next, we will address the more horizontal and generic EU policies with respect to quality and safety that follow from the mandate to support, coordinate or supplement national policies (Article 2.5 TFEU). Finally, we will draw conclusions on the different ways in which EU integration and policy touch upon quality in healthcare and how the approach has evolved over time.

4.3.1 Internal market-based legislation to ensure quality and safety

This first subsection will systematically scan the various areas where quality and safety are addressed through secondary European legislation that institutes the fundamental principles of free movement of goods, services and citizens in the field of health. Under free movement of goods different "healthcare products" can be distinguished: pharmaceuticals, medical devices, blood products, human tissues and cells, as well as organs. Free movement of citizens covers the mobility of both health professionals and patients. It is also closely connected with the free provision of health services.

Based on the above-mentioned provisions in the Treaty on the Functioning of the European Union (TFEU), which sets out the scope of the EU's competence in various policy areas, EU regulation has further detailed how free movement is to be implemented while preserving public health standards. This is mostly done through Directives which – contrary to EU Regulations – need to be transposed into national law first before they can become applicable. The main sources of EU legislation for the specific areas are listed in Table 4.4.

4.3.1.1 Healthcare products

Based on the principle of free movement of goods, the EU has taken legislative action to achieve the dual objective of creating an internal market whilst protecting public interests, in particular those of consumers. Harmonized regulatory standards promulgated at EU level and applicable in all Member States have been developed for different types of health product.

Table 4.4   *EU legal sources of quality and safety requirements in healthcare*

Focus	Legal basis	Main legal instruments
Pharmaceuticals	Internal market / Public health Article 114 and Article 168(4)(c) TFEU	The body of European Union legislation in the pharmaceutical sector is compiled in "The rules governing medicinal products in the European Union" (EudraLex). It consists of ten volumes that contain both the basic legislation and a series of supporting guidelines, including: Directive 2001/83/EC of 6 November 2001 on the Community code relating to medicinal products for human use (Consolidated version: 16/11/2012). Regulation (EC) No. 726/2004 of 31 March 2004 laying down Community procedures for the authorization and supervision of medicinal products for human and veterinary use and establishing a European Medicines Agency (Consolidated version: 05/06/2013).
Medical devices	Internal market / Public Health Article 114 and Article 168(4)(c) TFEU	Regulation (EU) 2017/745 of 5 April 2017 on medical devices, amending Directive 2001/83/EC, Regulation (EC) No. 178/2002 and Regulation (EC) No. 1223/2009 and repealing Council Directives 90/385/EEC and 93/42/EEC Regulation (EU) 2017/746 of 5 April 2017 on in vitro diagnostic medical devices and repealing Directive 98/79/EC and Commission Decision 2010/227/EU
Blood and blood components	Public health Article 168(4) TFEU	Directive 2002/98/EC of 27 January 2003 setting standards of quality and safety for the collection, testing, processing, storage and distribution of human blood and blood components and amending Directive 2001/83/EC Commission Directive 2004/33/EC of 22 March 2004 implementing Directive 2002/98/EC of the European Parliament and of the Council as regards certain technical requirements for blood and blood components Commission Directive 2005/61/EC of 30 September 2005 implementing Directive 2002/98/EC of the European Parliament and of the Council as regards traceability requirements and notification of serious adverse reactions and events Commission Directive 2005/62/EC of 30 September 2005 implementing Directive 2002/98/EC as regards Community standards and specifications relating to a quality system for blood establishments
Tissues and cells	Public health Article 168(4) TFEU	Directive 2004/23/EC of 31 March 2004 on setting standards of quality and safety for the donation, procurement, testing, processing, preservation, storage and distribution of human tissues and cells Commission Directive 2006/17/EC of 8 February 2006 implementing Directive 2004/23/EC of the European Parliament and of the Council as regards certain technical requirements for the donation, procurement and testing of human tissues and cells Commission Directive 2006/86/EC of 24 October 2006 implementing Directive 2004/23/EC as regards traceability requirements, notification of serious adverse reactions and events and certain technical requirements for the coding, processing, preservation, storage and distribution of human tissues and cells

Table 4.4   *EU legal sources of quality and safety requirements in healthcare [continued]*

Focus	Legal basis	Main legal instruments
Organs	Public health Article 168(4) TFEU	Directive 2010/45/EU of 7 July 2010 on standards of quality and safety of human organs intended for transplantation Directive 2013/55/EU of 20 November 2013 amending Directive 2005/36/EC on the recognition of professional qualifications and Regulation (EU) No. 1024/2012 on administrative cooperation through the Internal Market Information System
Health professionals	Internal market Articles 46, 53(1) and 62 TFEU	Directive 2005/36/EC of 7 September 2005 on the recognition of professional qualifications
Health services	Internal market / Public Health Articles 114 and 168 TFEU	Directive 2011/24/EU of 9 March 2011 on the application of patients' rights in cross-border healthcare

Pharmaceuticals

Starting in the 1960s, a comprehensive framework of EU legislation has gradually been put in place to guarantee the highest possible level of public health with regard to medicinal products. This body of legislation is compiled in ten volumes of "The rules governing medicinal products in the European Union" (EudraLex). All medicinal products for human use have to undergo a licensing procedure in order to obtain a marketing authorization. The requirements and procedures are primarily laid down in Directive 2001/83/EC and in Regulation (EC) No. 726/2004. More specific rules and guidelines, which facilitate the interpretation of the legislation and its uniform application across the EU, are compiled in volumes 3 and 4 of Eudralex. Since 1994 the European Medicines Agency (EMA) has coordinated the scientific evaluation of the quality, safety and efficacy of all medicinal products that are submitted to licensing. New pharmaceuticals can be licensed either by EMA or by authorities of Member States. More details about the regulation of pharmaceuticals are provided in Chapter 6.

The EMA is also responsible for coordinating the EU "pharmacovigilance" system for medicines. If information indicates that the benefit-risk balance of a particular medicine has changed since authorization, competent authorities can suspend, revoke, withdraw or change the marketing authorization. There is a EudraVigilance reporting system that systematically gathers and analyses suspected cases of adverse reactions to a medicine, which was further strengthened in 2010. The EMA has also released good pharmacovigilance practice guidelines (GVP) to facilitate the performance of pharmacovigilance activities in all Member States. In addition, Commission Implementing Regulation (EU) No. 520/2012 on the performance of pharmacovigilance activities stipulates operational details in relation to certain aspects of pharmacovigilance to be respected by marketing authorization holders, national competent authorities and the EMA.

In 2010 the EU's pharmacovigilance system was further improved. The main reform objectives were: making risk management more proactive and proportionate; increasing the quality of safety data; establishing stronger links between safety assessments and regulatory action; and strengthening transparency, communication and patient involvement. New legislation that became applicable in July 2012 (Regulation EU 1235/2010 and Directive 2010/84/EC) allows patients to report adverse drug reactions directly to the competent authorities. Additionally, reporting of adverse reactions is broadened to cover, for example, medication errors and overdose.

Further improvements introduced in 2013, following the Mediator scandal, provided for the creation of an automatic procedure of notification and assessment of safety issues, stricter transparency rules on the reasons for withdrawal, and increased surveillance of products that are subject to certain post-authorization safety conditions (Directive 2012/26/EU and Regulation 2012/1027/EU). The Commission also established a Black symbol to identify medicinal products that are subject to additional monitoring and to encourage patients and healthcare professionals to report unexpected adverse reactions through national reporting systems.

Also in 2013 new legislation on falsified medicines entered into force (Directive 2011/62/EU). It comprises measures such as an obligatory authenticity feature on the outer packaging of the medicines; a common EU-wide logo to identify legal online pharmacies; tougher rules on the controls and inspections of producers of active pharmaceutical ingredients; and strengthened record-keeping requirements for wholesale distributors. The Commission also published guidelines on Good Distribution Practice of medicinal products for human use.

Medical devices

Also for medical devices, EU regulation combines the double aim of ensuring a high level of protection of human health and safety with the good functioning of the Single Market. However, the scrutiny for product safety is not – as yet – so far advanced as in the case of pharmaceuticals (Greer et al., 2014). The legal framework in this area was developed in the 1990s with a set of three directives covering, respectively, active implantable medical devices (Directive 90/385/EEC), medical devices (Directive 93/42/EEC) and in vitro diagnostic medical devices (Directive 98/79/EC). They were supplemented subsequently by several modifying and implementing directives, including the last technical revision brought about in 2007 (Directive 2007/47/EC). Following recent safety problems with breast and hip implants, the European Commission in 2012 proposed a revision of the regulatory framework in order to increase patient safety protection (EC, 2012a). Two new regulations (Regulation (EU) 2017/745 and Regulation (EU) 2017/746) envisage among others a stronger supervision of the notified bodies, better traceability, updated risk classification rules, and better coordination between the national competent authorities and the Commission. However, they do not fundamentally change the core features of the system (Greer et al., 2014). Also, these new rules will only start to apply after the spring of 2020 and the spring of 2022, respectively.

To be marketed across the EU, devices have to obtain a European conformity marking (CE) from the national competent authority. The licensing requirements for medical devices vary according to the level of risk associated with their intended use. For the lowest-risk types conformity with relevant standards only needs to be declared. For more complex devices an explicit approval by the national notified body designated by the competent authority is needed. However, this assessment mainly looks at product performance and reliability. Specific requirements for pre-marketing clinical studies are vague and review data are not made publicly available, contrary to the US (Kramer, Xu & Kesselheim, 2012). The notified bodies are not really designed to act as public health agencies. As private companies they also retrieve their income from fees levied upon the manufacturers. Furthermore, the enforcement of the harmonized legislation concerning medical devices is essentially decentralized at the level of the Member States. Differences in the responsibilities of the competent authorities and in interpretation of the EU legislation further weaken guarantees for a strong safety protection. Under the new rules, control of high-risk devices (for example, implants) is tightened and will involve panels of independent experts at EU level. Also a new system of risk classification will be applied for in vitro diagnostic medical devices. A single registration procedure at EU level and a coordinated assessment for clinical trials taking place in several Member States will allow more uniformity in the application.

Also in the post-marketing phase, safety monitoring is still mostly operated at national level. Manufacturers must report all serious adverse events to the national competent authorities. However, since May 2011 they now also have to report to the European Databank on Medical Devices (EUDAMED), which stores all information on manufacturers as well as data related to approvals and clinical studies. Under the Medical Device Vigilance System adverse incidents are to be evaluated and, where appropriate, information is disseminated in the form of a National Competent Authority Report (NCAR) and field safety corrective actions are taken. The national authorities can decide to withdraw an unsafe medical device from the market or take particular health monitoring measures.

The European Commission can make sure that these measures are then applied throughout the Union. The new rules provide for a mandatory unique device identifier to strengthen traceability and an implant card to improve information to patients.

Blood, tissues, cells and organs

Substances of human origin (blood and blood products, organs, tissues and cells) constitute a very specific and delicate class of healthcare products. Scandals concerning contaminated blood at the end of the 1980s pushed the EU to take action on public health grounds and eventually led to the creation of a legal base for enacting binding legislation in this field (Article 168.4 TFEU). The scope of the legal mandate is essentially focused at setting minimum standards for quality and safety for substances of human origin, including ensuring traceability and notification of any adverse events that might occur. However, European action has traditionally taken a broader approach, such as in the case of organ transplantation with increasing organ availability and enhancing efficiency and accessibility of transplantation systems. With the exception of promoting the non-profit character within which the donation and procurement of substances of human origin should take place, the EU refrains from addressing other ethical considerations, such as the use of human cells for human cloning. Also, given the cultural and legal differences with respect to donation, these aspects remain the responsibility of the Member States, as is also reminded in Article 168, 7 in fine.[3]

EU regulation is aimed at protecting both donors and recipients of **blood and blood components** throughout the whole blood transfusion chain, in particular to prevent the transmission of diseases. Directive 2002/98/EC sets the standards of quality and safety for the collection, testing, processing, storage and distribution of human blood and blood components, irrespective of their final destination. This was complemented by Directive 2005/62/EC defining Community standards and specifications relating to a quality system for blood establishments. Member States have to designate and set up competent authorities, inspection systems, control measures and haemovigilance systems. They have to license blood establishments and organize inspections and appropriate control measures at least every two years. The traceability from donor to recipient must be guaranteed at all times. Blood and blood components imported from third countries should meet equivalent Community standards and specifications. In case of serious adverse events the competent authority must be notified and a procedure for the efficient withdrawal from distribution of the affected blood or blood components has to be executed by the blood establishment or hospital

---

3   The measures referred to in paragraph 4(a) shall not affect national provisions on the donation or medical use of organs and blood. (Article 168, 7, in fine).

blood bank. In addition to the national vigilance systems in place, a new EU Rapid Alert platform for human blood and blood components was set up in 2014 to allow Member States to quickly exchange information on incidents that may have cross-border implications. Strict rules apply to donations and donors. Donors are subject to an evaluation procedure based on specific criteria relating to the physical condition and the context of donation. To this effect information has to be obtained from the donor before giving blood. The donor should also receive information and the confidentiality of his data should be protected.

EU regulation is also setting quality and safety standards for the donation, procurement, testing, processing, preservation, storage and distribution of **human tissues and cells**. Directive 2004/23/EC, complemented by three implementing Directives, defines the obligations of Member States and technical requirements to be followed. Member States are required to set up competent authorities that maintain a publicly accessible register of tissue establishments, which are accredited, designated or authorized by them. These tissue centres have to implement a quality control system that records all their activities and operating procedures. Conditions of processing and storage have to meet strict requirements and have to be performed by qualified and experienced personnel. They have to report annually to the competent authorities. Inspections and checks are operated by the competent authorities at least every two years. In case the requirements are not met, the licence can be suspended or revoked. Member States have to ensure traceability from donor to recipient and vice versa of all tissues and cells that are procured, processed, stored or distributed on their territory. To this end they have to implement a donor identification system. This should ultimately lead to a single European coding system (Reynolds et al., 2010). Imports and exports of human tissues and cells from and to third countries have to equally comply with these standards. A notification and information system must be in place to detect and communicate any incident linked to the procurement, testing, processing, storage, distribution and transplantation of tissues and cells. The evaluation and selection of donors follow strict standards. Consent of both donors and recipients (or their next of kin) is required and their privacy has to be guaranteed. Member States have to observe that procurement of tissues and cells is carried out on a non-profit basis.

The legislation for **organ donation** (opt-in or opt-out) and the way waiting lists are managed remain the prerogative of the Member States. However, the EU is setting a common framework to ensure the quality and safety standards for human organs intended for transplantation. In addition, some EU Member States are collaborating in European organ exchange organizations, such as Eurotransplant set up in 1967. Directive 2010/45/EU regulates the different stages of the chain from donation to transplantation, including procurement, testing, characterization, transport and use of organs. It is complemented by one implementing Directive laying down information procedures for the exchange of organs between Member States. Member States have to designate competent authorities that are in charge of supervising the facilities licensed for this purpose, as well as exchanges with other Member States and third countries. Procurement organizations, European organ exchange organizations and transplantation centres are required to follow common standard operating procedures. Member States have to put in place a reporting system for any adverse event that might occur following organ transplantation. To protect the health of donors and recipients, the traceability of all organs on the territory needs to be ensured at all times and all stages of the process. The selection and evaluation of donors is subject to clear criteria and based on detailed information regarding the donor. Living donors are entitled to comprehensive information about the purpose of the donation and the risks involved. It must be voluntary and unpaid. Their anonymity should be guaranteed.

4.3.1.2 Health professionals

The free movement of workers is an economic imperative and a civil right enshrined in the treaties and supported by secondary legislation (Buchan, Glinos & Wismar, 2014). This also comprises health professionals, who either as salaried or self-employed workers can move to another Member State to take up or pursue activities, either on a permanent or temporary basis. However, mobility of health professionals raises concerns with respect to quality and safety (Abbing, 1997). In "exporting" countries it is felt that free movement of health professionals may have negative effects on the ability of health systems to maintain standards of quality and safety due to the growing regional or local shortage of health professionals and the loss of skilled professionals. In "host" countries professional mobility has led to concerns over quality and safety linked to professional skills and language knowledge of migrant health professionals and their integration into the host country's health system (Wismar et al., 2011). More specifically, these concerns can relate to differences in training content, competencies and national regulatory approaches but also variation in language proficiency or risks related to professional misconduct or unfitness to practise – but there is surprisingly little evidence on the subject (Maier et al., 2011).

While the regulation of professions is a national prerogative (*see also* Chapter 5), subject to principles of non-discrimination and proportionality, since the 1960s the EU has established a framework for the mutual recognition of professional qualifications between Member States. Each Member State is in principle required to also accept workers with a qualification that was obtained in another Member State. However, they can make this access subject to certain conditions and guarantees. Health professionals were among the first to be covered by this European legislation. In fact, the Treaty makes a special provision for the medical and allied and pharmaceutical professions, indicating that the progressive abolition of restrictions (to free movement) shall be dependent upon coordination of the conditions for their exercise in the various Member States (Article 53.2 TFEU).

Traditionally two coordination systems were combined to achieve equivalence between qualifications from different countries. The so-called "sectoral system" is based on a minimum harmonization of training requirements. Under this system Member States are obliged to automatically recognize a diploma without any individual assessment or imposing any further condition. It applies to specific regulated professions that are explicitly listed. Five of the seven professions falling under the sectoral system of automatic recognition are health professions: doctors (including specialists), nurses responsible for general care, dentists (including specialists), midwives and pharmacists. Other health professions (for example, specialist nurses, specialist pharmacists, psychologists, chiropractors, osteopaths, opticians) fall under the "general system". As under this system training requirements were not harmonized, Member States can require certain compensating measures to recognize a diploma from another Member State, such as an aptitude test or an adaptation period (Peeters, 2005).

The legislative framework regarding the mutual recognition of qualifications was revised for the first time in 2005. The various sectoral and general Directives were merged and consolidated into Directive 2005/36/EC on the recognition of professional qualifications. A second major revision took place in 2013 with Directive 2013/55. This revision aimed to modernize the legal framework and to bring it in line with the evolving labour market context. While clearly these consecutive revisions were aimed at making free movement of professionals simpler, easier and quicker – not least by cutting red tape and speeding up procedures through the use of e-government tools (cf. the European professional card) – they were also motivated by an ambition to better safeguard public health and patient safety with respect to health professions (Tiedje & Zsigmond, 2012).

One element has been the modernization of the minimum training requirements under the automatic recognition procedure. Next to the specification and updating of the minimum duration of training and the knowledge as well as skills and training subjects that have to be acquired, the possibility of adding a common list of competences was introduced (as was done for nurses under Article 31.7). The reform also made it possible to expand automatic recognition to professions falling under the general system (or specialties of a sectoral profession) that are regulated in at least one third of Member States by developing common training principles, a detailed set of knowledge, skills and competences. However, doubts are raised as to whether this would really improve quality and safety (cf. Council of European Dentists, 2015). Although there is no minimum harmonization, some would argue that the general system offers more possibilities for quality assurance as it allows the host Member State to require compensation measures and to more quickly respond to changes in clinical practice – in particular, the emergence of new specialties (Peeters, McKee & Merkur, 2010). Finally, the revised Directive also introduced an obligation for Member States to organize continuous professional development (CPD) – at least for the sectoral professions – so that professionals can update their knowledge, skills and competences.

The revisions also strengthened the rules concerning the "pursuit" of the profession. Indeed, equivalence of standards of education and training alone does not as such provide sufficient guarantees for good quality medical practice (Abbing, 1997). In principle, Member States can make authorization to practise subject to certain conditions, such as the presentation of certain documents (a certificate of good standing, of physical or mental health) and/or an oath or solemn declaration, or the applicability of national disciplinary measures.

Two main patient safety concerns prevailed in this context: language proficiency and professional malpractice. Since communication with patients is an important aspect of quality assurance in health care, improper language assessment and induction of inflowing health professionals could compromise patient safety (Glinos et al., 2015). Therefore, the revised professional qualification Directive clarified that for professions with implications for patient safety, competent authorities can carry out systematic language controls. However, this should only take place after the recognition of the qualification and should be limited to one official or administrative language of the host Member State. Any language controls should also be proportionate to the activity to be pursued and be open to appeal (Article 53). Another serious public health risk derives from professionals "fleeing" to another country after they have been found guilty of professional misconduct or considered unfit to practise. On several accounts the voluntary exchange of information between Member States as foreseen in the qualifications Directive was judged far from optimal. This is why in the last reform the duties in terms of information exchange were strengthened with a particular emphasis on health professionals. The revised Directive introduced a pro-active alert mechanism under the Internal Market Information system (IMI), with an obligation for competent authorities of a Member State to inform the competent authorities of all other Member States about professionals who have been banned, even temporarily, from practising.

Even if it is commonly accepted that national regulation of health professionals is needed to protect public health and to ensure quality of care and patient safety, any conditions imposed should be non-discriminatory and not unduly infringe on the principles of free movement. In the past, the European Court of Justice found that certain national measures that were taken to protect public health were unjustified and disproportionate, such as the requirement to cancel registration in the Member State of origin, the obligation to have a pharmacist run a pharmacy, and restrictions on operating chains of pharmacies (Baeten & Palm, 2011). Following a mutual evaluation exercise run in 2015–2016 that revealed that Member States repeatedly failed to demonstrate the necessity or the proportionality of certain rules, the Commission in 2017 issued a proposal for a Directive instituting an ex-ante proportionality test for any new regulation that is likely to restrict access to or the pursuit of a profession (Council of the European Union, 2017). As this draft targets measures commonly used in the health sector to ensure quality and safety (for example, CPD, language knowledge), it raises concerns and recalls former attempts towards deregulation (Baeten, 2017).

Finally, it should be noted that besides the professional qualifications Directive other secondary EU legislation also contains measures that could indirectly contribute to quality and safety in healthcare provision. A good example is the European Working Time Directive, 2003/88/EC, which is essentially meant to protect the health and safety of health professionals but indirectly would also contribute to ensuring quality and patient safety.

4.3.1.3 Healthcare services

In a way the free movement of health services is complementary to the free movement of health professionals covered under the previous section. As well as healthcare providers establishing themselves in another Member State, providers can also on a temporary and occasional basis treat patients in another Member State. Their right to freely provide services in another Member State (Article 56 TFEU) is also covered by the professional qualifications Directive. In principle, imposing a double regulatory burden on professionals can be considered as an impediment to free movement that needs to be justified and proven to be necessary and proportional (Ghekiere, Baeten & Palm, 2010). However, some of the quality and safety concerns mentioned before apply even more so in the case of temporary mobility (for example, "blitz aesthetic surgery"). While Member States can fully apply the same professional rules and standards to these incoming providers, they can also require to be notified in advance when they move for the first time and to provide them with proofs of nationality, establishment, qualification and liability cover in the home state. More specifically for regulated professions that have public health or patient safety implications, additional documents can be requested such as an attestation confirming absence of any professional suspension or criminal conviction, and a declaration of the applicant's knowledge of the language necessary for practising the profession in the host Member State. For non-sectoral health professions Member States can run a prior check and require an aptitude test if there is a risk of serious damage to the health or safety of the service recipient due to a lack of professional qualification of the service provider (Article 7.4).

Another dimension of free movement of health services is mobility of patients. The right of citizens to seek healthcare in another Member State was already acknowledged by the European Court of Justice in the cases *Luisi* and *Carbone* and *Grogan*.[4] That this right would also apply to health services provided within the context of statutory health systems – irrespective of the type of healthcare or health system – was subsequently confirmed in the cases *Kohll*, *Smits-Peerbooms* and *Watts*,[5] which dealt with the situation of patients requesting reimbursement for healthcare they obtained in another Member State. In this context quality of health services came up first as a justification ground for refusing reimbursement. The Luxembourg government, joined by other Member States, argued that requiring prior authorization for cross-border care was a necessary measure to protect public health and guarantee the quality of care that was provided abroad to its citizens. However, the Court rejected this on the grounds that the EU's minimum training requirements for doctors and dentists established equivalence and required that health professionals in other Member States should be treated equally.[6] Even though a similar framework based on the mutual recognition principle is lacking for hospitals, the Court in the *Stamatelaki* case (in which the Greek authorities refused to pay for treatment in a London-based private hospital) followed the same reasoning, arguing that private hospitals in other Member States are also subject to quality controls and that doctors working in those hospitals based on the professional qualifications Directive provide the same professional guarantees as those in Greece.[7]

In the discussion on how to codify the case law around cross-border care, quality and patient safety gradually gained importance. Perceived national differences in quality of healthcare – and in policies to guarantee quality and patient safety – were identified as both a driver for and an obstacle to patient mobility. Eurobarometer surveys on cross-border health services have repeatedly demonstrated that receiving better quality treatment was the second main reason to consider travelling to another Member State for care (after treatment that is not available at home) (EC, 2015). Also long waiting times have systematically come out as an important motivation for patients to seek care abroad. At the same time, lack of information about the quality of medical treatment abroad and patient safety was considered a major deterrent for considering the option

---

4   Joined Cases 286/82 and 26/83, Luisi and Carbone v. Ministero del Tesoro [1984] ECR 377; Case C-159/90, The Society for the Protection of Unborn Children Ireland Ltd v. Grogan [1991] ECR I-4685

5   Case C-158/96, Kohll v. Union des Caisses de Maladie [1998] ECR I-1931; Case C-157/99, Geraets-Smits and Peerbooms [2001] ECR I-5473; Case C-372/04, Watts [2006] ECR I-4325

6   Case C-158/96, Kohll, para. 49

7   Case C-444/05, Stamatelaki [2007] ECR I-3185, paras. 36–7

of cross-border care. One of the main conclusions drawn from the public consultation that the European Commission organized in 2006 to decide on what Community action to take in this field was that the uncertainty that deterred patients from seeking treatment in another Member State was not only related to their entitlements and reimbursement but also linked to issues of quality and safety (EC, 2006). This is also why the Commission finally opted for a broader approach that would not only tackle the financial aspects around cross-border care (as was initially proposed in the Services Directive) but would also address these other uncertainties (Palm et al., 2011). Only then would patients feel sufficiently confident to seek treatment across the Union.

The Directive 2011/24/EU on the application of patients' rights in cross-border[8] healthcare aims to facilitate access to safe and high-quality cross-border healthcare (Article 1). In line with this, each Member State is given the responsibility to ensure on their territory the implementation of common operating principles that all EU citizens would expect to find – and structures to support them – in any health system in the EU (Council of the European Union, 2006). This includes in the first place the obligation for the Member State providing treatment to guarantee cross-border patients access to good-quality care in accordance with the applicable standards and guidelines on quality and safety (Article 4.1 (b)). In addition, they are also entitled to obtain the provision of relevant information to help them make rational choices (Article 4.2(a) and (b)), as well as recourse to transparent complaint procedures and redress mechanisms (Article 4.2(c)), and systems of professional liability insurance or similar arrangements (Article 4.2(d)). Finally, they also have the right to privacy protection with respect to the processing of personal data (Article 4.2(e)), as well as the right to have and to access a personal medical record (Article 4.2(f)).

In its current form the Directive does not contain any obligation for Member States to define and implement quality and safety standards. It only states that if such standards and guidelines exist they should also apply in the context of healthcare provided to cross-border patients. The Commission's initial proposal was more ambitious: it wanted to set EU minimum requirements on quality and safety for cross-border healthcare. However, this was considered by the Member States as overstepping national competence to organize healthcare and was reframed into an obligation to – only – inform patients about the applicable quality and safety standards and guidelines. Member States are also required to mutually assist each other for implementing the Directive, in particular on standards and guidelines on quality and safety and the exchange of information (Article 10.1). Under Chapter IV of the Directive Member States are encouraged

---

8   Directive 2011/24/EU of 9 March 2011 on the application of patients' rights in cross-border healthcare, OJ L88/45–65

to develop cooperation in specific areas. Some of these are particularly relevant for improving the quality of healthcare in Member States, such as European reference networks (Article 12), rare diseases (Article 13), and Health Technology Assessment (Article 15). European reference networks are expected to encourage the development of quality and safety benchmarks and to help develop and spread best practice within and outside the network (Article 12.2 (g)).

While on the one hand the subsidiarity principle was used to weaken the guarantees for quality and safety in the cross-border care Directive, on the other hand, based on the absence of a minimum level of safety and quality throughout the Union, Member States claimed the possibility of maintaining prior authorization as a condition for reimbursing cross-border care if it is provided by a healthcare provider that could give rise to serious and specific concerns relating to the quality or safety of the care (Article 8.2(c)). If these concerns relate to the respect of standards and guidelines, including provisions on supervision, prior authorization can be refused (Article 8.6 (c)). The position of Member States can be considered somewhat inconsistent and paradoxical (Palm & Baeten, 2011). However, despite this watering-down, Member States are encouraged to make systematic and continuous efforts to ensure that quality and safety standards are improved in line with the Council Conclusions and take into account advances in international medical science and generally recognized good medical practices as well as new health technologies (recital 22). Also, since the Directive applies to all healthcare providers without distinction,[9] it might provoke the debate in some Member States about the application of standards and guidelines in private hospitals and the distinctive policies towards statutory and private care providers (Peeters, 2012).

In principle, differences in quality or safety standards are not accepted as a justified reason for claiming the right to be treated in another Member State and obtain reimbursement for it. Member States can continue to make reimbursement subject to prior authorization for types of care that are subject to planning and involve overnight stay or the use of costly, highly specialized infrastructure or equipment (Article 8.2). They can refuse to grant this authorization if the treatment is either not part of the benefit basket in the state of affiliation or it can be provided on its territory within a time limit which is medically justifiable (Article 8.6(d)). So unacceptably long waiting times are an important dimension of quality for which EU law grants an unconditional right to free movement (Palm & Glinos, 2010). The decision as to what has to be considered "undue delay" is to be based case by case on an objective medical assessment of the patient's medical condition, the history and probable course of the patient's illness, the degree of the patient's

---

9   See Article 3g; *"healthcare provider"* means any natural or legal person or any other entity legally providing healthcare on the territory of a Member State.

pain and/or the nature of the patient's disability at the time when the request for authorization was made or renewed (Article 8.5). However, the European Court of Justice made clear that the state of the health system also has to be taken into account. In the *Petru* case it held that if a patient cannot get hospital treatment in good time in his own country because of a lack of medication and basic medical supplies and infrastructure, reimbursement of medical expenses incurred in another Member State cannot be refused.[10] But also access to more advanced (better-quality) therapies has been a recurring point of discussion as to whether it would justify reimbursement. In the *Rindal* and *Slinning* case the EFTA Court held that when it is established according to international medicine that the treatment abroad is indeed more effective, the state may no longer justify prioritizing its own offer of treatment.[11] And in the *Elchinov* case the European Court of Justice stated that if the benefit basket of a country would only define the types of treatment covered but not specify the specific method of treatment, prior authorization could not be refused for a more advanced treatment (i.e. proton therapy for treating an eye tumour) if this was not available within an acceptable time period (Sokol, 2010).

4.3.2 Soft law strategies to promote a more integrated approach on quality and safety

Although many of the measures and legal instruments listed in the previous subsection have had a significant impact on increasing quality and safety standards in Member States within the different categories, the quality focus in these actions was often not a goal in itself but rather a precautionary measure of public health protection to secure free movement in the Single Market.

Still, an overarching approach that would coordinate the various dimensions of healthcare quality was missing. This is why complementary EU action and incentive measures can be developed to support national policies towards improving public health, and strengthening quality and safety (Article 168.1, §2 and 168.5 TFEU). Under this soft law approach, a broad scope of activities (including instruments like recommendations, guidelines, EU-funded projects, joint actions, etc.) can be organized, which can cover a wide range of topics and dimensions that relate to quality of health services: prevention and screening, patient safety, health literacy, innovation in healthcare, antimicrobial resistance, etc. (*See* Box 4.2 for an example on quality of cancer policies.)

In 1998, under the Austrian EU Presidency, the EU health ministers agreed to start collaborating on quality. On this occasion a summary of quality policies

---

10   Case C268/13, Elena Petru v. Romanian National Health Insurance Agency
11   EFTA Court, Joined Cases E-11/07 and E-1/08 – Olga Rindal and Therese Slinning v. Staten v./ Dispensasjons, para 84

Box 4.2 *Soft law instruments to improve quality of cancer control policies in the EU*

A good example is the action undertaken in the field of the fight against cancer. As one of the first areas where a specific Community initiative on health was launched, over time the political focus gradually expanded from one that essentially promoted cooperation in research and prevention to a more horizontal and integrated approach that covers all aspects of prevention, treatment and follow-up of cancer as a chronic disease. Following the "Europe against Cancer" programme that was started in 1985, the Council of Health Ministers in 2003 adopted a Council Recommendation on cancer screening, setting out principles of best practice in the early detection of cancer and calling for action to implement national population-based screening programmes for breast, cervical and colorectal cancer (Council of the European Union, 2003). To ensure appropriate quality assurance at all levels, the Commission, in collaboration with WHO's International Agency for Research on Cancer (IARC), produced European guidelines for quality assurance in respectively cervical, breast cancer and colorectal cancer screening and diagnosis. The European Partnership for Action against Cancer (EPAAC) that was launched in 2009 also marked the identification and dissemination of good practice in cancer-related healthcare as one of its core objectives (EC, 2009). This focus on integrated cancer care services is also reflected in the Cancer Control Joint Action (CanCon). As a next step, under the European Commission Initiative on Breast Cancer (ECIBC) launched in 2012, a ground-breaking project was started to develop a European quality assurance scheme for breast cancer services (BCS) underpinned by accreditation and referring to high-quality, evidence-based guidelines.*

* http://ecibc.jrc.ec.europa.eu/

---

in the Member States was published, followed by a similar report on the EU accession countries (Federal Ministry of Labour, Health and Social Affairs, 1998; Federal Ministry of Social Security and Generations, 2001). However, also inspired by the WHO Global Alliance for Patient Safety and the Council of Europe's 2006 Recommendation on patient safety and prevention of adverse events in healthcare, EU action also started to gradually focus on patient safety as a particular aspect of quality. In 2005 both the Luxembourg and UK EU Presidencies identified patient safety as a key priority. It was also picked up by the High Level Group on Health Services and Medical Care (2004) that created a specific working group to explore ways of stepping-up cooperation between Member States' health systems in the context of increasing patient mobility (Bertinato et al., 2005). This led to the publication in 2008 of a Commission's Communication and the adoption in 2009 of a Council Recommendation on patient safety, including the prevention and control of healthcare-associated infections (2009/C 151/01) (EC, 2008b; Council of the European Union, 2009). Both instruments envisaged coming to an integrated, overarching EU strategy that would support Member States in implementing their own national and regional strategies for patient safety, maximize the scope for cooperation and mutual support across the EU and improve patients' confidence by improving information on safety in health systems. The recommendations were mainly aimed at fostering a patient safety culture and targeted health professionals, patients, healthcare managers and policy-makers. Some of the measures proposed in the Recommendation (for example, information to patients about patient safety standards, complaint in case a patient is harmed while receiving healthcare, remedies and redress) were also included in the safety provisions of the 2011 cross-border healthcare Directive (*see above*). Two consecutive implementation reports published in 2012 and 2014 demonstrated the significant progress that was made in the development of patient safety policies and programmes as well as of reporting and learning systems on adverse events (EC, 2012b, 2014c). Still, more efforts are needed for educating and training health professionals[12] and empowering patients (*see also* chapter 11). This again pushed towards looking at other quality aspects than only safety.

The work on patient safety paved the way to broadening the scope of EU collaborative action to the full spectrum of quality in healthcare. With a somewhat more relaxed EU mandate on health systems, which was reflected in the EU health strategy (2008) and later confirmed in the Council Conclusion on the reflection process on modern, responsive and sustainable health systems (2011), the Commission could start to develop a Community framework for safe, high-quality and efficient health services that would support Member States in making their health systems more dynamic and sustainable through coordinated action at EU level (Council of the European Union, 2011). Some of the preparatory work was entrusted to the Working Group (then the Expert Group) on Patient Safety and Quality of Healthcare, which supported the policy development by the European Commission until 2017. Also the Joint Action on patient safety and quality of healthcare (PaSQ), which was launched in 2012, helped to further strengthen cooperation between EU Member States, international organizations and EU stakeholders on issues related to quality of healthcare, including patient safety. In 2014 the Commission's Expert Panel on Effective Ways of Investing in Health (EXPH) was asked to produce an opinion on the future EU agenda on quality. The report emphasized the important role that the European Commission can play in improving quality and safety in healthcare – either through the Health Programme or the Research Framework Programme (*see* Table 4.5) – by supporting the development of guidelines and sharing of good practices, boosting research in this area, promoting education and training of both patients and health professionals, further encouraging cooperation on HTA, collecting the

---

12 This was addressed under the 2010 Belgian EU Presidency: see Flottorp SA et al. (2010). Using audit and feedback to health professionals to improve the quality and safety of health care. Copenhagen: WHO Regional Office for Europe and European Observatory on Health Systems and Policies

necessary data, etc. It also proposed the creation of an EU Health Care Quality Board to coordinate EU initiatives in this field and the development of an HSPA framework to compare and measure impacts (Expert Panel on Effective Ways of Investing in Health, 2014). In 2014, under the Italian EU Presidency, Council Conclusions were adopted that invited the Commission and Member States to develop a methodology of establishing patient safety standards and guidelines, and to propose a framework for sustainable EU collaboration on patient safety and quality of care. Moreover, the Commission was invited to propose a recommendation on information to patients on patient safety. However, the EU activities on patient safety and quality of care were discontinued in 2015 and to date none of the recommendations made by the Expert Panel or the Council Conclusions has been taken forward.

Especially since the EU increased its role in monitoring the financial sustainability and performance of health systems, quality of healthcare has become embedded within the context of health system performance measurement and improvement. In order to ensure the uptake of the health theme in the European Semester process, the Council called for translating the concept of "access to good quality healthcare" into operational assessment criteria (Council of the European Union, 2013). The 2014 Commission's Communication on modern, responsive and sustainable health systems also marked quality as a core element of health systems' performance assessment (HSPA) (EC, 2014a). As a result the Expert Group on HSPA that was set up in 2014 as a first strand produced a report on quality (EC, 2016). The goal of this report was not so much to compare or benchmark quality between Member States but rather to support national policy-makers by providing examples, tools and methodologies for implementing or improving quality strategies. This should not only help to optimize the use of resources but also to improve information on quality and safety as required under Directive 2011/24.

4.4 Conclusions

This chapter has tried to show how international frameworks can help foster and support quality initiatives in countries. The international dimension is particularly important to raise political awareness, to share experience and practice and to provide tools (conceptual frameworks, standards, models, assessment frameworks) for implementing quality measures and policies at national and regional level. The legal status and binding nature of the various international instruments differ. Most legally binding instruments are to be found at EU level, but their prime purpose is often facilitating free movement rather than ensuring quality. Also non-binding instruments have shown to be effective in pushing policy-makers at country level towards putting quality in healthcare on the political agenda.

The various international organizations have been cooperating with each other on quality, and also complementing one another's work. As an example, EU pharmaceutical legislation makes direct reference to the Council of Europe's European Pharmacopoeia, and the European Medicines Agency (EMA) and the European Directorate for the Quality of Medicines and Healthcare (EDQM) work closely together.

Quality became more recently an international political priority and rapidly gained importance as a significant lever to the international community for pushing health system reform, complementing the objective of universal health coverage. The efforts made by international organizations, such as WHO, to support national actors with guidance, information, practical tools and capacity building have paid off and contributed to launching a global movement advocating for monitoring and improving quality and safety in healthcare worldwide.

Next to the importance of quality from a public health perspective, and its close ties with fundamental patient rights, there is also an important economic dimension. In a context of increasing mobility and cross-border exchange in healthcare, quality can constitute both a driver of and an impediment to free movement. This is also why at EU level the attention for quality initially was rather indirect, as a precautionary measure to ensure the realization of the internal market, mostly the free movement of medical goods and health professionals. When the European Court of Justice in 1998 had to deal with the first cases on cross-border care it explicitly referred to the framework of mutual recognition of professional qualifications to dismiss the argument put forward by Member States that differences in quality would justify denying reimbursement of medical care provided in another Member State (Ghekiere, Baeten & Palm, 2010). However, the principle of mutual recognition, which is one of the cornerstones of the EU Single Market as it guarantees free movement without the need to harmonize Member States' legislation (Ghekiere, Baeten & Palm, 2010), is not always considered sufficient to guarantee high quality and safety standards. Also, the attempts at EU level to submit national regulation to a proportionality test and to develop an industry-driven kind of standardization in healthcare provision are met with some criticism and concern of the health sector.

Hence, the awareness grew that a more integrated approach was needed for promoting and ensuring quality in healthcare, with the case law on patient mobility as a turning point. The 2003 High Level Process of Reflection on Patient Mobility and Healthcare Developments in the European Union called for more systematic attention and information exchange on quality issues as well as for assessment of how European activities could help to improve quality (EC, 2003). The High Level Group on Health Services and Medical Care that started to work in 2004 further elaborated quality-related work in various areas, which eventually also made its way into the EU's horizontal health strategy (EC, 2007). Where initially the focus was very much concentrated on safety, it gradually broadened to include other aspects of quality, such as patient-centredness.

The added value of cross-border cooperation in specific areas, such as quality and safety, and sharing experiences and information about approaches and good practice is widely recognized. While it is not considered appropriate to harmonize health systems, the development of quality standards or practice guidelines at EU level was always something that was envisaged as a way to further make health systems converge (Cucic, 2002). Even if Directive 2011/24/EU on the application of patients' rights in cross-border healthcare finally did not include any obligation for Member States to introduce quality and safety standards, it did provide a clear mandate for the European Commission to claim more transparency around quality and safety, from which domestic patients would also benefit (Palm & Baeten, 2011).

This illustrates how the EU's involvement in healthcare quality has gradually evolved. Besides a broadening of its scope, we have also seen a move from merely fostering the sharing of information and best practices towards standardization and even the first signs of enforcement (Vollaard, van de Bovenkamp & Vrangbæk, 2013).

Table 4.5 *A selection of EU-funded projects on quality and/or safety*

HCQI (Health Care Quality Indicators)	2002–	The OECD Health Care Quality Indicators project, initiated in 2002, aims to measure and compare the quality of health service provision in different countries. An Expert Group has developed a set of quality indicators at the health systems level, which allows the impact of particular factors on the quality of health services to be assessed.	HP	www.oecd.org/els/ health-systems/ health-care-quality- indicators.htm
QM IN HEALTH CARE (Exchange of knowledge on quality management in healthcare)	2003– 2005	The aim of the project was to facilitate and coordinate the exchange of information and expertise on similarities and differences among European countries in national quality policies, and in research methods to assess quality management (QM) in healthcare organizations at a national level.	FP5	
SImPatIE (Safety Improvement for Patients in Europe)	2005– 2007	The SImPatIE project gathered a Europe-wide network of organizations, experts, professionals and other stakeholders to establish a common European set of strategies, vocabulary, indicators and tools to improve patient safety in healthcare. It focused on facilitating free movement of people and services.	HP	
MARQuIS (Methods of Assessing Response to Quality Improvement Strategies)	2005– 2007	The MARQuIS project's main objective was to identify and compare different quality improvement policies and strategies in healthcare systems across the EU Member States and to consider their potential use for cross-border patients. Next to providing an overview of different national quality strategies, it described how hospitals in a sample of states applied them to meet the defined requirements of cross-border patients.	FP6	

HP = Health Programme FP = Framework Programme for Research

Table 4.5   *A selection of EU-funded projects on quality and/or safety [continued]*

EUnetHTA (European network for Health Technology Assessment)	2006–	EUnetHTA was first established as a project to create an effective and sustainable network for health technology assessment across Europe. After the successful completion of the EUnetHTA Project (2006–2008), the EUnetHTA Collaboration was launched in November 2008 in the form of a Joint Action. Under the cross-border health Directive it is being transformed into a permanent structure to help in developing reliable, timely, transparent and transferable information to contribute to HTAs in European countries.	FP7 HP	www.eunethta.eu
EUNetPaS (European Network for Patient Safety)	2008– 2010	The aim of this project was to encourage and improve partnership in patient safety by sharing the knowledge, experiences and expertise of individual Member States and EU stakeholders on patient safety culture, education and training, reporting and learning systems, and medication safety in hospitals.	HP	
VALUE+ (Value+ Promoting Patients' Involvement)	2008– 2010	The project's objective was to exchange information, experiences and good practices around the meaningful involvement of patients' organizations in EU-supported health projects at EU and national level and raise awareness on its positive impact on patient-centred and equitable healthcare across the EU.	HP	
ORCAB (Improving quality and safety in the hospital: the link between organizational culture, burnout and quality of care)	2009– 2014	This project sought to highlight the role of hospital organizational culture and physician burnout in promoting patient safety and quality of care. It aimed to profile and monitor the specific factors of hospital-organizational culture that increase burnout among physicians and their impact on patient safety and quality of care.	FP7	
EuroDRG (Diagnosis-Related Groups in Europe: Towards Efficiency and Quality)	2009– 2011	Based on a comparative analysis of DRG systems across 10 European countries embedded in various types of health system, this project wanted to improve the knowledge on DRG-based hospital payment systems and their effect on health systems performance. Since policy-makers are often concerned about the impact on quality, the project specifically assessed the relationship between costs and the quality of care.	FP7	www.eurodrg.eu
DUQuE (Deepening our Understanding of Quality improvement in Europe)	2009– 2014	This was a research project to study the effectiveness of quality improvement systems in European hospitals. It mainly looked at the relationship between organizational quality improvement systems, organizational culture, professional involvement and patient involvement in quality management and their effect on the quality of hospital care (clinical effectiveness, patient safety and patient experience). A total of 192 hospitals from eight countries participated in the data collection. Seven measures for quality management were developed and validated.	FP7	www.duque.eu

HP = Health Programme   FP = Framework Programme for Research

Table 4.5   *A selection of EU-funded projects on quality and/or safety [continued]*

QUASER (Quality and safety in EU hospitals: a research-based guide for implementing best practice and a framework for assessing performance)	2010– 2013	This translational multilevel study was designed to investigate organizational and cultural factors affecting hospital quality improvement initiatives, and to produce and disseminate a guide for hospitals to develop and implement organizational-wide quality and safety improvement strategies, and a guide for payers to assess the appropriateness of a hospital's quality improvement strategy.	FP7	
QUALICOPC (Quality and costs of primary care in Europe)	2010– 2014	This study analysed and compared how primary healthcare systems in 34 countries performed in terms of quality, costs and equity. It aimed to show which configurations of primary healthcare are associated with better outcomes.	FP7	www.nivel.nl/en/ qualicopc
InterQuality (International Research Project on Financing Quality in Health Care)	2010– 2014	This project investigated the effects of financing systems on the quality of healthcare.	FP7	
Research on Financing Systems' Effect on the quality of Mental health care (REFINEMENT)	2011– 2013	REFINEMENT conducted the first-ever comparative and comprehensive overview of links between the financing of mental health care in Europe and the outcomes of mental health services.	FP7	www. refinementproject. eu
Joint Action on Patient Safety and Quality of Care (PaSQ)	2012– 2016	The objective of this Joint Action was to support the implementation of the Council Recommendation on Patient Safety through cooperation and sharing of information, experience and the implementation of good practices. The main outcome was the consolidation of the permanent network for patient safety established under EUNetPaS.	HP	www.pasq.eu
Costs of unsafe care and cost-effectiveness of patient safety programmes	2015– 2016	This study provided a comprehensive picture of the financial impact of poor patient safety, including poor prevention and control of healthcare-associated infections, on health systems. Based on an analysis of patient safety programmes implemented in EU/EEA Member States, it assessed the cost-effectiveness and efficiency of investing in patient safety programmes.	HP	

HP = Health Programme FP = Framework Programme for Research

References

Abbing HDCR (1997). The right of the patient to quality of medical practice and the position of migrant doctors within the EU. *European Journal of Health Law*, 4:347–60.

Alarcón-Jiménez O (2015). The MEDICRIME Convention – Fighting against counterfeit medicines. *Eurohealth*, 21(4):24–7.

Baeten R (2017). Was the exclusion of health care from the Services Directive a pyrrhic victory? A proportionality test on regulation of health professions. OSE Paper Series, Opinion Paper 18. Brussels. Available at: http://www.ose.be/files/publication/OSEPaperSeries/Baeten_2017_OpinionPaper18.pdf , accessed 3 December 2018.

Baeten R, Palm W (2011). The compatibility of health care capacity planning policies with EU Internal Market Rules. In: Gronden JW van de et al. (eds.). Health Care and EU Law.

Bertinato L et al. (2005). Policy brief: Cross-border health care in Europe. Copenhagen: WHO Regional Office for Europe.

Buchan J, Glinos IA, Wismar M (2014). Introduction to health professional mobility in a changing Europe. In: Buchan J et al. (eds.). Health Professional Mobility in a Changing Europe. New dynamics, mobile individuals and diverse responses. Observatory Studies Series. WHO Regional Office for Europe.

Charter of fundamental rights of the European Union, 2002, Article 35.

Cluzeau F et al. (2003). Development and validation of an international appraisal instrument for assessing the quality of clinical practice guidelines: the AGREE project. Quality and Safety in Health Care, 12(2003):18–23.

Committee of Ministers (2001). Recommendation Rec(2001)13 of the Committee of Ministers to Member States on developing a methodology for drawing up guidelines on best medical practices, adopted by the Committee of Ministers on 10 October 2001 at the 768th meeting of the Ministers' Deputies.

Committee on Quality of Health Care in America, IoM et al. (1999). To err is human: Building a safer health system. Washington, DC: National Academy Press.

Council of Europe (1997). The development and implementation of quality improvement systems (QIS) in health care. Recommendation No. R(97)17 adopted by the Committee of Ministers of the Council of Europe on 30 September 1997 and explanatory memorandum. Strasbourg: Council of Europe.

Council of European Dentists (2015). Cf. Statement by the Council of European Dentists, Common training principles under Directive 2005/36/EC. Available at: http://www.eoo.gr/files/pdfs/enimerosi/common_training_principles_under_dir_2005_36_en_ced_doc_2015_023_fin_e.pdf , accessed 3 December 2018.

Council of the European Union (2003). Council Recommendation of 2 December 2003 on cancer screening (2003/878/EC), OJ L 327/34–37.

Council of the European Union (2006). Council Conclusions on Common values and principles in European Union Health Systems, (2006/C 146/01). *Official Journal of the European Union*, C-146:1–3. Available at: http://eur-lex.europa.eu/LexUriServ/LexUriServ.do?uri=OJ:C:2006:146:0001:0003:EN:PDF, accessed 3 December 2018.

Council of the European Union (2009). Council Recommendation of 9 June 2009 on patient safety, including the prevention and control of healthcare associated infections. *Official Journal of the European Union*, C151.

Council of the European Union (2011). Council conclusions "Towards modern, responsive and sustainable health systems". Luxembourg.

Council of the European Union (2013). Council conclusions on the "Reflection process on modern, responsive and sustainable health systems".

Council of the European Union (2017). Proposal for a directive of the European Parliament and of the Council on a proportionality test before adoption of new regulation of professions – General approach.

Cucic S (2000). European Union health policy and its implication for national convergence. *International Journal for Quality in Health Care*, 12(3):224.

Directive 2005/36/EC on the recognition of professional qualifications. *Official Journal of the European Union*, L255.

Directive 2011/24/EU of 9 March 2011 on the application of patients' rights in cross-border healthcare. *Official Journal of the European Union*, L88:45–65.

Directive 2013/55/EU of 20 November 2013 amending Directive 2005/36/EC on the recognition of professional qualifications and Regulation (EU) No. 1024/2012 on administrative cooperation through the Internal Market Information System ('the IMI Regulation'). *Official Journal of the European Union*, L354.

EC (2003). High Level Process of Reflection on Patient Mobility and Healthcare Developments in the European Union, Outcome of the Reflection Process. HLPR/2003/16. Available at: http://ec.europa.eu/health/ph_overview/Documents/key01_mobility_en.pdf, accessed 3 December 2018.

EC (2006). Commission Communication SEC (2006) 1195/4: Consultation regarding Community action on health services.

EC (2007). Together for Health: A Strategic Approach for the EU 2008–2013. COM (2007) 630 final. Available at: http://ec.europa.eu/health/ph_overview/Documents/strategy_wp_en.pdf, accessed 3 December 2018.

EC (2008b). Communication on patient safety, including the prevention and control of healthcare-associated infections, 15 December 2008. COM (2008) 837 final.

EC (2009). Communication of 24 June 2009 on Action against Cancer: European Partnership. COM (2009) 291 final.

EC (2011). A strategic vision for European standards: moving forward to enhance and accelerate the sustainable growth of the European economy by 2020. COM(2011) 311. Brussels.

EC (2012a). Communication on safe, effective and innovative medical devices and in vitro diagnostic medical devices for the benefit of patients, consumers and healthcare professionals. COM (2012) 540 final. Luxembourg: Publications Office of the European Union.

EC (2012b). Report from the Commission to the Council on the basis of Member States' reports on the implementation of the Council recommendation (2009/C 151/01) on patient safety, including the prevention and control of healthcare associated infections. COM (2012) 658 final.

EC (2014a). Communication on modern, responsive and sustainable health systems. COM (2014) 215 final.

EC (2014c). Report from the Commission to the Council. The Commission's Second Report to the Council on the implementation of Council Recommendation 2009/C 151/01 on patient safety, including the prevention and control of healthcare associated infections. COM (2014) 371.

EC (2015). Flash Eurobarometer 210. Cross-border health services in the EU, June 2007; Special Eurobarometer 425 – Patients' rights in cross-border healthcare in the European Union.

EC (2016). So What? Strategies across Europe to assess quality of care. Report by the Expert Group on Health Systems Performance Assessment. European Commission (EC). Brussels: European Commission.

ECIBC (2014). European Commission Initiative on Breast Cancer: background and concept. Available at: https://ec.europa.eu/jrc/sites/jrcsh/files/ECIBC%20background%20and%20 concept.pdf.

European Commission Joint Research Centre (2013). Round table European Forum for Science and Industry. "Putting Science into Standards: the example of Eco-Innovation".

European Hospital and Healthcare Federation et al. (2016). Joint letter of 6 July 2016. Available at: http://www.epsu.org/sites/default/files/article/files/

HOPE%2BCPME%2BCED%2BEPSU%2BETUC-Letter-Standardisation-06.07.16.pdf, accessed 2 February 2017.

Expert Panel on Effective Ways of Investing in Health (2014). Future EU Agenda on quality of health care with a special emphasis on patient safety.

Federal Ministry of Labour, Health and Social Affairs (1998). Quality in health care: opportunities and limits of co-operation at EU level. Report of meeting of European Union Health Ministers on quality in healthcare. Vienna: Federal Ministry.

Federal Ministry of Social Security and Generations (2001). Quality policy in the health care systems of the EU accession candidates. Vienna: Federal Ministry.

Ghekiere W, Baeten R, Palm W (2010). Free movement of services in the EU and health care. In: Mossialos E et al. (eds.). Europe: the role of European Union law and policy. Cambridge: Cambridge University Press, pp. 461–508.

Glinos IA et al. (2015). How can countries address the efficiency and equity implications of health professional mobility in Europe? Adapting policies in the context of the WHO Code of Practice and EU freedom of movement. *Policy Brief*, 18:13.

Greer SL, Vanhercke B (2010). The hard politics of soft law: the case of health. In: Mossialos E et al. (eds.). Europe: the role of European Union law and policy. Cambridge: Cambridge University Press, pp. 186–230.

Greer SL et al. (2014). Everything you always wanted to know about European Union health policies but were afraid to ask.

Kramer DB, Xu S, Kesselheim AS (2012). Regulation of medical devices in the United States and European Union. *New England Journal of Medicine*, 366(9):848–55.

Legido-Quigley H et al. (eds.) (2013). Clinical guidelines for chronic conditions in the European Union.

Maier CB et al. (2011). Cross-country analysis of health professional mobility in Europe: the results. In: Wismar M et al. (eds.). Health professional mobility and health systems. Evidence from 17 European countries. Observatory Studies Series. WHO Regional Office for Europe, p. 49.

Nys H, Goffin T (2011). Mapping national practices and strategies relating to patients' rights. In: Wismar M et al. (eds). Cross-Border Healthcare: Mapping and Analysing Health Systems Diversity. Copenhagen: World Health Organization on behalf of the European Observatory on Health Systems and Policies, pp. 159–216.

OECD (2017). Caring for quality in health: Lessons learnt from 15 reviews of health care quality. Paris: Organisation for Economic Co-operation and Development.

Palm W, Baeten R (2011). The quality and safety paradox in the patients' rights Directive. European Journal of Public Health, 21(3):272–4.

Palm W, Glinos I (2010). Enabling patient mobility in the EU: between free movement and coordination. In: Mossialos E et al. (eds.). Health systems governance in Europe: the role of European Union law and policy. Cambridge: Cambridge University Press, pp. 509–60.

Palm W et al. (2011). Towards a renewed community framework for safe, high-quality and efficient cross-border health care within the European Union. In: Wismar M et al. (eds.). Cross-border health care in the European Union: Mapping and analysing practices and policies. Observatory Studies Series. WHO Regional Office for Europe.

Peeters (2005). Free movement of medical doctors: the new Directive 2005/36/EC on recognition of professional qualifications. *European Journal of Health Law*, 12:373–96.

Peeters M (2012). Free movement of patients: Directive 2011/24 on the application of patients' rights in cross-border healthcare. *European Journal of Health Law*, 19:1–32.

Peeters M, McKee M, Merkur S (2010). EU law and health professionals. In: Baeten R, Mossialos E, Hervey T (eds.). Health Systems Governance in Europe: the Role of EU Law and Policy. Health economics, policy and management. Cambridge: Cambridge University Press, p. 599.

Reynolds M et al. (2010). European coding system for tissues and cells: a challenge unmet? *Cell and Tissue Banking*, 11:353–64.

Shaw C, Kalo I (2002). A background for national quality policies in health systems. Copenhagen: WHO Regional Office for Europe.

Shaw CD (2015). How can healthcare standards be standardised? *BMJ Quality and Safety*, 24:615–19.

Sokol T (2010). Rindal and Elchinov: a(n) (impending) revolution in EU law on patient mobility. *Croatian yearbook of European law & policy*, 6(6):167–208.

Tiedje J, Zsigmond A (2012). How to modernise the professional qualifications Directive. *Eurohealth*, 18(2):18–22.

Vollaard H, van de Bovenkamp HM, Vrangbæk K (2013). The emerging EU quality of care policy: from sharing information to enforcement. *Health Policy*, 111(3):226–33.

White Paper: Together for health: a strategic approach for the EU 2008–2013.

WHO (2002). World Health Assembly Resolution WHA55.18: Quality of care: patient safety.

WHO (1998). Health for All in the 21st Century, WHA51/5. Available at: http://apps.who.int/gb/archive/pdf_files/WHA51/ea5.pdf, accessed 3 December 2018.

Wismar M et al. (2011). Health professional mobility and health systems in Europe: an introduction. In: Wismar M et al. (eds.). Health professional mobility and health systems. Evidence from 17 European countries. Observatory Studies Series. WHO Regional Office for Europe, p. 11.

Part II

Chapter 5

Regulating the input: health professions

Anika Kreutzberg, Christoph Reichebner,
Claudia Bettina Maier, Frederic Destrebecq, Dimitra Panteli

Summary

What are the characteristics of the strategy?

Health professionals are both a health system input and an active component of the functions that the health system performs. As such, the performance of the health workforce is directly linked to the quality of health services. Regulation is essential to define a clear framework within which health professionals acquire and maintain the competence needed to provide health services that are of high quality, i.e. that are safe, effective and patient-centred. This chapter describes strategies that regulate health professionals, including: (a) strategies to develop professional competence (including training structure and contents, curriculum development and the accreditation of institutions for health education); (b) strategies that regulate the entry of physicians and nurses into their professions (for example, licensing and registration); (c) mechanisms to maintain competence (for example, continuing professional development); and (d) levers to address instances when fitness to practise comes into question.

What is being done in European countries?

The national regulation of professions in Europe is guided by the EU Directives on the recognition of professional qualifications; these aim to ensure comparability and equivalence of diplomas mainly by regulating the minimum duration of training. The detailed regulation of health *professional education* lies within national responsibility, leading to considerable variation in health professional training across countries. For most health professionals, training consists of basic undergraduate education and subsequent specialized training combined with on-the-job learning. Only a few countries allow physicians to practise after finishing undergraduate studies; usually, further specialization is required before they are allowed to deliver patient care. The pathway to becoming a medical specialist is very different among countries in Europe and worldwide. Nursing education is even less uniform, with varying levels of regulation. Across Europe, nursing education is usually subdivided into basic education, which offers the qualifications required to practise as a professional nurse, and subsequent specialty training. Developments in the design of training contents and curricula for medical and nursing education in recent decades have been moving towards outcome-based education. Several national bodies responsible for designing medical education in European countries have developed frameworks to describe the desired outcomes of medical education and define the competencies that graduates should possess to enter the profession. Countries differ in their requirements of what is required to be **granted the right to practise**. At a minimum, professionals have to successfully finish basic professional education. Licensing is often combined with mandatory registration in a health professional register. Registers serve as a tool to inform the public as well as potential employers about the accredited qualifications and scopes of practice of a certain health professional. Licensing and registration for doctors are mostly regulated at national level. In the majority of countries in Europe licensing and registration are also required in order to practise as a nurse. Closely linked to the process of licensing and registration are schemes for actively **maintaining professional competence**. Overall, continuing education for specialist doctors has become increasingly mandatory within the European Union, with 21 countries operating obligatory systems. In countries with voluntary structures, continuing education is at least actively supported. Continuing education and licence renewal is less regulated for the nursing professions. Finally, there is little consistency in how **events questioning competency and qualities** of medical professionals are handled across Europe. Considerable diversity exists in the range of topics addressed by regulatory bodies, with almost all covering healthcare quality and safety, and some also exploring themes around reputation and maintaining the public's trust in the profession.

What do we know about the effectiveness and cost-effectiveness of the strategy?

An umbrella review on the effectiveness of different curricular and instructional design methods in medical curricula found that most studies reported on learning outcomes such as knowledge and skill acquisition, while fewer than half reported on patient or organizational outcomes. Evidence seemed overall to be inconclusive and showing mixed effects, not least due to a lack of rigorous qualitative and quantitative research. In nursing, research has shown that the shift towards higher education can be beneficial for patient outcomes. Advanced knowledge and skill acquirement during undergraduate nursing training was shown to be effective in improving perceptions of competence and confidence. There is only little research regarding the effects of licensing on the quality of care; it suggests that additional performance points achieved in the national licensing examinations in the US were associated with small decreases in mortality. A review of reviews on the effectiveness of continuing medical education on physician performance and patient health outcomes found that continuing education is effective on all fronts: in the acquisition and retention of knowledge, attitudes, skills and behaviours as well as in the improvement of clinical outcomes, with the effects on physician performance being more consistent than those on patient outcomes across studies. No empirical evidence of good quality was identified on the cost-effectiveness of licensing for physicians or nurses.

How can the strategy be implemented?

In most countries regulating training contents and curricula of health professionals aims to ensure uniformity across educational programmes in an ever-changing society and body of clinical knowledge. Highly developed countries have experienced a notable trend towards an increase in health professional regulation over the last twenty years, especially for physicians. At the same time, an overly excessive degree of standardizing medical education puts innovation and advancements in curricula at stake. The key lies in finding the right degree of regulating educational standards that guarantee minimum levels of competency whilst at the same time allowing for flexibility and innovation. As learning in cooperation with others has been shown to be more effective than learning alone, interactive training approaches should be further endorsed. The health professional education system, particularly at undergraduate level, should ensure that students acquire a lifelong learning strategy, by means of both problem-based and simulation-based learning strategies integrated in undergraduate curricula. Effective continuing education involves learning (why?) and being fit to practise (how?) as well as putting both into practice; its funding remains an obstacle and should be independent from potential conflicts of interest. Safeguards and guidelines to regulate the contents of continuing education materials introduced by healthcare authorities can facilitate this process, as can collaborative initiatives.

Conclusions for policy-makers

It is important to invest in critically appraising healthcare-related curricula and supporting research into optimal learning modalities both in terms of scope and didactic approach. Existing evidence may be encouraging to continue developing and implementing outcome-based training concepts, but initiatives need to be accompanied with mechanisms for the critical appraisal of its benefits using sound research methods. A combination of problem-based and simulation-based learning strategies integrated in undergraduate curricula could help professionals overcome skill-based barriers to lifelong learning, thus fostering success in other regulatory components, such as continuing professional development education. Regulating entry to the profession (for example, by licensure and/or registration) in a manner that is adaptable to the changing landscape of healthcare and fit-for-purpose also merits consideration, as does (further) developing the mechanisms to maintain professional competence during practice, including guidance on content and modalities of continuing education, and accounting for the balance between activities to maintain competence and clinical practice.

5.1 Introduction: health professional regulation and its contribution to healthcare quality

Health professionals are a prerequisite for the delivery of healthcare services. Prevention, health promotion and medical interventions require an adequate mix of primary care and highly specialized health professionals who have the medical and technical expertise to perform high-quality care and possess the right skills in the right place for tailored, personal interactions and teamwork (OECD, 2016; WHO, 2016). Reaching the health-related Sustainable Development Goals, including universal access, is closely linked to the availability and accessibility of a country's health workforce (WHO, 2016). Health professionals represent both a health system input and an active component of the functions that the system itself performs (Diallo et al., 2003). As such, the performance of the health workforce is directly linked to the quality of health services (WHO, 2006). In WHO's model for health system strengthening, the health workforce is recognized as an important building-block: "A well-performing health workforce is one that works in ways that are responsive, fair and efficient to achieve the best health outcomes possible, given available resources and circumstances (i.e. there are sufficient staff, fairly distributed; they are competent, responsive and productive)" (*see* Chapter 1, and WHO, 2007). Investing in a country's health workforce has received increased policy attention in recent years with the creation of the High-Level Commission on Health Employment and Economic Growth (WHO, 2016), which highlighted the need for investing in a workforce of adequate numbers and skill-mix at country level. Such a workforce not only directly contributes to improved health, but in turn reduces unemployment and can stimulate economic growth.

Indeed, the competence and availability of health professionals, for instance doctors, nurses and midwives, affect health outcomes in many areas, such as maternal and infant mortality, independently of other determinants (Anand & Bärnighausen, 2004). A lower supply of general practitioners has been found to be associated with increased hospitalizations (Gulliford, 2002), while a higher proportion of nurses and more hours of care provided by nurses are associated with better care for hospitalized patients (Needleman et al., 2002). At the same time, a higher nursing workload, as measured by the patient-to-nurse ratio, is correlated with an increased 30-day mortality (Aiken et al., 2014).

In line with the general approach of this book, this chapter looks at the contribution of professional regulation to the quality of health services. We therefore focus on the role of policy and regulation in particular on the development and upkeep of professional competence. Although the planning of skill-mix and staffing levels is also crucial for health system performance, it is beyond the scope of this chapter. Indeed, as illustrated in Fig. 5.1, quality in health services requires competent – that is well-educated, trained and skilled – health professionals. This in turn is linked to the potential of improved population health outcomes. "Competence" describes the ability of individuals to repeatedly apply their skills and knowledge to achieve outcomes that consistently satisfy predetermined standards of performance. Beyond skills and knowledge, it therefore involves an individual's self-conception, personal characteristics and motivation (WHO, 2006).

Fig. 5.1   *Relationship between human resources actions and health outcomes and focus of this chapter (highlighted in blue)*

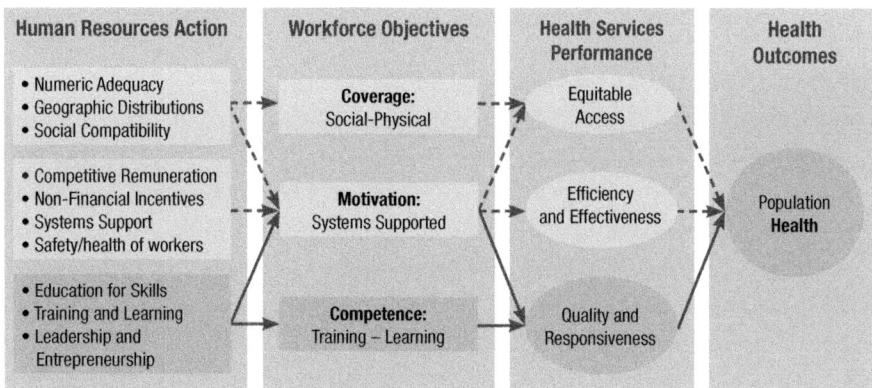

Source: based on WHO, 2006

Regulation is essential to define a clear framework within which health professionals acquire and maintain the competence needed to provide health services that are of high quality, i.e. that are safe, effective and patient-centred (*see* also the first lens of the quality framework described in Chapter 2). Regulation refers to laws or bylaws defining the conditions for health professionals' minimum educational requirements, entry to practice, title protection, scope-of-practice and other measures, such as the regulation of continuing professional development.

Countries are free to decide whether to regulate a specific profession or not. The decision is usually based on the level of complexity of the professional's role and its implications for patient safety. For some health professionals, such as healthcare assistants, countries may choose not to regulate the titles or scopes-of-practice by law, but to entrust the assurance of quality to other governance levers, such as employer-based mechanisms or protocols. In most European countries the primary aim of health professional regulation is to ensure quality and safety of care – this is mirrored in professional codes of conduct, which usually define quality of care as their main focus (Struckmann et al., 2015).

It is important to distinguish between the different regulatory mechanisms that can be used to ensure quality in the health and social sectors (command and control; meta-regulation; self-regulation; and market mechanisms – *see* Schweppenstedde et al., 2014). Professional self-regulation (as reflected in professional codes of conduct, for example) plays an important role in the regulation of health professionals. The professions are often involved in defining what standards constitute good professional practice (WHO, 2006). Striking the optimal balance between autonomy of the profession and regulation through command and control can be challenging. The roles of different regulatory bodies should be well balanced with clearly defined and transparent boundaries between them and public authorities. The interpretation of this balance differs considerably between countries, resulting in diverse national systems of health professional regulation.

Given the complexity of healthcare provision, the overall group of health professionals consists of numerous individual professions with different and complementary job profiles and skill requirements. WHO distinguishes two main groups of health professionals: (a) health service providers, encompassing all workers whose daily activities aim at improving health, including doctors, nurses, pharmacists, dentists and midwives working for hospitals, medical clinics or other community providers as well as for organizations outside the health sector (for example, factories or schools); and (b) health system workers, who do not provide health services directly but ensure that health service providers can do their jobs, like staff working in ministries of health, managers, economists, or specialists for information systems (WHO, 2006).

The diversity of the health workforce is in turn reflected in highly multifaceted and complex regulatory procedures for the different professions, and this chapter does not attempt to give an exhaustive overview of related mechanisms for all individual health professions. Although all health professionals are essential for a national health system to function, the following sections focus on health service providers as the ones directly involved with the delivery of healthcare services to the population. Specifically, this chapter looks at the regulation of physicians and nurses as two large health professional groups. It provides an overview of strategies that aim to regulate the acquisition and maintenance of competence among health professionals, discussing generic systems which are well established in many European countries but also outlining the diversity among countries when it comes to the detailed definition and practical application of these systems.

Following the general approach of this volume, this chapter is structured as follows: it first describes strategies that regulate health professionals along with current practice in European countries for each strategy. These include: (a) strategies to develop professional competence (including training structure and contents, curriculum development and the accreditation of institutions for health education); (b) strategies that regulate the entry of physicians and nurses into their professions (for example, licensing and registration); (c) mechanisms to maintain competence (for example, continuing professional development); and (d) levers to address instances when fitness to practise comes into question. The interplay of these strategies is shown in Fig. 5.2. The chapter then summarizes available evidence on the effectiveness and cost-effectiveness of the described strategies and subsequently derives implications for their implementation.

Tables 5.9 and 5.10 at the end of the chapter respectively provide an overview of the national bodies responsible for regulating physicians and nurses in selected European countries.

5.2 What is being done in Europe? Strategies to develop professional competence

As mentioned in the introduction, the key to linking the development of the workforce to quality of care is competence. Competence encompasses an "array of abilities across multiple domains or aspects of performance in a certain context" (Englander et al., 2017) and integrates knowledge, skills and attitudes; it is closely linked with professionalism. Moving forward in this chapter, we understand competence as a capacity that can be applied to a relatively wide range of contexts. Competencies of health professionals are related to a specific activity and can be measured and assessed to ensure their acquisition (Frank et al., 2010; Englander et al., 2017).

According to the OECD, a skill is usually a unit of competence that is relevant to a specific context (OECD, 2018) and represents its practical dimension (whereas knowledge refers to the theoretical dimension of competence, and attitude reflects

Fig. 5.2   *Strategies for regulating health professionals (in this chapter)*

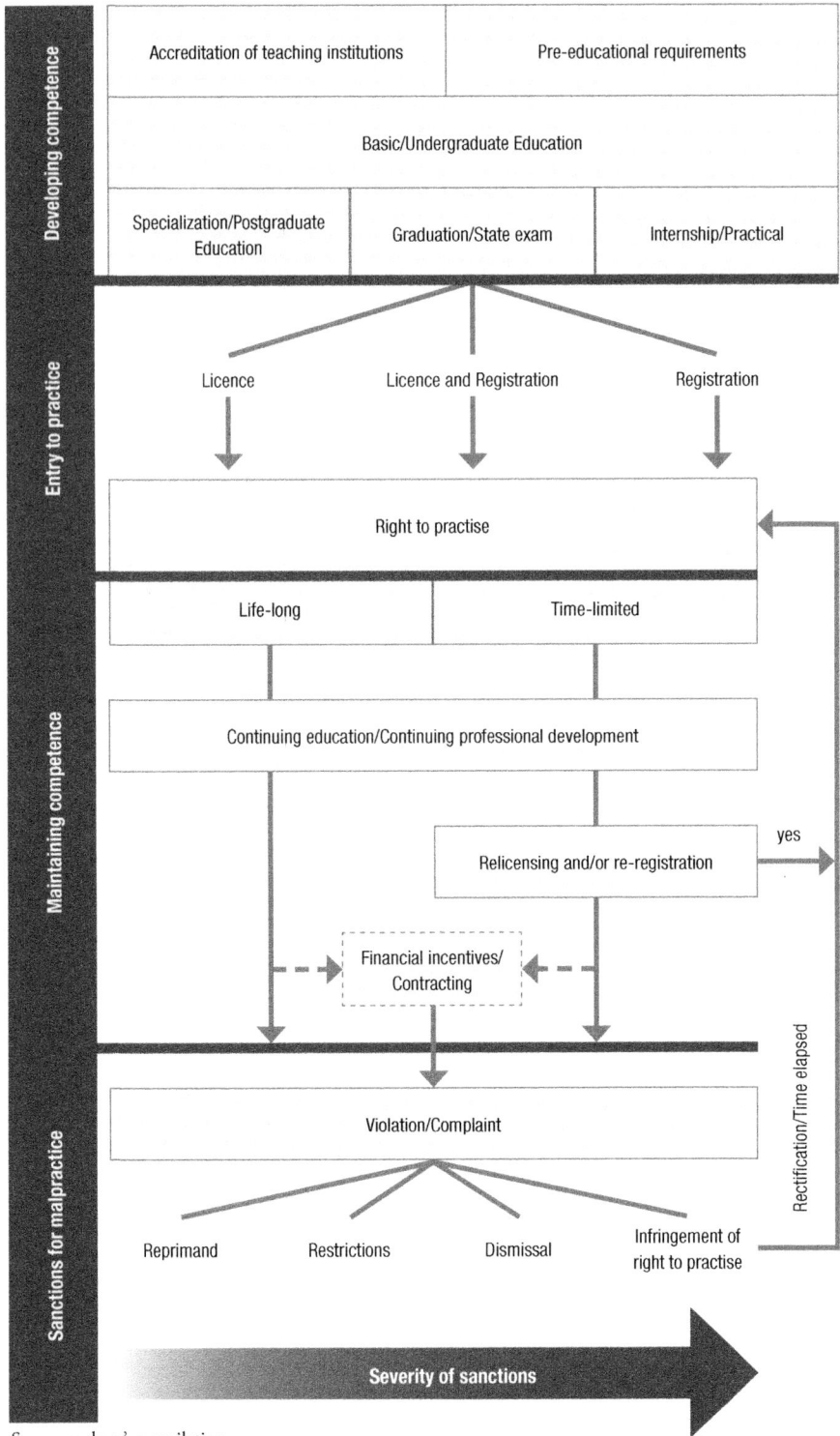

Source: authors' compilation

an individual's beliefs, dispositions and values). Skills can broadly be categorized into cognitive and non-cognitive or physical and learning skills (*see* Fig. 5.3). Transversal (or core/'soft') skills are relevant to a broad range of occupations and are considered to be necessary for the effective application of job-specific skills and knowledge. They have been gaining importance as a result of the ongoing transition from a disease-centred clinical care delivery approach towards person-centred, value-based and personalized models of care (OECD, 2018).

Fig. 5.3   *Various domains of skills*

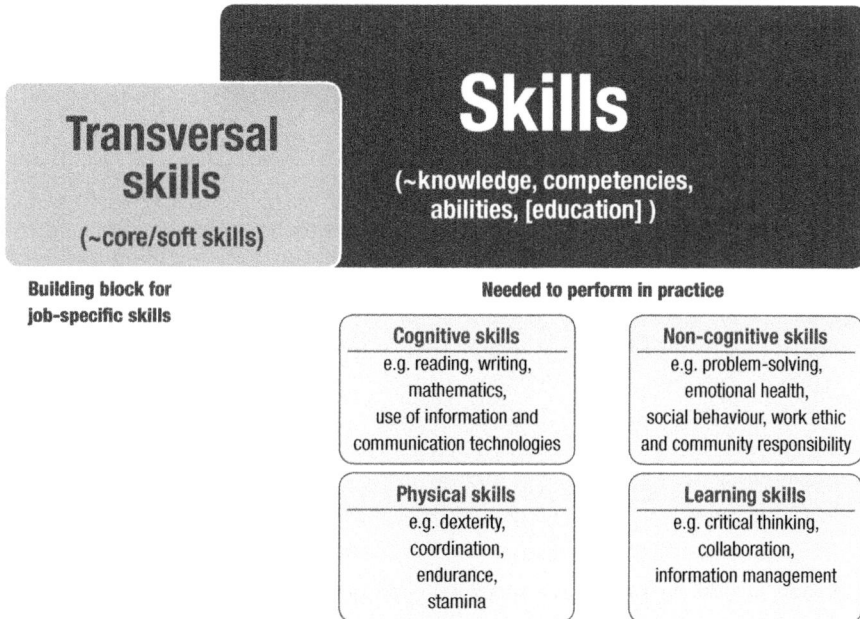

Skills
(~knowledge, competencies, abilities, [education])

Transversal skills
(~core/soft skills)

Building block for job-specific skills

Needed to perform in practice

Cognitive skills	Non-cognitive skills
e.g. reading, writing, mathematics, use of information and communication technologies	e.g. problem-solving, emotional health, social behaviour, work ethic and community responsibility

Physical skills	Learning skills
e.g. dexterity, coordination, endurance, stamina	e.g. critical thinking, collaboration, information management

Source: authors' compilation based on OECD, 2018

5.2.1 Regulating training duration and content

The cornerstone of building competence for health professionals is education and training. In most countries the regulation of training content and curricula for health professionals aims to ensure uniformity across educational programmes (Woodward, 2000). Arguably, building a competent health workforce starts with the requirements and selection procedures for students to access related higher education. A-level grades and grade-weighted lotteries, tailored entry tests and personal interviews are all used alone or in combination in European countries. For example, Austria operates a standardized admission examination for medical studies (EMS) at public universities (Bachner et al., 2018). Germany, in contrast, distributes study places centrally according to academic records, waiting times and interviews by the universities (Busse & Blümel, 2014; Zavlin et al., 2017).

Admission criteria for basic nursing education range from a minimum number of general education years and selection exams to the requirement of a medical certification (Humar & Sansoni, 2017).

For most health professionals training consists of basic undergraduate education and subsequent specialized training combined with on-the-job learning. Accordingly, physicians usually complete undergraduate studies in medicine at university level and in most cases require additional (postgraduate) training at a hospital in order to practise (WHO, 2006). The national regulation of professions in Europe is guided by the EU Directives on the recognition of professional qualifications (*see* Box 5.1).

Box 5.1 *Developments at EU level to ensure quality of care given the mobility of health professionals*

Increasing mobility of health professionals and patients across Europe challenges national regulations of qualification standards. Specifically, in the European Union and European Economic Area (EU/EEA) mobility is facilitated by the principle of freedom of movement. Mobility is catalysed by growing shortages in certain health professions or rural/underserved regions and countries, which lead national organizations to actively recruit staff to fill vacancies. Increasing professional migration has led to the realization that broader EU-level legislative changes need to be considered in the development of the healthcare workforce within EU Member States (Leone et al., 2016).

Several efforts at European level have aimed to ensure quality (and, therein, safety) of care in light of the mobility of health professionals. The Bologna Process, launched in 1999, had an enormous impact on the homogenization of education. Directive 2013/55/EU of 20 November 2013 amending Directive 2005/36/EC of the European Parliament and of the Council of 7 September 2005 form the legal foundation for the mutual recognition of professional qualifications in EU and EEA countries. The framework ensures that health professionals can migrate freely between EU Member States and practise their profession. The new Directive came into effect in January 2016. It introduced the possibility for responsible authorities to have professionals undergo language tests, a warning system to identify professionals who have been banned from practice, and a European professional card as an electronic documentation tool to attest a professional's qualifications and registration status (Ling & Belcher, 2014).

However, some important issues remain under the EU framework, such as the widely variable standards for accreditation of specialist training. Additional initiatives have been contributing to a change in this direction. For example, the European Union of Medical Specialists (UEMS) was founded in 1958 as the representative organization of all medical specialists in the European Community. Its mission is to promote patient safety and quality of care through the development of standards for medical training and healthcare across Europe. The UEMS outlined guiding principles for a European approach of postgraduate medical training in 1994 with the intention to provide a voluntary complement to the existing national structures and ensure the quality of training across Europe. More recently, the UEMS established the European Council for Accreditation of Medical Specialist Qualifications (ECAMSQ®), which developed a competence-based approach for the assessment and certification of medical specialists' competence across Europe. This framework is underpinned by the European Accreditation Council for Continuing Medical Education (EACCME®), established in 1999, which provides the mutual recognition of accreditation of EU-wide and international continuing medical education and continuing professional development activities.

To date, initiatives such as the EACCME® or ECAMSQ® have remained voluntary, complementing what is provided and regulated by the national authorities and/or training institutions. As such, their added value is predicated on the recognition provided by these national bodies. The aim of UEMS remains to encourage the harmonization of specialist training across Europe with the ambition to promote high standards of education, and in consequence high-quality healthcare, but also to facilitate recognition of qualifications.

The EU Directives aim to ensure comparability and equivalence of diplomas mainly by regulating the minimum duration of training. For example, undergraduate medical education requires a minimum of five years of university-based theoretical and practical training. The detailed regulation of health professional education beyond its minimum length still lies within national responsibility, leading to considerable variation in health professional training across countries. In countries with federal structures additional variations can exist among federal states. Undergraduate medical education is mostly regulated at national level, with governmental agencies of higher education being responsible for defining relevant standards. In contrast, subsequent specialist training or residency programmes are often subject to professional self-regulation, with the medical associations of the corresponding specialty being in charge of defining details of curricula, teaching approaches and assessment methods.

Fig. 5.4 provides a simplified visualization of the different pathways of medical education in selected countries in Europe as well as the USA and Canada. Nara, Suzuki & Tohda (2011) identified three types of medical education system. In type 1 – which can be found in countries such as Germany, the Netherlands, Belgium, Spain and Scotland – medical schools accept high school leavers. Undergraduate medical education lasts five (Scotland) to seven (Belgium) years. To enter medical school in type 2 systems (USA and Canada) a bachelor's degree from a non-medical college is required. Undergraduate education lasts four years in this type. Type 3 (for example, England and Ireland) represents a mix of types 1 and 2. That means some medical schools accept high school leavers or college graduates only, while others accept both, and the length of education varies accordingly.

Moreover, the detailed structure of undergraduate medical education may vary. For example, the six years in Germany are subdivided into a two-year preclinical component (Vorklinik) and a four-year clinical component (Klinik) (Zavlin et al., 2017). Progressing into the clinical component requires the successful completion of a first state board exam (Staatsexamen). A second state board exam is usually completed after the fifth year of education. In Bulgaria the six years are split into five years of theoretical and one year of practical training (Dimova et al., 2018). France distinguishes two phases, of which only the second, four-year, phase combines theoretical and clinical training (Chevreul et al., 2015). Most countries require some sort of supervised training (for example, internships of one to two years), which may be a prerequisite for or integrated with specialist training. For example, Austria requires nine months of clinical training for graduates (Bachner et al., 2018). In Portugal medical graduates undergo a 12-months internship (Ano Comum) in both the primary care and the hospital setting (Simões et al., 2017). The UK operates a two-year foundation programme which is predominantly based in hospital settings (Cylus et al., 2015; Rashid & Manek, 2016).

Fig. 5.4   *Visualization of the medical education systems in selected European countries and the USA/Canada*

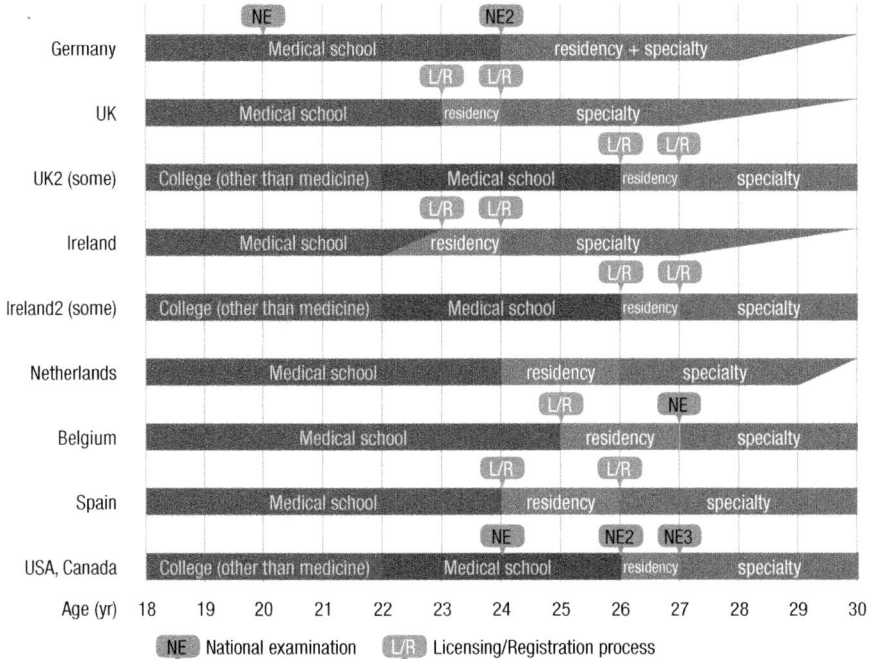

Source: adapted from Nara, Suzuki & Tohda, 2011

Only a few countries allow physicians to practise after finishing undergraduate studies. Most often, further specialization is required before they are allowed to deliver patient care. The pathway to becoming a medical specialist is, however, very different among countries within Europe and worldwide. Variation exists in admissions policy, duration, scope, terminology and significance of diplomas, and general structure of residency training (Weggemans et al., 2017). The length of specialist training can vary from a minimum of two years up to more than nine years. In Norway, for example, specialization requires at least five years of study with an average of nine years (Ringard et al., 2013). General practice (or family medicine) has become a specialty in its own right in most countries over the past years. The EU Directive requires specific training in general medical practice with at least three-year specialty and six months' practice training at both a hospital and a general practice in the community. In fact, most European countries operate a training programme for general medicine of at least three years.

Nursing education is even less uniform across countries, with varying levels of regulation. Some countries have regulations at national, others at subnational level. As can be seen in Table 5.10 at the end of the chapter, responsible authorities vary from government ministries, typically those concerned with health or education, to national nursing organizations and independent statutory bodies. Across Europe nursing education is usually subdivided into basic education, which offers the qualifications required to practise as a professional nurse,[1] and subsequent specialty training in a variety of fields in clinical practice, teaching and management. However, some countries allow direct entry routes into selected specialties even after basic nurse education.

The education of professional nurses across all countries participating in the EU's single market is regulated to the extent that a minimum requirement of 2 300 hours each of theory and practice has been set (Directive 36/2005/EC). Moreover, the Bologna process has instigated the move of nursing education to the academic level. Over the past decade most countries introduced (Bachelor's) degree level programmes provided by higher education institutions that run additionally to the traditional vocational education (Ousy, 2011; Humar & Sansoni, 2017). Different levels of basic nurse education in turn qualify professionals to take over different sets of tasks and responsibilities. For example, in the Netherlands nurses can develop their qualification from nurse or social care associate to a Bachelor's degree in Nursing. Responsibilities range accordingly from less complex to very complex tasks such as case management. Table 5.1 provides an overview of the available nurse categories and key features of the educational requirements in selected European countries. Some countries have

---

1   Also referred to as registered nurses. Because not all countries mandate the registration of their nurses, we use the term "professional nurse" in this chapter

Table 5.1 *Nurse categories and key elements of basic nursing education for selected European countries*

Country	Degree	Educational institution	Length	ECTS
Austria	1) Bachelor of Science	University of Applied Science	3 years	180
	2) Diploma	Nursing school		
Finland	1) Bachelor of Arts	University or University of Applied Science	3.5 to 4 years	210 to 240
Germany	1) Bachelor of Arts or Science	University of Applied Science	>3 years	>180
	2) Diploma	Nursing school	3 years	
Netherlands	1) Bachelor of Nursing	University of Applied Science or Nursing school	4 years	240
United Kingdom	1) Bachelor of Arts	University	3 to 4 years	180

Source: based on Riedel, Röhrling & Schönpflug, 2016

started to move nursing education entirely to the graduate level. The UK, for example, introduced the Bachelor's degree as the minimum level of education for professional nurses in 2013 (Riedel, Röhrling & Schönpflug, 2016). Austria is considering restricting nursing education exclusively to the university level by 2024 (Bachner et al., 2018).

In turn, the increasing importance of degree-level nursing education further triggered the specialization of nurses and the expansion of their roles. The majority of European countries offer some form of specialized training with varying titles, levels and length of education (Dury et al., 2014). Nurse specialists may be qualified to care for certain patient groups such as chronically ill patients (Riedel, Röhrling & Schönpflug, 2016). The number of recognized specializations (for example, theatre nursing, paediatric nursing, anaesthesia, mental health, public health or geriatrics) can vary considerably between countries. Also, Master's degrees in Advanced Practice Nursing are increasingly available. Within Europe, Finland, the Netherlands, Ireland and the UK have established nursing roles at an advanced practice level, for example, Nurse Practitioners at Master's level. They have considerably expanded the scope of practice of Nurse Practitioners, changing the professional boundaries between the medical and nursing professions (Maier & Aiken, 2016). This change in skill-mix has implications for whether and how to regulate changes to the division of tasks and responsibilities between professions.

5.2.2 Curriculum development: outcome-/competency-based education

An important change in the way professional education is approached has been under way in recent decades. Conventional education was criticized for being structure- and process-based with a focus on knowledge acquisition. However, the hands-on application of this knowledge was rarely assessed; this introduced the risk that trainees were not necessarily appropriately prepared for independent practice (Cooney et al., 2017). It was widely recognized that training needed to be linked more directly to job performance and the tasks that professionals would be expected to perform rather than to rest on ingrained assumptions about the curricula that should be taught (WHO, 2006). Thus, developments in the design of training contents and curricula have been based on the notion that the application of knowledge and practical skills, rather than knowledge alone, is the key to a competent health workforce. That is, quality patient care can only occur when health professionals acquire and apply competencies effectively (Swing, 2007). The concept of outcome-based education was first introduced into medical curricula in the 1970s and has been disseminated and adapted internationally since the late 1990s (Morcke, Dornan & Eika, 2013; Bisgaard et al., 2018). It requires a clear definition of predetermined outcomes which inform all curricular decisions.

Outcome-based medical and nursing education focuses on defined competencies which are required for practice. A similar concept discussed in this context is competency-based education. While both approaches differ in their detailed definition, they are based on the same idea: education should be guided by predetermined outcomes (Morcke, Dornan & Eika, 2013; Frank et al., 2010; Pijl-Zieber et al., 2014). These competencies are derived from the current challenges healthcare is facing and the corresponding societal and patient needs (Touchie & ten Cate, 2016). Outcome-based education constituted a paradigm shift in medical education: it put greater emphasis on accountability, flexibility and learner-centredness (Frank et al., 2010). Within its context, curricula and teaching approaches are designed on the basis of what learners should know, understand and demonstrate, and how to adapt this knowledge to life beyond formal education (Tan et al., 2018). Table 5.2 provides a comparison of key elements between the traditional structure-based approach and the outcome-based concept.

So-called "entrustable" professional activities and milestones are main features of outcome-based education (Touchie & ten Cate, 2016; Carracio et al., 2017). They are broad units of professional practice which describe the tasks or responsibilities a professional can be entrusted with once specific competences have been acquired through training (Touchie & ten Cate, 2016). Outcome-based

Table 5.2 *Comparison of structure-based versus outcome-based educational programmes*

Variable	Structure- and process-based	Outcome-based
Driving force for curriculum	Content-knowledge acquisition	Outcome-knowledge application
Driving force for process	Teacher	Learner
Path of learning	Hierarchical (teacher → student)	Non-hierarchical (teacher ↔ student)
Responsibility for content	Teacher	Student and teacher
Goal of educational encounter	Knowledge acquisition	Knowledge application
Typical assessment tool	Single subjective measure	Multiple objective measures ("evaluation portfolio")
Assessment tool	Proxy	Authentic (mimics real task)
Setting for evaluation	Removed (gestalt)	Direct observation
Evaluation	Norm-referenced	Criterion-referenced
Timing of assessment	Emphasis on summative	Emphasis on formative
Programme completion	Fixed time	Variable time

Source: based on Carracio et al., 2002

education intends to promote cumulative learning along a continuum of increasing professional sophistication (Ross, Hauer & van Melle, 2018). Milestones are a tool to reflect the fact that competence progresses over time as learners advance on their way to the explicit outcome goal of the training (Frank et al., 2010). They can be defined as an "observable marker of an individual's ability along a developmental continuum" (Englander et al., 2017). The developmental process is accompanied by reflection on experiences (Leach, 2002).

Many national bodies responsible for designing medical education have developed frameworks to describe the desired outcomes of medical education and define the competencies that graduates should possess to enter the profession (Hautz et al., 2016). These national outcome frameworks are very diverse in content and scope. Based on its publication "Tomorrow's Doctors" in 1993, the General Medical Council in the UK defines seven curricular outcome domains (good clinical care, maintaining good medical practice, relationships with patients, working with colleagues, teaching and training, probity, health) all medical graduates are required to achieve (Rubin & Franchi-Christopher, 2002). The Scottish Deans' Medical Curriculum Group agreed on common learning outcomes that are based on the three essential elements of the competent and reflective medical practitioner: (1) technical intelligence (what are doctors able to do?); (2) intellectual, emotional, analytical and creative intelligence (how does the doctor approach her/his practice?); and (3) personal intelligence (the doctor as a professional) (Simpson et al., 2002). In Germany the National Competence Based Catalogue of Learning Objectives for Undergraduate Medical Education

(NKLM) was released in April 2015 (Steffens et al., 2018). The catalogue defines a total of 234 competencies and 281 subcompetencies. Primarily, the NKLM serves as recommendation for the restructuring of medical curricula. Medical faculties are encouraged to compare their existing curricula with the catalogue and gather practical experience before it becomes mandatory for medical education in Germany.

Competency-based requirements for post-graduate medical training on the other hand are implemented only in a few European countries (Weggemans et al., 2017). In the UK specialty training programmes define standards of knowledge, skills and behaviours according to the General Medical Council's framework "Good Medical Practice" (General Medical Council, 2013). In the Netherlands assessment during postgraduate medical education is competence-based; competencies for specialty training are increasingly described at national level to ensure all specialists possess all necessary competencies. All starting residents work on a portfolio which documents the progression on pre-defined competency domains and builds the basis for progress evaluations. Postgraduate training in Germany is not yet competency-based but some initiatives are under way. For instance, the working group on post-graduate training at the German Society of Primary Care Paediatrics defined guidelines (PaedCompenda) for educators in paediatric medicine (Fehr et al., 2017). At the European level ECAMSQ®, established by the UEMS (*see* Box 5.1), is developing a common framework for the assessment and certification of medical specialists' competence based on the core curricula developed by the specialist sections of the UEMS.

Outside Europe, in 1998 the Accreditation Council on Graduate Medical Education (ACGME) in the United States defined six domains of clinical competence for graduate medical education programmes that reliably depict residents' ability to care for patients and to work effectively in healthcare delivery systems (Swing, 2007). The competencies were refined in 2013 alongside the definition of milestones towards achieving them. Similarly, the Royal College of Physicians and Surgeons in Canada introduced the Canadian Medical Educational Directives for Specialists (CanMEDS) framework,[2] which groups the abilities that physicians require to effectively meet healthcare needs under seven roles (professional, communicator, collaborator, leader, health advocate, scholar and the integrating role of medical expert). The CanMEDS framework was subsequently also adopted in the Netherlands as of 2005–2006. In Australia the Confederation of Postgraduate Medical Education Councils (CPMEC) launched the (outcome-based) Australian Curriculum Framework for Junior Doctors in October 2006 (Graham et al., 2007).

---

2   http://www.royalcollege.ca/rcsite/canmeds/canmeds-framework-e.

Despite having originated in the education and training of doctors, outcome-based approaches are also increasingly used in nursing education (Gravina, 2017; Pijl-Zieber et al., 2014; Tan et al., 2018). At European level the amendment of the EU Directive on mutual recognition of professional qualifications in 2013 (*see* Box 5.1) included a set of eight competencies as mandatory minimum educational requirements for general practice nurses (Article 31). Based on this set of competencies, the European Federation of Nurses (EFN) developed the EFN Competency Framework which aims to help National Nurses Associations to engage and guide nursing schools in the implementation process of Article 31 (EFN, 2012).

Centrally developed outcome frameworks like the ones described above usually serve as guidance for medical and nursing schools to establish objectives for their own programmes (Swing, 2007). Schools are still free to decide what degree of emphasis and level of detail to place on each outcome, and which learning and teaching methods to use. Therefore education institutions still play a major role in the acquisition of competence for health professionals. They are responsible for providing the foundations for developing knowledge and skills that are necessary for safe and effective practice. In some countries the accreditation of health education facilities has been established as a formal process to assess and recognize whether educational programmes are designed to produce competent graduates (Greiner & Knebel, 2003). The process is carried out periodically either by the government or by a recognized non-governmental institution (Woodward, 2000). It may be voluntary or compulsory and financial incentives may be in place to promote voluntary accreditation. In the European Community national authorities are responsible for the recognition of health education institutions and teachers in their jurisdiction. However, UEMS (*see* Box 5.1) has established the Network of Accredited Clinical Skills Centres in Europe (NASCE) which aims to evaluate and accredit institutions of medical education within Europe to ensure high standards of medical education and promote patient safety.

5.2.2.1 Regulating entry to practise

Despite the move towards more outcome-based curricula, formal training alone is not sufficient in itself to ensure good performance of health professionals in practice. At the same time the general public does not have sufficient information to judge a health professional's qualifications or competence (Greiner & Knebel, 2003). To protect patients from the potential consequences of this information asymmetry, formal processes have been developed to recognize an individual as being qualified to belong to a particular health profession, using criteria based on education and experience (Woodward, 2000). Procedures to acknowledge a health professional's right to practise are discussed under various terms such as credentialling, licensing, registration or certification (WHO, 2006). Definitions of the concepts partly overlap and terms are used interchangeably in different national contexts. But all of them have in common that they build the link between the more academic component of education and good performance in practice. These processes may bestow a lifelong or time-limited right to enter the profession, depending on the underlying principle for maintaining competence (*see* next section).

WHO defines licensing as "a process by which a statutory authority grants permission to an individual practitioner or health care organization to operate or to engage in an occupation or profession" (WHO, 2006). Licensing is based on a set of minimum standards of competence for holding a professional title accompanied by regulations to govern the behaviour of such professionals (Woodward, 2000). It may not only protect the use of the professional title but also define the scope of practice the professional is entitled to when holding the licence, in what settings the licensee can practise, and what oversight is required (Greiner & Knebel, 2003).

Countries differ in their requirements of what is necessary to be granted the right to practise. At a minimum, professionals have to successfully finish basic professional education. For example, in Estonia doctors are authorized to practise medicine after the successful completion of six years undergraduate medical education. In the Netherlands licensure is granted upon graduation from medical school. In Australia and the UK medical school graduates first need to complete one or two years of clinical work before they are fully licensed (Weggemans et al., 2017).

Licensing usually requires the successful completion of an examination. In some countries this is integrated in the examinations required to obtain the academic degree. So-called national licensing examinations are large-scale examinations usually taken by medical doctors close to the point of graduation from medical school (Price et al., 2018; Weggemans et al., 2017). In general, graduating medical students wishing to practise in their national jurisdiction must pass a national licensing exam before they are granted a licence to practise. Requirements for graduates wishing to practise in a different country than the one in which they obtained their degrees (international graduates) may vary. Table 5.3 provides an overview of current national licensing exam practices in selected European countries. Computerized or written multiple-choice examinations have traditionally been the main method by which professionals are initially licensed or certified. However, these tools are not sufficient to reflect the range of complexity and degree of uncertainty encountered in practice. Thus, a variety of other mechanisms, such as peer review, professional portfolio, clinical examination,

Table 5.3 *Overview of national licensing exams for medical graduates in selected European countries*

Country	Title	Components	Examinees
Finland	Professional Competence Examination	Written exam in: (1) medicine (2) healthcare management (3) oral examination in clinical setting (with patient)	International medical graduates (if qualifications both acknowledged to be comparable)
France	Epreuves Classantes Nationales (NCE)	Written test for national ranking	National medical graduates, international medical graduates can apply (only EU/EEA, separate test for non-EU/EEA with limited space)
Germany	Staatsexamen	(1) Physikum (preclinical medicine) after two years (2) Written MCQs and oral practical (clinical phase)	National medical graduates Non-EU/EEA may take knowledge test to prove equivalence to German standards
Ireland	Pre-Registration Examination system (PRES)	(1) Applicants are assessed and documents verified (2) Computer-based examination (MCQs) (3) Clinical skill assessment via Objective Structural Clinical Examination and paper-based interpretation skill test	International medical graduates Medical council examination for non-EU/EEA graduates may be required (unless exempted)
Poland	State Physician and Dental Final Exam (SP/DE)	Written test about medical knowledge, specific medical processes, analysis of medical records and establishing medical diagnoses (MCQs)	National medical graduates and non-EEA candidates
Portugal	Exame Nacional de Seriacao	Written test about internal medicine (MCQs)	National medical graduates Communication skill test for international medical graduates
Spain	Médicos Internos Residentes (MIR)	Written test (MCQs)	National medical graduates
United Kingdom	Professional and Linguistic Assessments Board (PLAB) test	(1) 200 single answer questions (2) 18 Objective Structural Clinical Examination scenarios	Non-UK, EEA or Switzerland (no EC rights, approved sponsor, approved postgraduate qualification)
Switzerland	Federal Licensing Examination	(1) Written exam (MCQs) (2) Objective Structured Clinical Examination of clinical skill	National medical graduates (and international medical graduates if they wish to practise independently) For non-EU/EEA qualification is assessed at Kanton (state) level

Source: based on Price et al., 2018. Note: MCQs = multiple choice questions

patient survey, record review and patient simulation, can be used to measure professional performance.

Licensing is often combined with mandatory registration in a health professional register. Registers serve as a tool to inform the public as well as potential employers about the accredited qualifications and scope of practice of a certain health professional. Registers can also be used to monitor staff numbers and to estimate the future demand of the various professions, as well as corresponding training capacities. Most European countries operate a register for doctors, dentists and nurses, and increasingly also for other health professionals. In Estonia all doctors, nurses, midwives and dentists have to be registered with the Health Board which issues registration certificates after verifying their training and qualifications (Habicht et al., 2018). In France registration in the national information system on health professionals (ADELI) is mandatory for almost all health professionals (Chevreul et al., 2015). Often, registration is a prerequisite for providing healthcare under the Social Health Insurance System (for example, Germany) or to be employed within the National Health Service (for example, UK). Whereas in Slovenia, Hungary and the UK registration and licensing must be actively completed to practise independently, Belgium assigns a licence ("visa") automatically after graduation. However, doctors still need to register on the "cadastre" of the healthcare professions to obtain the right to practise. Registration into the Health Care Professional Register in Austria became compulsory for previously exempted healthcare professional groups, such as nurses, physiotherapists and speech therapists, in 2018.

Licensing and registration for doctors are mostly regulated at national level (Kovacs et al., 2014). Countries with federal structures may still partly delegate processes to bodies at the federal level (for example, Germany). National bodies vary from governmental ministries to self-regulating professional bodies, with varying degrees of statutory control. Medical chambers represent key stakeholders in this process in most countries. In Romania and Malta licensing and registration are undertaken by the national medical associations. In Denmark, Estonia, Finland and Hungary both are governed by public institutions. In the UK the General Medical Council issues licences and is responsible for maintaining a doctor's registration.

In the majority of countries in Europe licensing and registration are also required in order to practise as a nurse (*see* Table 5.4). One of the few exceptions is Germany, where there is no national system of registration. However, recently there have been developments to establish registries in selected federal states (*Länder*), situated in newly set-up Nursing Chambers. To date, 3 of the 16 Länder have a Nursing Chamber and registry in place. The licensing and registration of nurses are usually handled by different responsible bodies and regulated by different actors than doctors (*see* Table 5.10 at the end of the chapter). Most countries have either established a regulatory body for nursing and/or nursing representation at governmental level.

Table 5.4 *Overview of licensing and registration procedures for nurses in selected European countries*

Country	Mandatory Licensing	National Register	Nursing order or regulatory body	Nursing representation at governmental level
Austria	-	no	no	yes
Belgium	yes	yes	yes	yes
Bulgaria	no	yes	yes	no
Cyprus	yes	yes	yes	yes
Denmark	yes	yes	yes	yes
Finland	yes	yes	no	yes
France	yes	yes	yes	no
Germany	yes	no	yes	yes
Ireland	yes	no	yes	no
Italy	yes	yes	yes	no
Lithuania	yes	yes	yes	yes
Malta	yes	yes	yes	no
Norway	yes	yes	no	no
Poland	yes	yes	yes	yes
Romania	yes	yes	yes	yes
Slovenia	yes	yes	yes	yes
Spain	no	no	yes	yes
Sweden	yes	yes	yes	yes
Switzerland	-	no	no	no

Source: based on Humar & Sansoni, 2017

An additional tool to recognize a health professional's knowledge in a particular profession is certification. Certification is defined as "a process by which an authorized (governmental or non-governmental) body evaluates and recognizes either an individual or an organization as meeting predetermined requirements or criteria" (WHO, 2006). Certification can add to the process of licensing, if licensing is understood as the assurance of a minimal set of competencies (Greiner & Knebel, 2003). Professionals can be certified for clinical excellence if they voluntarily meet additional requirements, such as completing advanced education and training or passing a certifying examination beyond the minimum competencies required for licensure, thus ensuring that they meet the highest standards in an area of specialization.

5.2.2.2 Mechanisms to maintain professional competence

Closely linked to the process of licensing and registration are schemes for actively maintaining professional competence (*see also* Fig. 5.2). Whereas licensing and registration ensure that health professionals fulfill the requirements to independently practise their profession, it is not guaranteed that their competence and practice performance resulting from education and training remain up to the expected standards throughout their careers. Not least due to the rapid expansion in health-related knowledge, accompanied by the continuing development of new technologies and ongoing changes in the healthcare environment, health professionals are required to not only maintain but also update their skills and knowledge constantly (Greiner & Knebel, 2003).

On the one hand, one could rely on the expectation that health professionals will maintain their competence without the need to comply with externally enforced explicit standards or obligations. In countries such as Austria, Finland, Estonia and Spain it has traditionally been the responsibility of the individual health professional to ensure that they are fit to practise (Solé et al., 2014). Other countries have introduced more formalized requirements to demonstrate continued competence. Formal mechanisms to demonstrate sustained professional competence can encompass elements such as mandatory continuing education, mandatory relicensing, peer review and external inspection (Solé et al., 2014). Particularly in systems where licensing or registration are time-limited, the idea of continuous demonstration of competence is already implemented through procedures of periodic relicensing or re-registration. The renewal of a licence usually requires the demonstration of continuing education or lifelong learning activities (*see* Table 5.5).

Continuing education encompasses all training activities that enable health professionals to keep their level of knowledge and skills up-to-date from the time of licensure to the end of their career (IOM, 2010). The aim is to ensure that health professionals continue to provide the best possible care, improving patient outcomes and protecting patient safety throughout their career. Well-known concepts of continuing education in the field of medicine are Continuing Medical Education (CME) and Continuing Professional Development (CPD). Whereas CME refers to medical education and training with the purpose of keeping up-to-date with medical knowledge and clinical developments, CPD also includes the development of personal, social and managerial skills (Solé et al., 2014). Although the idea of continuing education appears intuitively sound, the challenge lies in defining formal standards that ensure that training activities are effective in maintaining competence to practise and are not just a bureaucratic requirement that does not influence "business as usual". CME/CPD has often been criticized regarding the duration and content of courses, as well as

Table 5.5   *Key considerations and components of relicensing strategies*

Key considerations of relicensing	Components
Assessment extent	• Competency domain(s), professional practice domain(s)
	• Use of meta-level framework
	• Individual needs
	• Focus: process of care
	• Focus: patient outcome (including patient satisfaction)
Frequency of assessment	• Yearly
	• Every 2–3 years
	• Every 4–5 years
	• Every >5 years
	• No time frame
Assessment methods	• Miler's assessment pyramid (cognition versus performance)
	• Self-assessment
	• Portfolios
	• Credit collection through course participation
	• (Standardized) examinations
	• Simulations
	• Clinical audits
	• Multisource feedback
Assessment mode	• Voluntary or mandatory
	• Legal or professional obligation
Assessment goal	• Voluntary or mandatory
	• Legal or professional obligation
Consequences of non-compliance	• Licence loss
	• Financial sanctions
	• Follow-up
	• Work under supervision
	• Feedback

Source: based on Sehlbach et al., 2018

the factors motivating clinicians in choosing them (for example, attractiveness of the location of offered courses, see Woodward, 2000). This leads to the essential question of which activities get approved for credit.

The growing influence of outcome-based education approaches described previously in this chapter has also affected developments in continuing education. There has been a shift from simply improving knowledge to improving skills, performance and patient outcomes through modifying clinician practice behaviours (Ahmed et al., 2013). New educational methods such as multimedia, multitechnique and multiple exposure approaches have emerged to increasingly engage clinicians in learning activities beyond didactic lectures (*see* Table 5.6).

Table 5.6   *Overview of methods for Continuing Medical Education*

Educational methods	Definition
Academic detailing	Service-oriented outreach education provided by an institution (medical governing bodies or industry) or hospital.
Audience response systems	Type of interaction associated with the use of audience response systems. It addresses knowledge objectives (used in combination with live lectures or discussion groups).
Case-based learning	An instructional design model which addresses high order knowledge and skill objectives (actual or authored clinical cases are created to highlight learning objectives).
Clinical experiences	Clinical experiences address skill, knowledge, decision-making and attitudinal objectives (preceptorship or observership with an expert to gain experience).
Demonstration	Involves teaching or explaining by showing how to do or use something. It addresses skill or knowledge objectives (live video or audio media).
Discussion group	Addresses knowledge, especially application or higher order knowledge (readings, or another experience).
Feedback	Addresses knowledge and decision-making (the provision of information about an individual's performance to learners).
Lecture	Lecture addresses knowledge content (live, video, audio).
Mentor or preceptor	Personal skill developmental relationship in which an experienced clinician helps a less experienced clinician. It addresses higher order cognitive and technical skills. Also used to teach new sets of technical skills.
Point of care	Addresses knowledge and higher order cognitive objectives (decision-making). Information that is provided at the time of clinical need, integrated into chart or electronic medical record.
Problem-based learning or team-based learning	PBL is a clinician-centred instructional strategy in which clinicians collaboratively solve problems and reflect on their experiences. It addresses higher order knowledge objectives, meta-cognition, and some skill (group work) objectives (clinical scenario/ discussion).
Programmed learning	Aims to manage clinician learning under controlled conditions. Addresses knowledge objectives (delivery of contents in sequential steps).
Readings	Reading addresses knowledge content or background for attitudinal objectives (journals, newsletters, searching online).
Role play	Addresses skill, knowledge and affective objectives.
Simulation	Addresses knowledge, team working, decision-making and technical skill objectives (full simulation; partial task simulation; computer simulation; virtual reality; standardized patient; role play).
Standardized patient	Addresses skill and some knowledge and affective objectives. Usually used for communication and physical examination skills training and assessment.
Writing and authoring	Addresses knowledge and affective objectives. Usually used for assessment purposes.

Source: based on Ahmed et al., 2013

For example, problem-based learning exposes participants to contextualized, real world but paper-based situations that they are expected to solve in small groups. Learners are made aware of their gaps in knowledge and skills and develop strategies of independent self-directed learning. Simulation-based learning is also a small group learning activity in which a simulated problem is presented to participants who actively participate in resolving it. Learners experience immediate clinical responses and results as consequences of their actions or inactions (Koh & Dubrowski, 2016).

Table 5.7 shows the configuration of processes to demonstrate continued competence in selected European countries. The frequency of relicensing varies between one and five years. While in some countries (for example, Germany) evidence of undertaking continuing education is sufficient to maintain a licence to practise, in others renewal requires a combination of mandatory continuing education with other measures, such as peer review in the form of audit and feedback, to encourage health professionals to follow standards of care (*see* Ivers et al., 2012; and Chapter 10 of this volume). For example, in the UK all physicians not only have to demonstrate participation in approved continuing education activities but also must undergo detailed annual appraisals including surveys of colleagues and patients, and a review of compliments and complaints ("revalidation"; *see* Solé et al., 2014).

Overall, continuing education for specialist doctors has become increasingly mandatory within the European Union, with 21 countries operating obligatory systems. In countries with voluntary structures, continuing education is at least actively supported (Simper, 2014). Most frequently, the professional associations decide about which continuing education activities get accredited and monitor the participation of their members. In several countries validated events are allocated a certain number of points and physicians must collect a specified total number within a given timeframe, regardless of which events they choose to participate in (*see also* Table 5.7). There is an increasing variety of approved activities. Consequences for non-compliance involve removal of the licence to practise or to contract with social insurance funds (Germany). Belgium is one of a few countries which positively incentivize physicians to participate in continuing education activities. Doctors who participate voluntarily in continuing education can earn up to €15 000 through increased fees and one-off payments (Solé et al., 2014).

Continuing education is usually provided by a number of different organizations such as scientific societies, medical institutions, professional bodies, academic centres or private companies. The pharmaceutical industry is the largest sponsor of continuing medical education worldwide, financing 75% of all activities in certain European countries (Ahmed et al., 2013). Due to the criticism arising from this commercial influence on medical practice, many countries are in the process of reforming their continuing education systems. The previously mentioned activities of the EACCME® (*see* Box 5.1) aim to support these reformation processes by providing quality requirements and accreditation for Continuing

Table 5.7   *Relicensing strategies of physicians in selected European countries*

Country	Relicensing purpose	Relicensing focus	Mandatory	Required credits / Period of time	Assessment methods
Denmark	Quality of care Patient safety	Practice performance	No	NA 1 year	CPD courses; clinical audit
Germany	Quality of care; maintenance of doctors' knowledge and skills	Lifelong learning	Yes	250 credits 5 years	General and specialty-specific CPD courses; individual learning; conference attendance; research and scientific publications; E-learning; time as visiting professional
Hungary	Patient safety	Lifelong learning	Yes	250 credits 5 years	General and specialty-specific CPD courses; research and scientific publications; E-learning; time as visiting professional; portfolio; minimum hours of patient contact; mandatory intensive course
Ireland	Maintenance of doctors' knowledge and skills	Lifelong learning; practice performance	Yes	50 credits 1 year	General CPD course; individual learning; conference attendance; research and scientific publications; clinical audit
Poland	Maintenance of doctors' knowledge and skill	Lifelong learning	Yes	200 credits 4 years	General and specialty-specific CPD courses; conference attendance; teaching; research and scientific publications; E-learning
Portugal	Career	Lifelong learning; practice performance	No	NA 5 years	Portfolio
Spain	Career	Lifelong learning; practice performance	No	NA 3 years	General CPD course; portfolio

Source: based on Sehlbach et al., 2018

Medical Education activities at the European level to ensure that they are free from commercial bias and follow an appropriate educational approach.

Continuing education and licence renewal are less regulated for the nursing profession (IOM, 2010). Belgium and the UK are among the few countries where nurses are required to demonstrate continuing education to re-register. In Belgium general nurses have to renew registration every three years, nurse specialists every six years (Robinson & Griffiths, 2007). In the UK nurses have to re-register annually and since 2016 they also have to revalidate their license. The Nursing and Midwifery Council requires revalidation every three years based on proof of participation in continuing education activities and reflection of their experiences among peers (Cylus et al., 2015). In other countries, such as the Netherlands, the responsibility of continuing education for nurses resides with the healthcare provider where the nurse is employed. However, nursing staff can voluntarily record their training and professional development activities online in the "Quality Register for Nurses" (Kwaliteitsregister). This offers individuals the chance to compare their skills with professionally agreed standards of competence (Kroneman et al., 2016).

5.2.2.3 Sanctions and withdrawal of the right to practise

The explicit demonstration of continued competence in a defined period of time can only be effective if failure to fulfil requirements has consequences for the right to practise. A relevant question when choosing the formal mechanisms to assess professional competence is what consequences result from non-compliance with minimum standards. Actions usually range from reprimands and financial penalties, to shortening of the registration period, to the temporary or permanent withdrawal of the right to practise. In serious cases, consequences beyond those pertaining to professional codes of conduct may also be in order and are governed by the corresponding legal entities. Traditionally, malpractice has been related to criminal convictions, problems with performance, substance abuse or unethical behaviour of health professionals.

Across Europe there is little consistency in how events questioning competency and qualities of medical professionals are handled. Considerable diversity exists in the range of topics addressed by regulatory bodies, with almost all covering healthcare quality and safety, and some also exploring themes around reputation and maintaining the public's trust in the profession (Risso-Gill et al., 2014). In most cases, patients or their relatives initiate complaints about the practice of a health professional (Struckmann et al., 2015), but cases can also be brought to the attention of regulatory bodies by specific organizations with an inspectorate role in the oversight of health professionals or by employers with monitoring tasks. Complaints may lead to disciplinary action in which it is investigated whether the professional's competence to practise is impaired. Table 5.8 summarizes the responsible bodies for sanctioning in cases of impaired fitness to practise for selected European countries. In the UK the Medical Act mandates the General Medical Council to investigate when serious concerns arise about a physician's fitness to practise. In the Netherlands the Dutch Health Care Inspectorate executes an inspector role in the oversight of physician's practices. The Austrian

Table 5.8 *Responsible institutions for the sanctioning of medical professionals in selected European countries*

Member State	Institution with main responsibility	Institution with responsibility for less severe sanctions	Institution with responsibility for severe sanctions
Austria	Federal Ministry of Health	Austrian Medical Chamber and the employer	Austrian Medical Chamber and the administrative court
Estonia	Ministry of Social Affairs (Estonian Health Board)	The employer	The court
Finland	Valvira (National Supervisory Authority for Welfare and Health)	Valvira and Regional State Administrative Agencies	Valvira and the court
Germany	LÄK (State Medical Chamber) and office for approbation	The professional court and medical chambers	Office for approbation and the administrative court
Hungary	Ministry of Health (Office of Health Authorization and Administrative Procedures) and National Institute for Quality and Organizational Development in Healthcare and Medicines	The court	The court
Malta	Medical Council of Malta	The employer	Court of Justice and Medical Council
The Netherlands	KNMG (The Royal Dutch Medical Association) and disciplinary boards	Inspectorate and the board of directors of a hospital	Disciplinary boards
Romania	CMR (Romanian College of Physicians)	Discipline Commission of the Romanian College of Physicians	Discipline Commission of the Romanian College of Physicians
Slovenia	Medical Chamber	Medical Chamber	The court of the Medical Chamber
Spain	Ministry of Health	The employer	The employer or the court
UK	GMC	The GMC case examiners	MPTS, IOP and MPTS FTP panel

CMR = Colegiul Medicilor din România; FTP = fitness to practise; GMC = General Medical Council; IOP = Interim Orders Panel; KNMG = Koninklijke Nederlandsche Maatschappij tot bevordering der Geneeskunst; LÄK = Landesärztekammer; MPTS = Medical Practitioners Tribunal Service

Source: based on Struckmann et al., 2015

Medical Chamber has established an Association for Quality Assurance and Quality Management in Medicine (ÖQMed) to oversee physicians practising in ambulatory care.

A physician's employer may also investigate complaints internally and take action at that level, which may lead to civil litigation proceedings. For example, in Hungary it is the employer (for example, the hospital) that first investigates complaints and moves the case to court only if the matter cannot be resolved within the hospital. In most countries disciplinary panels are mainly composed of legal experts and health professionals in related specialties. Some countries like Malta and the UK include lay people, while others such as Estonia, Finland, Hungary, Slovenia and Spain use external experts (Struckmann et al., 2015).

The diverse sanctioning procedures at national level are also challenged by the increasing mobility of health professionals. Health professionals banned from practice may move to another country and continue practising if no adequate cross-border control mechanisms are in place. Under the revised EU Directive on the mutual recognition of professional qualifications (*see* Box 5.1), an alert mechanism was established to enable warnings across Member States when a health professional is banned or restricted from practice, even temporarily. This idea came out of an earlier collaboration between competent authorities under the "Health Professionals Crossing Borders" initiative led by the UK's GMC. Since the introduction of the mechanism in January 2016, and until November 2017, more than 20 000 alerts were sent by competent Member State authorities, mostly pertaining to cases of professionals who were restricted or prohibited from practice (very few alerts were related to the falsification of qualifications). Surveyed stakeholders found the alert system appropriate for its purpose and the Commission recognized the importance of continuous monitoring and adaptation of its use and functionalities (European Commission, 2018a, 2018b).

5.3 The effectiveness and cost-effectiveness of strategic approaches to regulation of professionals

This section summarizes available evidence on the effectiveness and cost-effectiveness of the main strategies aiming to ensure that health professionals attain and maintain the necessary competence to provide safe, effective, patient-centred care, as described above. It largely follows the sequence of presentation set out in the previous section.

5.3.1 Effectiveness of education approaches on professional performance

Overall, research on the impact of curricular design in undergraduate medical education on outcomes, be it at patient level or in regard to broader organizational effects, is of limited scope and quality. An umbrella review on the effectiveness of different curricular and instructional design methods (including early clinical and community experience, inter-professional education, problem-based learning, etc.) found that most studies reported on learning outcomes such as knowledge and skill acquisition, while fewer than half reported on patient or organizational outcomes (Onyura et al., 2016). Evidence seemed to be inconclusive overall and showing mixed effects, not least due to a lack of rigorous qualitative and quantitative research.

One concept used to describe the "effectiveness" of medical education is preparedness to practise. Effective education has to ensure that graduates are prepared for the complexity and pressures of today's practice (Monrouxe et al., 2018). Despite constant developments in medical education, the self-perceived preparedness of doctors at various stages of their career is still lagging behind. Graduates feel particularly unprepared for specific tasks including prescribing, clinical reasoning and diagnosing, emergency management or multidisciplinary team working (Monrouxe et al., 2017; Geoghegan et al., 2017; General Medical Council, 2014). Also, senior doctors and clinical supervisors are concerned that patient care and safety may be negatively affected as graduate doctors are not well enough prepared for clinical practice (Smith, Goldacre & Lambert, 2017; Vaughan, McAlister & Bell, 2011).

The concept of preparedness can be used to measure the effect of new training approaches, such as interactive training in small groups (for example, problem-based or simulation-based training), compared to traditional training techniques based on lectures and seminars. Empirical evidence on the effectiveness of problem-based training approaches in undergraduate medical education is mixed. On the one hand, some UK-based studies have shown a beneficial effect of problem-based curricula on medical graduates' preparedness (O'Neill et al., 2003; Cave et al., 2009), reflected in better skills related to recognizing limitations, asking for help and teamwork (Watmough, Garden & Taylor, 2006; Watmough, Taylor & Garden, 2006). On the other hand, some more recent studies observed no relation between the perceived, self-reported preparedness of medical graduates and the type of training they received. For example, Illing et al. (2013) found that junior doctors from all training types in the UK felt prepared in terms of communication skills, clinical and practical skills, and teamwork. They felt less prepared for areas of practice based on experiential learning such as ward work, being on call, management of acute clinical situations, prescribing, clinical prioritization and time management, and dealing with paperwork. Also, Miles, Kellett & Leinster (2017) found no difference in the overall perceived preparedness for clinical practice and the confidence in skills when comparing problem-based training with traditional discipline-based and lecture-focused curricula. However, graduates having undergone problem-based training felt better prepared for tasks associated with communication, teamwork and paperwork than graduates from traditional training. Overall, more than half of all graduates felt insufficiently prepared to deal with neurologically or visually impaired patients, write referral letters, understand drug interactions, manage pain and cope with uncertainty, regardless of curriculum type. Further evidence has shown that a shift from multiple-choice-based assessment methods towards open-ended question examinations results in better student performance. Students attributed the improved performance in learning towards the conceptual understanding of learning material in contrast to the simple memorization of facts (Melovitz Vasan et al., 2018).

A remaining question in this context is whether observed differences in outcomes between training types are indeed caused by the medical training mode or rather by the personal characteristics and preferences of students. For instance, certain students may respond better to problem-based training approaches than others. Holen et al. (2015) found that students' personality traits and sociocultural background significantly determined preferences related to learning methods. Outgoing, curious, sociable and conscientious students, women and students who lived with other fellow students or with their partners or spouses were more positive towards problem-based learning methods. As effective problem-based learning requires small groups to function effectively – which in turn poses the challenge of understanding group dynamics – these results are perhaps not surprising. More insights into the nature of students' preferences may guide aspects of curriculum modifications and the daily facilitation of groups.

The accreditation of medical education institutions has been found to be associated with better performance of students in medical examinations. For example, the United States Medical Licensing Examination performance of graduates of international medical schools was better if graduates came from a country with an existing accreditation system. The strongest association was observed with performance in the basic science module of the exam; this is unsurprising, as this module's content corresponds to the focus of many accreditation criteria. However, performance in the clinical skills module was also better for graduates from accredited institutions. Next to the existence of an accreditation system, its quality (determined by the number of essential elements included) and, by proxy, the rigour of the accrediting institution, was positively associated with performance in both basic science and clinical skills (van Zanten, 2015).

To foster patient-centredness, a number of approaches have been discussed to tailor medical education already in the undergraduate phase. For instance, the concept of "patient educators", who interact with trainees from an early stage in their studies, has been successful in changing learner perspectives and achieving a new understanding of their role, beyond that of a medical expert (Fong et al., 2019).

In nursing, research has shown that the shift towards higher education described earlier in the chapter can be beneficial for patient outcomes. Every 10% increase in nurses with Bachelor degrees was associated with a reduced likelihood of mortality by 7% (Aiken et al., 2014). The nature of academic training has also been examined in conjunction with nurse staffing levels; it was estimated that mortality would be almost 30% lower in hospitals in which 60% of nurses had Bachelor's degrees and would care for an average of six patients compared to hospitals in which only 30% of nurses had Bachelor's degrees and cared for an average of eight patients (Zander et al., 2016). Advanced knowledge and skill acquirement during undergraduate nursing training was shown to be effective in improving perceptions of competence and confidence (Zieber & Sedgewick, 2018). In this context, the right balance between teaching hours and time for clinical practice in nursing education is critical. For example, a condensation of the weekly timetable for Bachelor students in nursing in order to extend time in clinical placements was found to be related to lower academic achievement and poorer quality in learning experience (Reinke, 2018).

Also, postgraduate-level nursing education can contribute to increased self-perceived competence and confidence among nurses (Baxter & Edvardsson, 2018). Nurses in Master programmes rate their competence higher than nurses in specialist programmes (Wangensteen et al., 2018). Furthermore, academic literacy is strongly related to the development of critical thinking skills which in turn are of relevance for professional practice (Jefferies et al., 2018). A study on nurse competencies in relation to evidence-based practice (which includes components such as questioning established practices towards improving quality of care, identifying, evaluating and implementing best available evidence, etc.) showed that the higher the level of education, the higher the perceived competence in such approaches (Melnyk et al., 2018). Benefits of Master-level education such as increased confidence and self-esteem, enhanced communication, personal and professional growth, knowledge and application of theory to practice, as well as analytical thinking and decision-making may positively affect patient care (Cotterill-Walker, 2012). However, quantitative evidence on whether Master-level nursing education makes a difference to patient outcomes is rare and lacks the development of measurable and observable evaluation.

Tan et al. (2018) recently reviewed the evidence on the effectiveness of outcome-based education on the acquisition of competencies by nursing students. The methodological quality of the few identified studies was moderate. Overall, outcome-based education seemed to predicate improvements in acquired nursing competencies in terms of knowledge acquisition, skills performance, behaviour, learning satisfaction and achieving higher order thinking processes. One study reported contradictory, negative outcomes. The authors conclude that the current evidence base is limited and inconclusive and more robust experimental study designs with larger sample sizes and validated endpoints (including patient outcomes) are needed, mirroring the findings by Onyura et al. (2016) on medical education. In the same direction, Calvert & Freemantle (2009) pointed out that "assessing the impact of a change in the undergraduate curriculum on patient care may prove difficult, but not impossible". They propose that competency-based outcomes be assessed using simulated or real patients, particularly for students nearing graduation, and that randomized designs should be used to produce robust evidence on cost-effectiveness that can guide practice (Calvert & Freemantle, 2009).

5.3.2 Effectiveness of licensing and registration

There is only little research regarding the effects of licensing on the quality of care. Norcini, Lipner & Kimball (2014) found that each additional performance point achieved in the national licensing examinations in the US was associated with a 0.2% decrease in mortality (Norcini, Lipner & Kimball, 2014). Work comparing the performance of US and international graduates by measuring differences in mortality rates found that, if anything, outcomes seemed to favour graduates with international education backgrounds and concluded that this was an indication of the proper functioning of selection standards for international medical graduates to practise in the US. However, they also point out that the general body of evidence on the issue, limited as it is, suggests that the quality of care provided by international graduates could depend on the specialty and/ or on the rigorousness of the licensure process in the issuing country (Tsugawa et al., 2017). Indeed, research in the performance of international graduates in different countries and settings has shown largely inconclusive results (Price et al., 2018).

In a seminal study, Sharp et al. (2002) reviewed the body of evidence on the impact of specialty board certification on clinical outcomes at the time. About half of identified studies demonstrated a significant positive association between certification status and positive clinical outcomes, while almost as many showed no association and few revealed worse outcomes for certified physicians. The methodology of included work was weak overall. Norcini, Lipner & Kimball (2002) found that successful certification in internal medicine or cardiology was associated with a 19% reduction in mortality among treated patients but was not associated with length of stay.

5.3.3 Effectiveness of continuing education

Continuing education aims to help professionals keep clinically, managerially and professionally up-to-date, thus ultimately improving patient care (*see* also Schostak et al., 2010). A review of reviews published in 2015 synthesized evidence on the effectiveness of continuing medical education on both physician performance and patient health outcomes (Cervero & Gaines, 2015). It found that continuing education is effective on all fronts: in the acquisition and retention of knowledge, attitudes, skills and behaviours as well as in the improvement of clinical outcomes, with the effects on physician performance being more consistent than those on patient outcomes across studies. The latter observation is intuitive: it is methodologically more challenging to determine the extent of the contribution of individual physicians' actions to observed outcomes, as these are also influenced by the healthcare system and the interdisciplinary team. Braido et al. (2012) found that a one-year continuing education course for general practitioners significantly improved knowledge. Training also resulted in pharmaceutical cost containment and greater attention to diagnosis and monitoring.

More research is needed on the mechanisms of action by which different types of continuing education affect physician performance and patient health. Although numerous studies exist, as reviewed by Cervero & Gaines (2015), the variable study objectives and designs hinder any generalizable conclusions. Bloom (2005) found that interactive methods such as audit and feedback, academic detailing, interactive education and reminders are most effective at improving performance and outcomes. More conventional methods such as didactic presentations and printed materials alone showed little or no beneficial effect. The superiority of interactive, multimedia or simulation-based methods over conventional approaches seems to be mirrored in other studies as well (Marinopoulos et al., 2007; Mazmanian, Davis & Galbraith, 2009). At the same time, there seems to be an overall agreement that a variety of strategies, or so called "multiple exposures", is necessary to achieve the desired effects of continuing education in an optimal manner.

5.3.4 Cost-effectiveness of strategies to regulate professionals

Studies on the cost-effectiveness of educational interventions in healthcare are rare. Cost savings may occur through various channels, such as the prevention of complications and improved patient outcomes, training doctors to use resources in professional practice most effectively, or achieving reduced costs of training for the same educational outcomes.

A number of studies investigating potential cost savings of outcome-based training methods for anaesthesia-related procedures through the effective reduction of complications and related costs estimated a return of investment from $63 000 over 18 months to $700 000 per year (Bisgaard et al., 2018). Other recent work investigated the link between medical training and future practice costs. The underlying idea is one of educational imprinting, i.e. that learners adapt behaviours and beliefs in practice that they witnessed during training, sometimes despite what they were taught, and hence practice costs mirror those of their teaching hospital regions. Phillips et al. (2017) showed that US physicians practising in low-cost hospital service areas were more likely to have trained in low-cost areas, and those practising in high-cost service areas were more likely to have trained in high-cost areas. Physicians trained in high-cost areas spent significantly more per patient than those trained in low-cost areas independent from the cost category, without a significance difference in quality outcomes. Tsugawa et al. (2018) found that US physicians who graduated from highly ranked medical schools had slightly lower costs of care than graduates of lower ranked schools. The authors comment that this is in line with previous findings showing that "practice patterns embedded in residency training are subsequently implemented into practice after physicians complete their residency", influencing costs of care. Finally, one feature of outcome-based education approaches are time-variable curricula. That is, students study as long as necessary to achieve the defined outcomes rather than being expected to complete a pre-defined duration of training. Van Rossum et al. (2018) investigated whether time-variable postgraduate medical education in gynaecology can lead to a better revenue-cost balance while maintaining educational quality. They found that while time-variable training structures can indeed help to shorten postgraduate training without sacrificing educational quality, this may lead to overall higher costs at the hospital level, as time can particularly be gained in activities where residents generate the highest revenues.

Overall, existing evidence on the cost-effectiveness of educational approaches is scarce and inconsistent in the approaches to costing, hindering the development of general conclusions. Most studies compare only one educational mode to a control group of standard care instead of measuring the relative cost-effectiveness between interventions to aid decisions about which intervention to favour.

On the cost-effectiveness of licensing, Price et al. (2018) point out that "the standard economic model for understanding the impact of occupational regulation rests on the notion that there is a trade-off between the cost of service provision and its quality, that is, licensing increases the costs but also the quality of service … although regulating professions does increase the overall costs of service provision, it decreases the marginal costs of providing a quality service as it encourages investment in human capital (i.e. better and more efficient training)". No empirical evidence of good quality was identified to test these hypotheses for physicians or nurses. Brown, Belfield & Field (2002) reviewed studies on the cost-effectiveness of continuing professional development activities. The calculated rates of return where the excess of benefit over costs is divided by the costs of the intervention ranged considerably from 39% to over 10 000%.

5.4 How can professional regulation strategies be implemented?

5.4.1 Health professional education

In most countries regulating training contents and curricula of health professionals aims to ensure uniformity across educational programmes in an ever-changing society and the evolving body of clinical knowledge. Highly developed countries have experienced a notable trend towards an increase in health professional regulation over the last twenty years, especially for physicians. At the same time, an overly excessive degree of standardizing medical education puts innovation and advancements in curricula at risk (Price et al., 2018). The key lies in finding the right degree of regulating educational standards that guarantees minimum levels of competency whilst at the same time allowing for flexibility and innovation.

Furthermore, there is a difference between preparing graduates for immediate practice and preparing them for careers in healthcare across a wide range of (sub)specialties in a highly dynamic healthcare environment. The complex and rapidly changing nature of clinical care stresses the importance of on-the-job training in addition to establishing safety precautions and preventive interventions, such as induction programmes and supervision (Monrouxe et al., 2018; Illing et al., 2013). Effective learning is not a matter of consuming information but of active processing of the information by the learner (van der Fleuten & Driessen, 2014). The shift towards outcome-based education models mirrors this fact. However, fundamental changes in how health professional education is to be approached are required. Competencies that are crucial for optimal patient care outcomes must be clearly defined and guide the design of all curricular elements. Outcome-based models can be implemented in several formats (Gravina, 2017). In the most radical approach, traditional time-based semester structures are removed completely and students only progress in the programme when learning is demonstrated without conventional grades or credit hours. However, elements of outcome-based education can also be implemented within traditional semester-based programmes where the completion of each semester is aligned with learning outcomes. Hybrid formats between the two extreme approaches can also be found in practice.

Outcome-based education further leads to a substantial redefinition of assessment practices as well as faculty and learner roles, responsibilities and relationships (Ross, Hauer & van Melle, 2018). The implications of these effects need to be weighed carefully when changes are considered. Although outcome-based education has been advocated and implemented in medical as well as nursing education, strong empirical evidence on the effectiveness of different competencies is still lacking. Existing evidence can be considered encouraging to continue developing and implementing outcome-based training concepts. But initiatives need to be accompanied with mechanisms for the critical appraisal of its benefits using sound research methods. The research focus should shift from comparing one curriculum to the other towards research that explains why things work in education under which conditions (van der Fleuten & Driessen, 2014). This involves the development of theories based on empirical evidence.

Learning in cooperation with others has been shown to be more effective than learning alone, which is why interactive training approaches are also increasingly applied in medical education (van der Vleuten & Driessen, 2014). Such approaches require students to take more responsibility for their learning and incorporate the dimension of personal traits and preferences into the design of training. Indeed, it has been argued that students' characteristics and preferences need to be acknowledged as important determinants in the effective design of curricula (Holen et al., 2015). This becomes even more relevant with the increasing international mobility of not only professionals but students who bring their diverse cultural background into their learning processes and group dynamics.

Finally, most barriers to lifelong learning (for example, lack of awareness of knowledge deficits, poor research skills, deficient communication and collaborative skills, unfamiliarity with availability of resources, inability to use existing resources efficiently, failure to self-reflect) were found to be skill-based barriers (Koh & Dubrowski, 2016). System level barriers, such as unavailability of resources and lack of opportunities for repeated practice, are mainly secondary. The health professional education system, particularly at undergraduate level, should ensure that students acquire a lifelong learning strategy. A combination of problem-based and simulation-based learning strategies integrated in undergraduate curricula could help physicians to overcome skill-based barriers to lifelong learning (Koh & Dubrowski, 2016), thus fostering success in other regulatory components, such as continuing professional development, by enabling, inter alia, adaptability to change and cooperation with professionals from other disciplines.

5.4.2 Entry to the profession and sustained competence to practise

National Licensing Exams are critical to ensure a minimum level of competency of graduates, but at the same time their design has been criticized as outdated and not in line with new modalities in learning and testing otherwise employed throughout medical schools and in practice (Price et al., 2018). Especially in light of increased professional mobility, staff shortages and political developments influencing the scope of application of the free movement of citizens within Europe, a first area of action would be to revisit how these requirements are set out and where the potential for improvement lies, facilitated by cross-country learning. Detailed work on the status quo would build the necessary foundation for such an initiative. This is probably best viewed in combination of the (desired) shift in curricular design described in the previous paragraphs.

There is no doubt that continuing education and lifelong learning are important components of the healthcare professions and keeping knowledge and skills up-to-date is crucial to quality healthcare. The challenge lies in the development of effective relicensing and continuing education strategies, which focus on elements relevant for current practice. The effectiveness of continuing education has been questioned mostly because of the way standards have been implemented in the past. Overall, the tendency has been to focus on meeting regulatory requirements rather than identifying individual knowledge gaps and choosing programmes to address them (IOM, 2010). However, effective continuing education involves learning (why?) and being fit to practice (how?) as well as putting both into action. This means moving away from "tick-box" approaches where time spent per se is accredited – professionals should rather determine their own learning needs through reflection and within the totality of their practice (Schostak et al., 2010). However, this comes with the risk that professionals stay within their comfort zone instead of using continuing education as a tool to uncover and address their knowledge gaps. Box 5.2 summarizes the main criticisms for the established continuing education paradigm as discussed by the Institute of Medicine (2010).

Additional barriers to continuing education reported by clinicians were the limited availability of opportunities to leave for study, costs, and difficulties to maintain work–life balance (Schostak, 2010; Ahmed et al., 2013). Indeed, funding remains an obstacle in implementing effective continuing education. In order to remain a reliable tool of independent lifelong learning, funding of continuing education must be independent from potential conflicts of interest. Safeguards

---

Box 5.2   *Challenges in the established continuing education paradigm*

1. Most responsible organizations enforce continuing education by setting minimal and narrowly defined criteria.
2. The didactic approach is most often limited to lectures and seminars in traditional classroom settings. More research is needed on which learning approaches are most effective.
3. Content is mainly teacher-driven with the danger that it lacks practical relevance.
4. Activities are mostly separated by profession and specialties and thus hinder the growing need for interdisciplinary knowledge and approaches.
5. Provision of and research on continuing education needs to be independent from the financing of pharmaceutical and medical device companies to prevent conflicts of interest.
6. Regulations vary considerably by specialty and by country.

Source: based on IOM, 2010

and guidelines to regulate the content of continuing education materials introduced by healthcare authorities can facilitate this process (Ahmed et al., 2013). Collaborative initiatives, such as the European Accreditation by the EACCME, should be strengthened and expanded. Effective continuing education standards should aim to develop approaches that enable professionals to critically appraise their knowledge gaps and own practices. Finally, the need for striking the balance between appropriate continuing education and/or relicensing requirements on the one hand, and not overburdening clinicians to the point where time and energy for actual clinical practice are compromised on the other, should inform any new policies on these instruments.

5.5 Conclusions for policy-makers

In Europe most countries have clear rules on work entry requirements and professional development for physicians and nurses. The necessary educational attainment for achieving professional qualification is influenced by the relevant European directives. However, evidence on the effectiveness and cost-effectiveness of different modalities at each level of health professional regulation is relatively sparse and mixed. The potential for knowledge exchange is vast and a common understanding of what constitutes competence to practise, its impairment and its potential impact on quality of care, is crucial, not least because other strategies discussed in this book encompass professional education as a vital tool for achieving their goals.

In 2006 WHO recognized a need to develop closer links between the education and training of health professionals and the needs of patients within the wider health system. At the same time, the evidence about how learning can be best supported in the context of health professional education and continuing education is still insufficient. The lack of definite conclusions about the effectiveness of specific methods of continuing education puts its overall value for health professionals in question. Systems to demonstrate the (continuing) competence of physicians and nurses in Europe are inconsistent in scope, coverage and content. In light of sizeable movement and workforce shortages as well as the fast-paced change in clinical practice developments, here as well the potential for knowledge exchange is substantial. However, standardization for standardization's sake has the inherent risk of stifling novelty in approaches and contributing to skill mismatch over time. National policy-makers should invest in critically appraising healthcare-related curricula and supporting research into optimal learning modalities in terms of both scope and didactic approach. Existing evidence may be encouraging to continue developing and implementing outcome-based training concepts, but initiatives need to be accompanied with mechanisms for the critical appraisal of its benefits using sound research methods. A combination of problem-based and simulation-based learning strategies integrated in undergraduate curricula could help professionals overcome skill-based barriers to lifelong learning, thus fostering success in other regulatory components, such as continuing professional development.

As Woodward (2000) points out, "many of the strategies [regulating health professionals] attempt to assure or control quality or facilitate a climate for quality improvement. They alone usually cannot directly change behavior – rather, they provide motivation for change". Indeed, there is an argument to be made that regulating health professionals should be viewed in a holistic manner, including an overview of all strategic components described in this chapter. It should also leverage the contributions of other strategies discussed in this book, such as clinical guidelines and audit and feedback. The aim should be to create learning systems of regulation that combine effective checks and balances with a flexible response to global needs for a competent, sufficient workforce.

With these considerations in mind and taking the described evidentiary limitations into account, a number of possible avenues can be considered, which should, however, be further evaluated in future research. These include:

- Creating competence through revisiting, evaluating and updating curricula, teaching methods and assessment procedures to ensure the attainment of knowledge and skills and attitudes necessary to practise;

- Regulating entry to the profession (for example, by licensure and/or registration) in a manner that is adaptable to the changing landscape of healthcare and fit-for-purpose;

- Mandating continuing professional development and other mechanisms to maintain professional competence during practice and providing guidance on content and modalities, as well as the balance between activities to maintain competence and clinical practice; and

- Establishing transparent systems of redress in cases of questionable fitness to practice.

Table 5.9 *Overview of national bodies that regulate physicians in selected European countries*

Country	National body	Responsibilities
Austria	Austrian Medical Chamber (Österreichische Ärztekammer)	• Grants permission to practise • Organizes continuing medical development • Releases medical code of ethics • Constitutes the Austrian medical academy (Akademie der Ärzte)
Belgium	Federal Public Service for Public Health, Food Chain, Safety and Environment (FPS) and Order of Physicians	• Licenses general practitioners • Grants permission to practise with registration at the Order of Physicians • Lists licensed doctors
Denmark	Danish Health and Medicines Authority (Sundhedsstyrelsen) Danish Patient Safety Authority	• Regulation of specialist training for medical doctors and dentists • Regulation of advanced education for nurses • Regulations of educational programmes for other healthcare professions • Registration of health professionals
Finland	National Supervisory Authority for Welfare and Health (Valvira)	• National Supervisory Authority for Welfare and Health (Valvira)
France	National Order of Doctors French National Authority for Health (Haute Autorité de santé)	• Coordination of CPD for all health professionals • Registration and accreditation of CPD providers • Regulation of the Medical Code of Ethics • Sanctioning for non-adherence
Germany	German Medical Association (Bundesärztekammer) and Federal State Chambers of Physicians (Landesärztekammern)	• Regulation of professional duties and principles for medical practice in all fields • Regulation of the professional code (Berufsordnung) and the specialty training regulations (Weiterbildungsordnung) • Promoting continuing medical education • Promoting quality assurance
Italy	Ministry of Health National Federation of Medico-Surgical and Dental Orders (Federazione Nazionale degli Ordini dei Medici-Chirurghi e degli Odontoiatri, FNOMCeo) and medical associations of the provinces	• License to practise the profession • Regulating continuing medical education • Registration of physicians • Responsible for establishing the code of conduct • Disciplinary authority over doctors registered with them
Netherlands	The Royal Dutch Medical Association (KNMG)	• Regulation of postgraduate training • Registration and recertification of specialists • Regulation of the recognition of training institutes and trainers for postgraduate education
Spain	General Council of Official Colleges of Physicians (CGCOM)	• Regulation of criteria for licensing • Regulation of registration • Promoting Continuing Medical Education • Regulation of the Medical Code of Ethics • Disciplinary authority

Table 5.9 *Overview of national bodies that regulate physicians in selected European countries [continued]*

Country	National body	Responsibilities
United Kingdom	General Medical Council (GMC)	• Recommendations about undergraduate medical education to the universities with medical schools • Monitoring of teaching and examination practices in medical schools • Operates the medical register, a list showing registration, training and other useful information

Source: authors' research

Table 5.10 *Overview of national bodies that regulate nurses and midwives in selected European countries*

Country	National body	Responsibilities
Belgium	Minister of Public Health (Ministere de la Sante Publique)	• Minister of Public Health (Ministere de la Sante Publique)
Denmark	Ministry of Education National Board for Health	• Regulation of standards for education • Registration and right to practise
Finland	Ministry of Education National Supervisory Authority for Welfare and Health (Valvira)	• Regulation of degree programmes • Registration and right to practise for both levels of nurses
France	Ministry of Health	• Approval of state certification
Germany	Ministry of Health Regional Health Authorities (Gesundheitsämter der Länder)	• Regulation of education • Regulation of right to practise (no national system of registration or regulatory nursing body)
Italy	Colleges of nursing in each province	• Registration and right to practise • No central control/validation of degree courses
Netherlands	Ministry of Education, Culture and Science Central Information Centre for Professional Practitioners in Health Care (CIBG)	• Regulation of standards for education • Registration of nurses
Spain	Ministry of Education General Council of Nursing	• Regulation of standards for education • Registration of nurses
United Kingdom	Health & Care Professions Council (HCPC) Nursing and Midwifery Council (NMC)	• Regulation of standards for education • Registration and right to practise • Monitoring fitness to practise Registration and revalidation

Source: based on Robinson & Griffiths, 2007; Riedel, Röhrling & Schönpflug, 2016

References

Ahmed K et al. (2013). The effectiveness of continuing medical education for specialist recertification. *Canadian Urological Association Journal*, 7(7–8):266–72.

Aiken LH et al. (2014). Nurse staffing and education and hospital mortality in nine European countries: a retrospective observational study. *Lancet*, 383(9931):1824–30.

Anand S, Bärnighausen T (2004). Human resources and health outcomes: cross-country econometric study. *Lancet*, 364(9445):1603–9.

Bachner F et al. (2018). Austria: Health system review. *Health Systems in Transition*, 20(3):1–256.

Baxter R, Edvardsson D (2018). Impact of a critical care postgraduate certificate course on nurses' self-reported competence and confidence: a quasi-experimental study. *Nurse Education Today*, 65:156–61.

Bisgaard CH et al. (2018). The effects of graduate competency-based education and mastery learning on patient care and return on investment: a narrative review of basic anesthetic procedures. *BMC Medical Education*, 18(1):154.

Bloom BS (2005). Effects of continuing medical education on improving physician clinical care and patient health: a review of systematic reviews. *International Journal of Technology Assessment in Health Care*, 21(3):380–5.

Braido F et al. (2012). Knowledge and health care resource allocation: CME/CPD course guidelines-based efficacy. *European Annals of Allergy and Clinical Immunology*, 44(5):193–9.

Brown CA, Belfield CR, Field, SJ (2002). Cost effectiveness of continuing professional development in health care: a critical review of the evidence. *BMJ*, 324:652–5.

Busse R, Blümel M (2014). Germany: health system review. *Health Systems in Transition*, 16(2):1–296.

Calvert MJ, Freemantle N (2009). Cost-effective undergraduate medical education? *Journal of the Royal Society of Medicine*, 102(2):46–8.

Carraccio C et al. (2002). Shifting Paradigms: From Flexner to Competencies. *Academic Medicine*, 77(5):361–7.

Carraccio C et al. (2017). Building a framework of Entrustable Professional Activities, supported by competencies and milestones, to bridge the educational continuum. *Academic Medicine*, 92(3):324–30.

Cave J et al. (2009). Easing the transition from student to doctor: how can medical schools help prepare their graduates for starting work? *Medical Teacher*, 31(5):403–8.

Cervero RM, Gaines JK (2015). The impact of CME on physician performance and patient health outcomes: an updated synthesis of systematic reviews. *Journal of Continuing Education in the Health Professions*, 35(2):131–8.

Chevreul K et al. (2015). France: Health system review. *Health Systems in Transition*, 17(3):1–218.

Cooney R et al. (2017). Academic Primer Series: key papers about competency-based medical education. *Western Journal of Emergency Medicine*, 18(4):713–20.

Cotterill-Walker SM (2012). Where is the evidence that master's level nursing education makes a difference to patient care? A literature review. *Nurse Education Today*, 32(1):57–64.

Cylus J et al. (2015). United Kingdom: Health system review. *Health Systems in Transition*, 17(5):1–125.

Diallo K et al. (2003). Monitoring and evaluation of human resources for health: an international perspective. *Human Resources for Health*, 1(1):3.

Dimova A et al. (2018). Bulgaria: Health system review. *Health Systems in Transition*, 20(4):1–256.

Dury C et al. (2014). Specialist nurse in Europe. *International Nursing Review*, 61:454–62.

EFN (2012). EFN Competency Framework for Mutual Recognition of Professional Qualifications Directive 2005/36/EC, amended by Directive 2013/55/EU. EFN Guideline to implement Article 31 into national nurses' education programmes. European Federation of Nurses Associations (EFN). Available at: http://www.efnweb.be/?page_id=6897, accessed 4 January 2019.

Englander R et al. (2017). Toward a shared language for competency-based medical education. *Medical Teacher*, 39(6):582–7.

European Commission (2018a). Assessment of stakeholders' experience with the European Professional Card and the Alert Mechanism procedures. Available at: https://ec.europa.eu/docsroom/documents/28671/attachments/1/translations/en/renditions/native, accessed 7 April 2019.

European Commission (2018b). Assessment of functioning of the European Professional Card and the Alert Mechanism procedure. Available at: http://www.enmca.eu/system/files/epc_alerts.pdf, accessed 7 April 2019.

Fehr F et al. (2017). Entrustable professional activities in post-licensure training in primary care pediatrics: necessity, development and implementation of a competency-based post-graduate curriculum. *GMS Journal for Medical Education*, 34(5):Doc67.

Fong S et al. (2019). Patient-centred education: how do learners' perceptions change as they experience clinical training? *Advances in Health Sciences Education. Theory and Practice*, 24(1):15–32. doi: 10.1007/s10459-018-9845-y.

Frank JR et al. (2010). Toward a definition of competency-based education in medicine: a systematic review of published definitions. *Medical Teacher*, 32:631–7.

General Medical Council (2013). Good medical practice. Version from 25 March 2013. Available at: https://www.gmc-uk.org/ethical-guidance/ethical-guidance-for-doctors/good-medical-practice, accessed 3 December 2018.

General Medical Council (2014). The state of medical education and practice in the UK. Version from November 2014. Available at: https://www.gmc-uk.org/about/what-we-do-and-why/data-and-research/the-state-of-medical-education-and-practice-in-the-uk/archived-state-of-medical-education-and-practice-in-the-uk-reports, accessed 3 December 2018.

Geoghegan SE et al. (2017). Preparedness of newly qualified doctors in Ireland for prescribing in clinical practice. *British Journal of Clinical Pharmacology*, 83(8):1826–34.

Graham IS et al. (2007). Australian curriculum framework for junior doctors. *Medical Journal of Australia*, 186(7):s14–s19.

Gravina EW (2017). Competency-based education and its effects on nursing education: a literature review. *Teaching and Learning in Nursing*, 12:117–21.

Greiner AC, Knebel E (2003). Health professions education: a bridge to quality. Committee on the Health Professions Education Summit; Board on Health Care Services; Institute of Medicine. Available at: http://nap.edu/10681, accessed 3 December 2018.

Gulliford MC (2002). Availability of primary care doctors and population health in England: is there an association? *Journal of Public Health Medicine*, 24:252–4.

Habicht T et al. (2018). Estonia: Health system review. *Health Systems in Transition*, 20(1):1–193.

Hautz SC et al. (2016). What makes a doctor a scholar: a systematic review and content analysis of outcome frameworks. *BMC Medical Education*, 16(119).

Holen A et al. (2015). Medical students' preferences for problem-based learning in relation to culture and personality: a multicultural study. *International Journal of Medical Education*, 6:84–92.

Humar L, Sansoni J (2017). Bologna process and basic nursing education in 21 European countries. *Annali di Igiene: Medicina Preventiva e di Comunita*, 29:561–71.

Illing JC et al. (2013). Perceptions of UK medical graduates' preparedness for practice: a multi-centre qualitative study reflecting the importance of learning on the job. *BMC Medical Education*, 13:34.

IOM (2010). Redesigning Continuing Education in the Health Professions. Committee on Planning a Continuing Health Care Professional Education Institute; Board on Health Care Services; Institute of Medicine. Available at: http://nap.edu/12704, accessed 3 December 2018.

Ivers N et al. (2012). Audit and feedback: effects on professional practice and healthcare outcomes (Review). *Cochrane Database of Systematic Reviews*, 2012(6):CD000259.

Jefferies D et al. (2018). The importance of academic literacy for undergraduate nursing students and its relationship to future professional clinical practice: a systematic review. *Nurse Education Today*, 60:84–91.

Koh J, Dubrowski A (2016). Merging Problem-Based Learning with Simulation-Based Learning in the Medical Undergraduate Curriculum: the PAIRED Framework for Enhancing Lifelong Learning. *Cureus*, 8(6):e647.

Kovacs E et al. (2014). Licensing procedures and registration of medical doctors in the European Union. *Clinical Medicine*, 14(3):229–38.

Kroneman M et al. (2016). The Netherlands: health system review. *Health Systems in Transition*, 18(2):1–239.

Leach DC (2002). Competence is a habit. *Journal of the American Medical Association*, 287(2):243–4.

Leone C et al. (2016). Nurse migration in the EU: a moving target. *Eurohealth incorporating Euro Observer*, 22(1):7–9.

Ling K, Belcher P (2014). Medical migration within Europe: opportunities and challenges. *Clinical Medicine (London)*, 14(6):630–2.

Maier CB, Aiken LH (2016). Task shifting from physicians to nurses in primary care in 39 countries: a cross-country comparative study. *European Journal of Public Health*, 26:927–34.

Marinopoulos SS et al. (2007). Effectiveness of continuing medical education. *Evidence Report/ Technology Assessment (Full Report)*, 149:1–69.

Mazmanian PE, Davis DA, Galbraith R (2009). Continuing Medical Education Effect on Clinical Outcomes: Effectiveness of Continuing Medical Education: American College of Chest Physicians Evidence-Based Educational Guidelines. *Chest*, 135(3):49s–55s.

Melnyk BM et al. (2018). The First U.S. Study on Nurses' Evidence-Based Practice Competencies Indicates Major Deficits That Threaten Healthcare Quality, Safety, and Patient Outcomes. *Worldviews on Evidence Based Nursing*, 15(1):16–25. doi: 10.1111/wvn.12269.

Melovitz Vasan CA et al. (2018). Analysis of testing with multiple choice versus open-ended questions: outcome-based observations in an anatomy course. *Anatomical Sciences Education*, 11(3):254–61.

Miles S, Kellett J, Leinster SJ (2017). Medical graduates' preparedness to practice: a comparison of undergraduate medical school training. *BMC Medical Education*, 17(1):33.

Monrouxe LV et al. (2017). How prepared are UK medical graduates for practice? A rapid review of the literature 2009–2014. *BMJ Open*, 7(1):e013656.

Monrouxe LV et al. (2018). New graduate doctors' preparedness for practice: a multistakeholder, multicentre narrative study. *BMJ Open*, 8(8):e023146.

Morcke AM, Dornan T, Eika B, (2013). Outcome (competency) based education: an exploration of its origins, theoretical basis, and empirical evidence. *Advances in Health Sciences Education*, 18:851–63.

Nara N, Suzuki T, Tohda S (2011). The Current Medical Education System in the World. *Journal of Medical and Dental Sciences*, 58:79–83.

Needleman J et al. (2002). Nurse-staffing levels and the quality of care in hospitals. *New England Journal of Medicine*, 346:1715–22.

Norcini JJ, Lipner RS, Kimball HR (2002). Certifying examination performance and patient outcomes following acute myocardial infarction. *Medical Education*, 36:853–9.

OECD (2016). Health workforce policies in OECD countries: right jobs, right skills, right places. OECD Health Policy Studies. Paris: OECD Publishing.

OECD (2018). Feasibility study on health workforce skills assessment. Supporting health workers achieve person-centred care. OECD Health Division team, February 2018. Available at: http://www.oecd.org/els/health-systems/workforce.htm, accessed 3 December 2018.

O'Neill PA et al. (2003). Does a new undergraduate curriculum based on Tomorrow's Doctors prepare house officers better for their first post? A qualitative study of the views of pre-registration house officers using critical incidents. *Medical Education*, 37:1100–8.

Onyura B et al. (2016). Evidence for curricular and instructional design approaches in undergraduate medical education: an umbrella review. *Medical Teacher*, 38(2):150–61. doi: 10.3109/0142159X.2015.1009019.

Ousy K (2011). The changing face of student nurse education and training programmes. *Wounds UK*, 7(1):70–6.

Phillips RL et al. (2017). The effects of training institution practice costs, quality, and other characteristics on future practice. *Annals of Family Medicine*, 15(2):140–8.

Pijl-Zieber EM et al. (2014). Competence and competency-based nursing education: finding our way through the issues. *Nurse Education Today*, 34(5):676–8.

Price T et al. (2018). The International landscape of medical licensing examinations: a typology derived from a systematic review. *International Journal of Health Policy and Management*, 7(9):782–90.

Rashid A, Manek N (2016). Making primary care placements a universal feature of postgraduate medical training. *Journal of the Royal Society of Medicine*, 109(12):461–2.

Reinke NB (2018). The impact of timetable changes on student achievement and learning experiences. *Nurse Education Today*, 62:137–42.

Riedel M, Röhrling G, Schönpflug K (2016). Nicht-ärztliche Gesundheitsberufe. Institute for Advanced Studies, Vienna. Research Report April 2016. Available at: http://irihs.ihs.ac.at/4112/, accessed 3 December 2018.

Ringard Å et al. (2013). Norway: Health system review. *Health Systems in Transition*, 15(8):1–162.

Risso-Gill I et al. (2014). Assessing the role of regulatory bodies in managing health professional issues and errors in Europe. *International Journal for Quality in Health Care*, 26(4):348–57.

Robinson S, Griffiths P (2007). Nursing education and regulation: international profiles and perspectives. Kings College London, National Nursing Research Unit. Available at: https://www.kcl.ac.uk/nursing/research/nnru/Publications/.../NurseEduProfiles, accessed 3 December 2018.

Ross S, Hauer K, van Melle E (2018). Outcomes are what matter: competency-based medical education gets us to our goal. *MedEdPublish*, 7(2):1–5.

Rubin P, Franchi-Christopher P (2002). New edition of Tomorrow's Doctors. *Medical Teacher*, 24(4):368–9.

Schostak J et al. (2010). Effectiveness of Continuing Professional Development project: a summary of findings. *Medical Teacher*, 32:586–92.

Schweppenstedde D et al. (2014). Regulating Quality and Safety of Health and Social Care: International Experiences. *Rand Health Quarterly*, 4(1):1.

Sehlbach C et al. (2018). Doctors on the move: a European case study on the key characteristics of national recertification systems. *BMJ Open*, 8:e019963.

Sharp LK et al. (2002). Specialty board certification and clinical outcomes: the missing link. *Academic Medicine*, 77(6):534–42.

Simões J et al. (2017). Portugal: Health system review. *Health Systems in Transition*, 19(2):1–184.

Simper J (2014). Proceedings from the second UEMS Conference on CME-CPD in Europe, 28 February 2014, Brussels, Belgium. *Journal of European CME*, 3(1), Article 25494.

Simpson JG et al. (2002). The Scottish doctor – learning outcomes for the medical undergraduate in Scotland: a foundation for competent and reflective practitioners. *Medical Teacher*, 24(2):136–43.

Smith F, Goldacre MJ, Lambert TW (2017). Adequacy of postgraduate medical training: views of different generations of UK-trained doctors. *Postgraduate Medical Journal*, 93(1105):665–70.

Solé M et al. (2014). How do medical doctors in the European Union demonstrate that they continue to meet criteria for registration and licencing? *Clinical Medicine*, 14(6):633–9.

Steffens S et al. (2018). Perceived usability of the National Competence Based Catalogue of Learning Objectives for Undergraduate Medical Education by medical educators at the Hannover Medical School. *GMS Journal for Medical Education*, 35(2):1–12.

Struckmann V et al. (2015). Deciding when physicians are unfit to practise: an analysis of responsibilities, policy and practice in 11 European Union member states. *Clinical Medicine*, 15(4):319–24.

Swing SR (2007). The ACGME outcome project: retrospective and prospective. *Medical Teacher*, 2007(29):648–54.

Tan K et al. (2018). The effectiveness of outcome based education on the competencies of nursing students: a systematic review. *Nurse Education Today*, 64:180–9.

Touchie C, ten Cate O (2016). The promise, perils, problems and progress of competency-based medical education. *Medical Education*, 50:93–100.

Tsugawa Y et al. (2017). Quality of care delivered by general internists in US hospitals who graduated from foreign versus US medical schools: observational study. *BMJ (Clinical research edition)*, 356:j273.

Tsugawa Y et al. (2018). Association between physician *US News & World Report* medical school ranking and patient outcomes and costs of care: observational study. *BMJ (Clinical research edition)*, 362:k3640.

van der Vleuten CP, Driessen EW (2014). What would happen to education if we take education evidence seriously? *Perspectives on Medical Education*, 3(3):222–32.

van Rossum TR et al. (2018). Flexible competency based medical education: more efficient, higher costs. *Medical Teacher*, 40(3):315–17.

van Zanten M (2015). The association between medical education accreditation and the examination performance of internationally educated physicians seeking certification in the United States. *Perspectives on Medical Education*, 4:142–5.

Vaughan L, McAlister, Bell D (2011). "August is always a nightmare": results of the Royal College of Physicians of Edinburgh and Society of Acute Medicine August transition survey. *Clinical Medicine*, 11:322–6.

Wangensteen S et al. (2018). Postgraduate nurses' self-assessment of clinical competence and need for further training. A European cross-sectional survey. *Nurse Education Today*, 62:101–6.

Watmough S, Garden A, Taylor D (2006). Pre-registration house officers' views on studying under a reformed medical curriculum in the UK. Medical Education, 40(9):893–9.

Watmough S, Taylor D, Garden A (2006). Educational supervisors evaluate the preparedness of graduates from a reformed UK curriculum to work as pre-registration house officers (PRHOs): a qualitative study. *Medical Education*, 40:995–1001.

Weggemans MM et al. (2017). The postgraduate medical education pathway: an international comparison. *GMS Journal for Medical Education*, 34(5):Doc63.

WHO (2006). Human resources for health in the WHO European Region. Available at: www.euro.who.int/__data/assets/pdf_file/0007/91474/E88365.pdf, accessed 3 December 2018.

WHO (2007). Strengthening health systems to improve health outcomes. WHO's framework for action. Available at: https://www.who.int/healthsystems/strategy/en/, accessed 3 December 2018.

WHO (2016). Working for health and growth. Investing in the health workforce. Report of the High-Level Commission on Health Employment and Economic Growth. Available at: https://www.who.int/hrh/com-heeg/reports/en/, accessed 2 December 2019.

Woodward CA (2000). Strategies for assisting health workers to modify and improve skills: developing quality health care – a process of change. World Health Organization, Issues in health services delivery, Discussion paper no. 1, WHO/EIP/OSD/00.1. Available at: www.who.int/hrh/documents/en/improve_skills.pdf, accessed 3 December 2018.

Zander B et al. (2016). The state of nursing in the European Union. *Eurohealth incorporating Euro Observer*, 22(1):3–6.

Zavlin D et al. (2017). A comparison of medical education in Germany and the United States: from applying to medical school to the beginnings of residency. *GMS German Medical Science*, 15:Doc15.

Zieber M, Sedgewick M (2018). Competence, confidence and knowledge retention in undergraduate nursing students – a mixed method study. *Nurse Education Today*, 62:16–21.

Chapter 6

Regulating the input – Health Technology Assessment

Finn Borlum Kristensen, Camilla Palmhøj Nielsen, Dimitra Panteli

Summary

What are the characteristics of the strategy?

Health Technology Assessment (HTA) is "a multidisciplinary process that summarizes information about the medical, social, economic and ethical issues related to the use of a health technology in a systematic, transparent, unbiased and robust manner" and is considered a policy-informing tool, usually linked to coverage decision-making. HTA has the potential to contribute to quality of care, equity in access and value for money by providing input to decision-making at different levels in the system and fostering both the adoption of valuable innovation and the removal of obsolete technologies in a robust manner. In conjunction with all the dimensions of the use of health technologies it captures, HTA can be described as encompassing four contributing streams: (i) policy analysis; (ii) evidence-based medicine; (iii) health economic evaluation; and (iv) social and humanistic sciences. Depending on whether HTA is applied to new or established technologies, it contributes to setting or updating standards for healthcare provision.

What is being done in European countries?

HTA programmes evolved organically in the majority of European countries; as a result, they differ considerably regarding process and methodology. However, assessments uniformly summarize (best) available evidence to provide the basis for decision-making on reimbursement and/or pricing, depending on the system. A recent overview of European practices (2018) found that in the last 20 years all EU Member States have started to introduce HTA processes at national or regional level. While there is some convergence in national HTA systems in Europe, there are also significant discrepancies concerning both process and methodology. Regulation proposed by the European Commission in January 2018 opts for mandating joint assessments of clinical elements (effectiveness and safety), while leaving the consideration of other domains such as the economic and organizational impact to national authorities. The proposal has been met with criticism from various sides, regarding the lack of flexibility for national assessments in light of different standard practices of care (which influence comparator therapies and choice of outcomes), the lack of an obligation for the industry to submit full trial data despite increased traction in transparency expectations in recent years and the loss of flexibility in decision-making at a national level in the presence of a binding assessment. However, there is general consensus that synergies emerging from increased collaboration can have a considerable impact in realizing the benefits of HTA at country level.

What do we know about the effectiveness and cost-effectiveness of the strategy?

HTA is defined as information input to policy and other decision-making in health-care. As such, its "effectiveness" is primarily evaluated based on its ability to support evidence-informed decisions. In general, the impact of HTA is variable and inconsistently understood. A major influencing factor is the directness of the relationship between an HTA programme, policy-making bodies and healthcare decisions. However, even when the reporting of HTA findings is followed by concrete changes, for example, in policy or use of a technology, it may be difficult to demonstrate the causal effect of the HTA on those changes. Historically, systematic attempts to document the dissemination processes and impacts of HTA programmes have been infrequent despite recognition that monitoring the impact of individual HTAs and HTA programmes is a key principle for the good practice of HTA. Along with the lack of generalizable evidence of the effectiveness of HTA, there has also been limited discussion on its cost-effectiveness. In countries where the results of evaluation directly inform pricing negotiations, the impact of HTA may be monetized more directly, but the scope of this is not generalizable.

How can the strategy be implemented?

Setting up a national HTA mechanism is a complicated and resource-intensive exercise that requires a given timeframe to mature and political commitment to be sustainable and effective. Even established HTA systems require a certain degree of flexibility to maintain their usefulness and appropriateness, especially in light of the emergence of new technologies that are increasingly accompanied by high price tags. Stakeholder involvement is an important part of enabling the establishment and continued usefulness of HTA processes. Key principles for best practice in national HTA programmes have been defined, but are only partially applied in reality. Recommendations on overcoming barriers for performing HTA and establishing HTA organizational structures were issued by EUnetHTA in 2011. More recent work (2019) shows that many good practices have been developed, mostly regarding assessment methodology and certain key aspects of HTA processes, but consensus on good practice is still lacking for many areas, such as defining the organizational aspects of HTA, use of deliberative processes and measuring the impact of HTA.

Conclusions for policy-makers

This chapter clearly demonstrates HTA's potential to contribute to quality improvement. Across Europe, different countries have to deal with different challenges, depending on the maturity of their HTA programmes and health system structures. However, it is clear that in the following months and years changes at country level will be influenced by European developments. Nevertheless, it is important for national policy-makers to maintain focus on the implementation of HTA findings to the extent that they contribute to quality of care by monitoring and ensuring impact and to explore potential synergies with other strategies, especially in the realm of evidence synthesis for knowledge translation. The (re)organization of HTA activities should draw on existing knowledge from the comprehensive experiences with establishing, running and improving the performance of HTA agencies in European countries.

6.1 Introduction: health technology regulation and health technology assessment

Health technologies are crucial inputs in any healthcare system and their attributes and utilization can have a direct influence on the quality of care received by patients. In a broad sense technology is defined as "knowledge of how to fulfill certain human purposes in a specifiable and reproducible way" (Brooks, 1980). Health technologies, as the application of scientific knowledge in the field of healthcare, may also be understood in this way and not only as physical artifacts.

One conceptualization differentiates between health technologies within the system, i.e. healthcare products like drugs, devices and procedures, and those applied to the system, i.e. governance, financial, organizational, delivery and implementation arrangements (Velasco-Garrido et al., 2010). Another also looks at the purpose of health technologies (for example, diagnostic, therapeutic or rehabilitative) as another factor affecting their characteristics and application (Banta & Luce, 1993), and thus potentially the specifics of any required regulation.

This chapter briefly introduces an overview of the different components of regulation for health technologies and proceeds to focus on health technology assessment (HTA) as a strategy contributing to quality of care. In the context of regulation, health technology is most often understood in its narrow sense as physical products, like pharmaceuticals and medical devices. Accordingly, most of the information in this chapter relates to these types of technologies; when system innovations are regulated, this is done more indirectly and in a less formalized and systematized manner.

In Europe markets for pharmaceuticals and medical devices are strongly regulated both at European and national levels. Policy-makers have had to introduce regulations to handle market approval, intellectual property rights and the pricing and reimbursement of health technologies to address a number of market failures stemming from information asymmetry, third party payer dilemmas and positive externalities associated with knowledge production in the field of health technologies. While requirements for market approval and intellectual property are mostly handled at supranational level, reimbursement and pricing are a national competence.

Fig. 6.1 shows the different stages of managing health technologies throughout their life-cycle, using the example of pharmaceuticals. Chapter 4 details the background and specifics of market entry regulations for pharmaceuticals and medical devices, along with European provisions for pharmacovigilance. In essence, the main considerations for patients and health professionals charged with selecting the technologies to use are that they are fit-for-purpose, safe, effective and of good quality. This is secured through a number of regulatory steps.

As a rule, marketing authorization is a fundamental requirement that needs to be fulfilled before medicines or devices can be made available and any decision-making on pricing or reimbursement can take place (*see* Chapter 4). In brief, the marketing authorization process aims to verify the safety and functionality of candidate products (Fig. 6.2); depending on technology type, requirements and process characteristics vary and the approval is carried out by competent authorities at national or European level. Safety is the main criterion for marketing authorization. A limited proof of efficacy (medicines) or performance (medical devices) based on often small sample sizes is usually sufficient. Submitted evidence consists of clinical trials carried out under optimized study conditions, usually without an active comparator and frequently reporting clinical (surrogate) outcome measures.

Thus, it is clear that obtaining marketing authorization does not require evidence that technologies provide benefit which is meaningful to patients in real world conditions. Patient-relevant benefit is examined in peri- and post-marketing evaluations, which have been established in the majority of European countries.

Fig. 6.1 *Regulating pharmaceuticals along the product life-cycle*

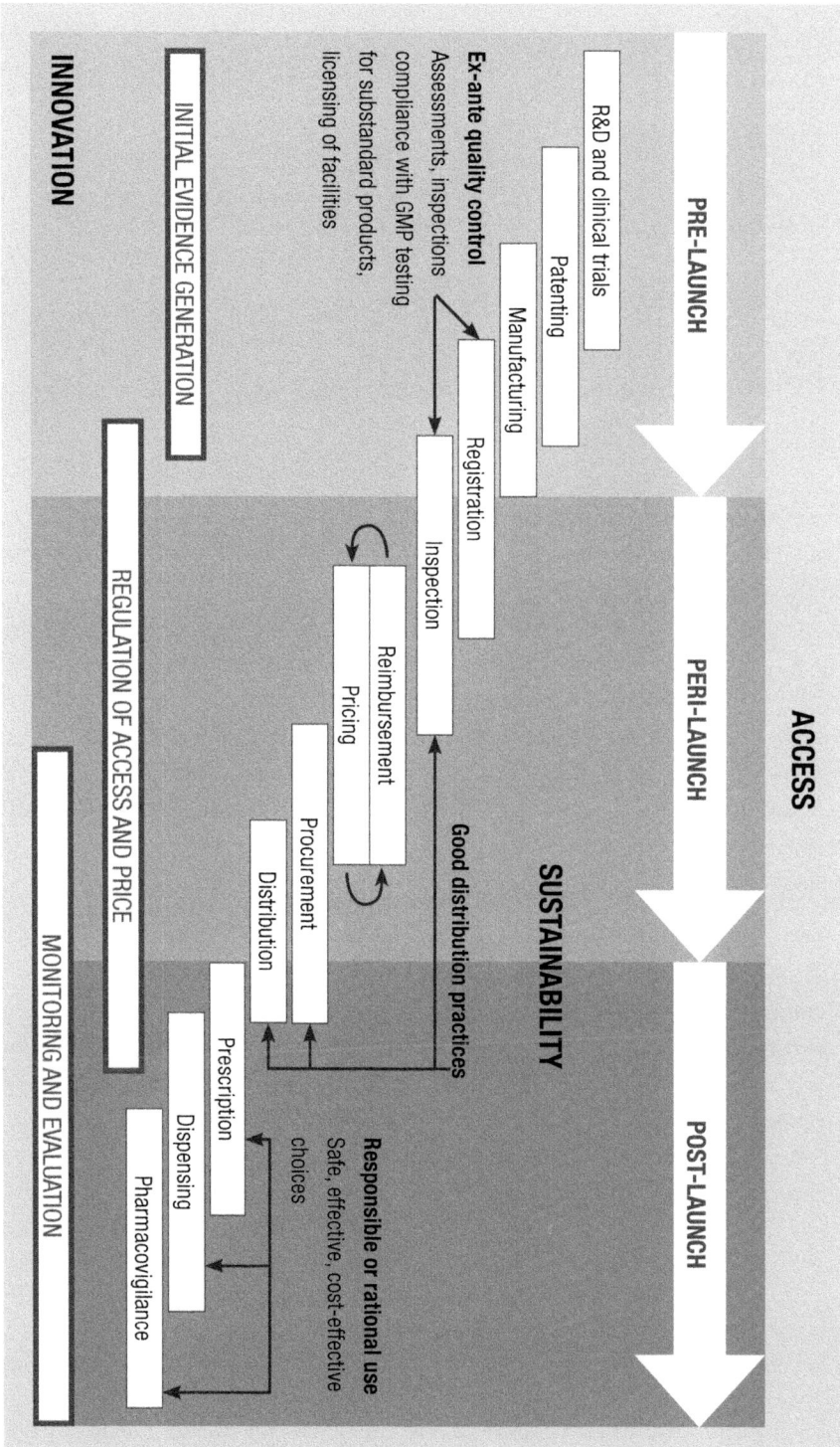

Source: Panteli & Edwards, 2018

Fig. 6.2   *Health technology regulation, assessment and management*

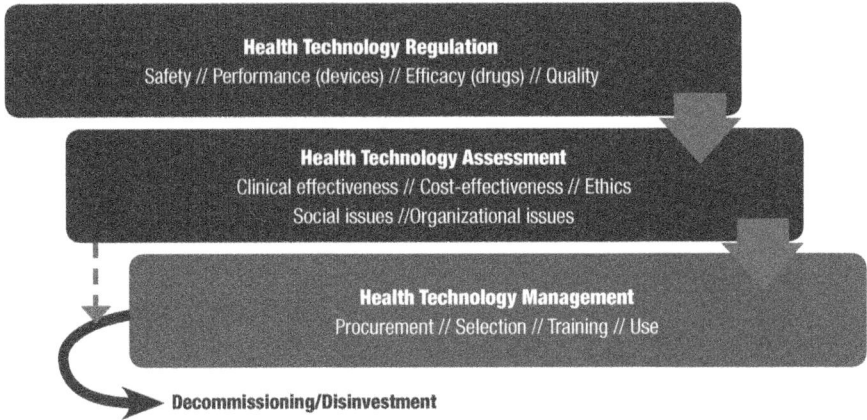

Health Technology Regulation
Safety // Performance (devices) // Efficacy (drugs) // Quality

Health Technology Assessment
Clinical effectiveness // Cost-effectiveness // Ethics
Social issues //Organizational issues

Health Technology Management
Procurement // Selection // Training // Use

Decommissioning/Disinvestment

Source: adapted from WHO, 2011

These evaluation systems usually serve to inform or determine the reimbursement eligibility and/or price of (new) pharmaceuticals or medical devices in the publicly financed (statutory) health system; they introduce the concept of effectiveness and often the concept of efficiency, or "value for money", as a criterion for prioritizing health technologies for coverage. As they are embedded in various decision-making structures at national or regional level in different countries, their configuration varies. However, a common characteristic – and the main difference from marketing authorization – is that their role is to provide recommendations and support informed decision-making. As such, their results are not necessarily mandatory in nature.

Post-marketing evaluations are usually based on the principles of HTA, that is "a multidisciplinary process that summarizes information about the medical, social, economic and ethical issues related to the use of a health technology in a systematic, transparent, unbiased and robust manner". As such, HTA is considered a policy-informing tool. According to the European Network for Health Technology Assessment (EUnetHTA), "the aim of HTA is to inform the formulation of safe and effective health policies that are patient-focused and seek to achieve best value". As per this definition, HTA can be understood as both a quality assurance and an efficiency mechanism. In the context of HTA, health technologies generally comprise pharmaceuticals, vaccines, medical devices, medical and surgical procedures, prevention and rehabilitation interventions, and the systems within which health is protected and maintained.

The origins of HTA can be traced to the establishment, in 1975, of the healthcare track at the Office of Technology Assessment (OTA) in the United States, following concerns about the diffuse and inefficient use of new medical technologies. OTA was founded with the aim of providing impartial input on the potential social, economic and legal implications of new technologies in order to guide public policy (O'Donnell et al., 2009). Its model of technology evaluation included, among others, elements of safety, effectiveness and cost, as well as socioeconomic and ethical implications, and was subsequently adapted by national HTA programmes in a number of European countries (*see* below).

In conjunction with all the dimensions of the use of health technologies it captures, HTA can be described as encompassing four contributing streams: (i) policy analysis; (ii) evidence-based medicine; (iii) health economic evaluation; and (iv) social and humanistic sciences (Kristensen et al., 2008). Although HTA is an instrument for informing primarily policy and more generally decision-making at different levels in the health system, it is since its inception by definition firmly rooted in good scientific practice ("in a systematic, transparent, unbiased and robust manner"). In its most robust version, scientific evidence synthesis takes the form of systematic reviews of interventions. However, as HTA has a broader perspective that includes considerations of value, especially when linked to coverage decision-making (*see also* Luce et al., 2010), participatory approaches are often necessary in addition to the systematic consideration of evidence from existing primary sources. Specifically, in the context of HTA, the exact scientific methods are chosen depending on the research question(s) and the issue at hand. The current gold standard, at least in Europe, underpinning the procedural and methodological understanding of conducting HTA is the HTA Core Model®, developed in an iterative process over 10 years by the EUnetHTA collaboration and Joint Actions (Kristensen et al., 2017).

Box 6.1 summarizes the content of the HTA Core Model®. It is important to note that not all domains of the model are necessarily meant to be addressed in all HTA reports; depending on the scope of evaluation foreseen in the decision-making process in which it is embedded (i.e. the HTA's purpose), the technology at hand and feasibility parameters, a narrower or broader perspective can be adopted. Quite often, reports focus on the clinical and economic implications only (Lee, Skott & Hansen, 2009). In any case, results from the analyses of the different domains in HTA are synthesized and reported in a way that aims to support decision-makers at various levels.

6.2 Why should HTA contribute to healthcare quality?

HTA has the potential to contribute to quality of care, equity in access and value for money by providing input to decision-making at different levels in the system. Its role is to provide a contextualized summary of the relevant evidence base for politicians, policy-makers, managers, clinicians, etc., to support the use of safe, effective technologies both by fostering the adoption of valuable innovation and

---

Box 6.1 *The HTA Core Model®*

From the EUnetHTA website: "The HTA Core Model® is a methodological framework for production and sharing of HTA information. It consists of three components, each with a specific purpose: 1) a standardised set of HTA questions (the ontology), which allow users to define their specific research questions within a hierarchical structure; 2) methodological guidance to assist in answering the research questions and 3) a common reporting structure for presenting findings in a standardised 'question-answer pair' format."

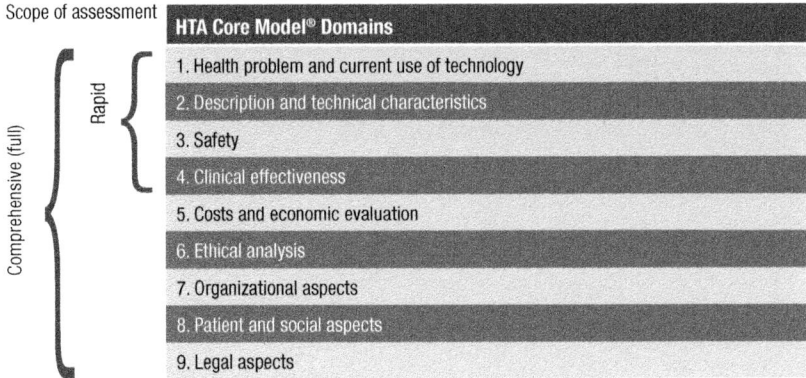

Scope of assessment

HTA Core Model® Domains

1. Health problem and current use of technology
2. Description and technical characteristics
3. Safety
4. Clinical effectiveness
5. Costs and economic evaluation
6. Ethical analysis
7. Organizational aspects
8. Patient and social aspects
9. Legal aspects

Rapid (domains 1–4), *Comprehensive (full)* (domains 1–9)

---

by enabling the removal of obsolete technologies ("disinvestment") in a robust manner (*see* Fig. 6.2).

Linking back to the conceptual framework of quality presented in Chapter 2, depending on whether HTA is applied to new or established technologies (the latter with potentially new alternatives) it contributes to setting or updating standards for healthcare provision. In the usual definition of technologies in an HTA context (*see* above), it ensures that structural components of healthcare, such as medicines or medical devices, are chosen based on the best available evidence. If organizational or system innovations are assessed, HTA can also directly address the process component of Donabedian's triad. Considering the dimensions of the application of a health technology evaluated in a full HTA (*see* Box 6.1), it can have an impact on not only the safety and effectiveness of care, but also its responsiveness to patient expectations, for instance by investigating ethical, social and organizational implications.

6.3 What is being done in Europe?

HTA activities take place all over the world – in April 2019 the International Network of Agencies for Health Technology Assessment (INAHTA) had 48 member organizations from around the world (INAHTA, 2019). Despite its US origins, a pivot of developments in HTA kicked off in Europe in the 1990s, where the first HTA institutions had started to develop in the 1980s. This comprised a combination of scientific, practical and political steps in countries with social insurance- or tax-based national health systems and in a region of the world that provides certain conditions that are conducive to collaboration – the European integration and the European Union (EU) (Kristensen, 2012). Box 6.2 summarizes the timeline of developments on HTA at the European level.

Regarding the institutions actually producing HTA reports, one can distinguish between agencies that serve the population of a whole nation or a region (i.e. national or regional) and those that are integrated into single hospitals or hospital trusts (hospital-based HTA). The focus of this chapter lies with the former, but the possibilities and particularities of the latter have also been studied comparatively at the European and international level (for example, Sampietro-Colom & Martin, 2016; Gagnon et al., 2014).

European HTA organizations can be classified into two main groups: those concentrating on the production and dissemination of HTA and those with broader mandates, which are often related to quality of care and include but are not limited to the production and dissemination of HTA reports (Velasco-Garrido et al., 2008). Variation is also observed in the degree to which HTA organizations (and their products) are linked to decision-making. This is largely dependent on whether there are formalized decision-making processes – most often established in relation to service coverage and reimbursement and most predominantly for pharmaceuticals. Indeed, HTA systems evolved organically in the majority of European countries; as a result, they differ considerably regarding process and methodology. The varying set-up of HTA systems in Europe has been well documented (for example, Allen et al., 2013; Allen et al., 2017; Panteli et al., 2015, Panteli et al., 2016, Fuchs et al., 2016).

The most recent overview of European practices stems from a background document (European Commission, 2018a) produced for the European Commission to inform the development of regulation (European Commission, 2018b) for strengthening EU cooperation beyond 2020. The latter included joint clinical assessment at European level as a part of the HTA process for certain technologies in the Member States (*see* Box 6.2 and below). This background work found that in the last 20 years all EU Member States have started to introduce HTA processes at national or regional level. National legal frameworks for HTA are already in place in 26 Member States while some Member States are only at the initial phase of establishing HTA systems and/or have dedicated only limited resources to HTA (European Commission, 2018a). The Commission's work confirmed previous findings, namely that while there is some convergence in national HTA systems in Europe, there are also significant discrepancies.

Box 6.2 *European developments in HTA (adapted from Panteli & Edwards 2018)*

The European Commission has supported collaboration in HTA across countries since the early 1990s. In 2004 it set HTA as a political priority, followed by a call towards establishing a sustainable European network on HTA. The call was answered by 35 organizations throughout Europe and led to the introduction of the European network for Health Technology Assessment (EUnetHTA) Project in 2005. The strategic objectives of the EUnetHTA Project were to reduce duplication of effort, promote more effective use of resources, increase HTA input to decision-making in Member States and the EU to increase the impact of HTA, strengthen the link between HTA and healthcare policy-making in the EU and its Member States, and support countries with limited experience in HTA (Kristensen et al., 2009; Banta, Kristensen & Jonsson, 2009).

In May 2008 the EUnetHTA partner organizations endorsed a proposal for a permanent collaboration. On the basis of the project's results, the European Commission has consistently funded a number of continuing initiatives: the EUnetHTA Collaboration 2009, the EUnetHTA Joint Action 2010–2012, EUnetHTA Joint Action 2 2012–2015 and EUnetHTA Joint Action 3 2016–2020. This research has mainly focused on developing joint methodologies for assessment, perhaps most importantly the so-called Core Models for different types of technologies, but also piloting them in carrying out joint assessments. It also maintains a database of planned and ongoing national HTA reports accessible to its member organizations.

Cross-border collaboration in HTA was anchored in EU law through Directive 2011/24/EU on the application of patients' rights in cross-border healthcare. According to article 15, "the Union shall support and facilitate cooperation and the exchange of scientific information among Member States within a voluntary network connecting national authorities or bodies responsible for health technology assessment designated by the Member States". The Directive sets out both the network's goals and activities for which additional EU funds may be requested. It also explicitly reinforces the principle of subsidiarity, stating that adopted measures should not interfere with Member States' competences in deciding on the implementation of HTA findings or harmonize any related laws or regulations at national level, while providing a basis for sustained Union support for HTA cooperation.

In October 2016 the European Commission launched a public consultation on strengthening EU cooperation on HTA. The European Commission's impact assessment offered different policy options ranging from maintaining the status quo of project-based collaboration to cooperation on the production of fully fledged joint HTA reports including the evaluation of cost-effectiveness and organizational aspects (which are more topical) along with clinical effectiveness and safety. The impact assessment was based on evidence from the EUnetHTA activities of previous years, which showed that collaboration in producing joint methodologies and assessments themselves can improve both the quality and quantity of produced assessments while avoiding duplication of work. However, evaluative research on these collaborative activities also highlighted challenges, particularly for the alignment of a joint HTA process with national needs and processes (European Commission, 2018a; Kleijnen et al., 2015). This primarily concerned the timely availability of joint assessments, the relevance of each jointly selected topic for individual HTA agencies and difficulties with integrating jointly produced reports in national templates and procedures. The consultation culminated in the new proposed regulation described in the main text.

Regarding their **procedural framework**, national HTA systems differ in the scope of health technologies that are being assessed. Most Member States have national HTA tracks for pharmaceuticals, and more than half (20) have a system for medical devices, although not always formalized. Other technologies are not evaluated as often. The main role of most HTA organizations is to carry out assessments and provide recommendations for decision-making (i.e. pricing and reimbursement decisions). Some are also tasked with developing quality standards and/or clinical guidelines, performing horizon scanning, managing registries or advising health technology developers. The vast majority of HTA organizations are public bodies, usually financed through the government's annual budget; however, the amount and types of resources dedicated to them varies considerably, with – for instance – the number of staff ranging from zero to 600. The initial evidence base for the assessment often consists of industry submissions for pharmaceuticals, while more Member States carry out their own assessments for medical devices. When industry dossiers are used, the extent of the review performed by HTA bodies varies and may include aspects such as missing evidence, errors in submitted evidence and internal and external validity of submitted evidence. Some HTA bodies also carry out their own additional evidence analyses. All Member States perform assessment of single technologies (for example, those entering the market) compared to standard of care, while several also perform assessments of multiple technologies in use for a particular indication. Variation is also evident in the number of assessments produced per year (ranging from five to up to 390), the time needed to complete the assessment (reflecting the choice between rapid vs. full assessment but also capacity), and stakeholder involvement (European Commission, 2018a).

Allen et al. (2013) have depicted further differences in the process of HTA among European countries by distinguishing between the scientific assessment of the evidence, be it regarding therapeutic or economic effects, and the appraisal of these findings in the context of the health system, as well as the stages of regulation (i.e. marketing authorization), evaluation (i.e. HTA) and final decision on coverage (i.e. pricing and reimbursement). Their typology is shown in Fig. 6.3. Following this distinction between scientific assessment, appraisal in context and final decision-making, it can generally be observed that assessment conclusions are the basis for but not the sole consideration informing the appraisal's recommendations, and the latter often deviate from replicating the scientific

Fig. 6.3 *Typology of HTA processes in European countries*

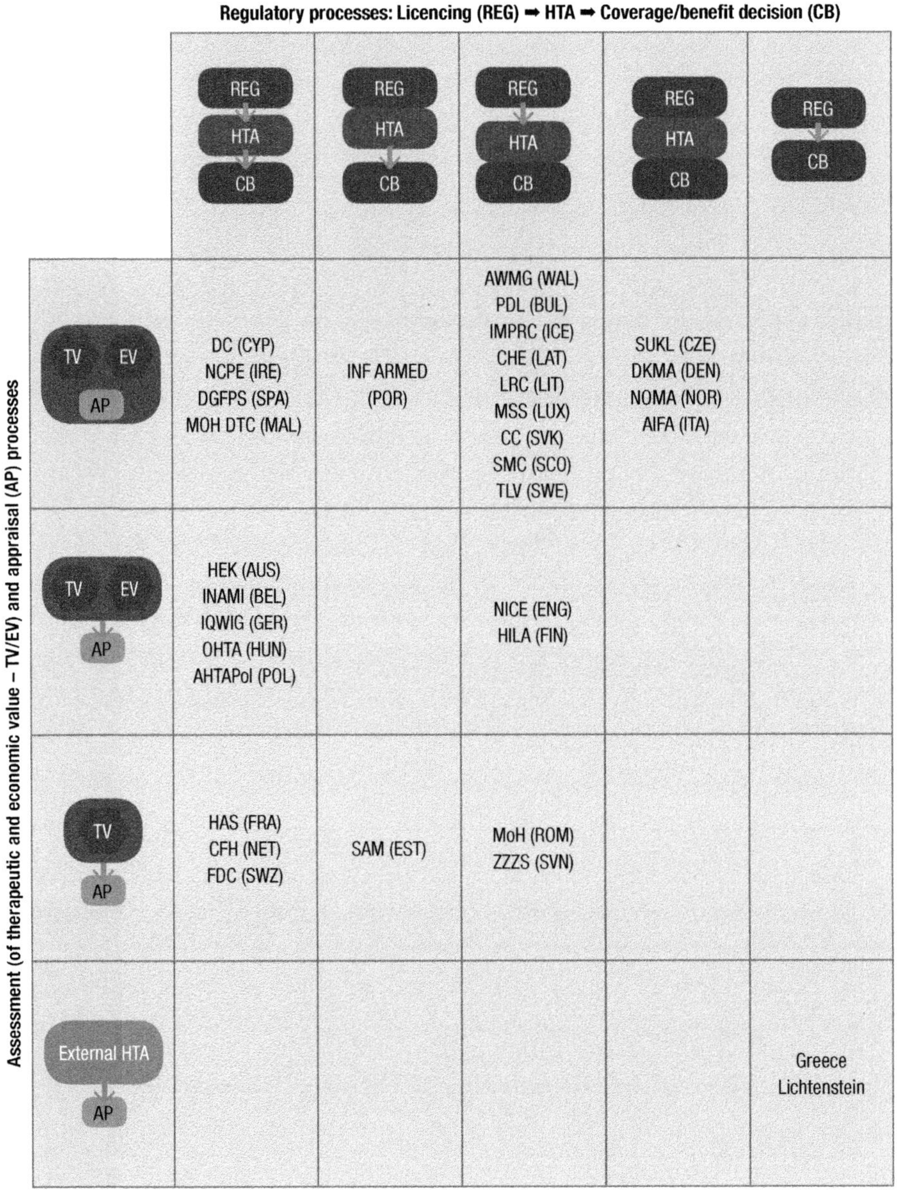

Regulatory processes: Licencing (REG) ➡ HTA ➡ Coverage/benefit decision (CB)

	REG→HTA→CB	REG→HTA→CB	REG→HTA→CB	REG→HTA→CB	REG→CB
TV EV / AP	DC (CYP) NCPE (IRE) DGFPS (SPA) MOH DTC (MAL)	INF ARMED (POR)	AWMG (WAL) PDL (BUL) IMPRC (ICE) CHE (LAT) LRC (LIT) MSS (LUX) CC (SVK) SMC (SCO) TLV (SWE)	SUKL (CZE) DKMA (DEN) NOMA (NOR) AIFA (ITA)	
TV EV / AP	HEK (AUS) INAMI (BEL) IQWIG (GER) OHTA (HUN) AHTAPol (POL)		NICE (ENG) HILA (FIN)		
TV / AP	HAS (FRA) CFH (NET) FDC (SWZ)	SAM (EST)	MoH (ROM) ZZZS (SVN)		
External HTA / AP					Greece Lichtenstein

Assessment (of therapeutic and economic value – TV/EV) and appraisal (AP) processes

Source: based on Allen, 2013

Notes: AP= appraisal, CB = decision on coverage, EV = economic value; TV = therapeutic value; REG = regulatory approval

conclusions. Furthermore, appraisal recommendations are usually not binding for decision-makers who can still diverge in their final call (although usually have to justify their choice if they do so) (Panteli et al., 2015).

Regarding **methodology**, the Commission's background work highlights three main areas of variation: the comparator used (for example, reflecting current healthcare practice and/or best evidence-based profile of efficacy and safety; the process for choosing the comparator also differs, potentially comprising manufacturer proposals and/or input from medical societies/healthcare professional organizations), the endpoints measured (for example, whether surrogate, composite and/or patient-reported outcomes are accepted), and the study design specifications (for example, types of studies accepted and restrictions on patients enrolled and duration) (European Commission, 2018a). These differences were often cited as concerns about the appropriateness of what may be perceived as formally "centralizing" HTA as foreseen in the Commission's proposal.

The proposed regulation issued by the Commission in January 2018 opts for mandating joint assessments of clinical elements (effectiveness and safety), while leaving the consideration of other domains such as economic and organizational impact to national authorities. In brief, the draft regulation proposes four main changes to current systems of post-marketing evaluations for medicines approved by the European Medicines Agency (EMA):

- Joint clinical assessments of new pharmaceuticals as well as certain medical devices and in vitro diagnostics. Following a phase-in period of three years, participation in the centralized assessments and use of the joint clinical assessment reports at Member State level will be mandatory.

- Joint scientific consultations: these will allow developers of pharmaceuticals and medical devices to seek advice from the Coordination Group of HTA agencies (newly instituted in the draft regulation and hosted by the Commission) on the data and evidence likely to be required as part of a potential joint clinical assessment in the future. These consultations can potentially be held in conjunction with scientific advice from the EMA. After the phase-in period, equivalent consultations at the Member State level are not to take place for technologies covered by the joint scientific consultation.

- Identification of emerging health technologies ("horizon scanning"): the Coordination group is to carry out an annual study to ensure that health technologies expected to have a major impact on patients, public health or healthcare systems are identified at an early stage in their development and are included in the joint work of the Coordination Group.

- Support for continuing voluntary cooperation and information exchange on non-clinical aspects of HTA.

Despite the general consensus that synergies emerging from increased collaboration can have a considerable impact in realizing the benefits of HTA at country level, the proposal has been met with criticism from various sides, regarding three main points: a) the lack of flexibility regarding (additional) national assessments in light of the aforementioned different standard practices of care which influence comparator therapies, and choice of outcomes, b) the lack of an obligation for the industry to submit full trial data despite increased traction in transparency expectations in recent years and c) the loss of flexibility in decision-making at national level in the presence of a binding assessment (see Panteli & Edwards 2018). In October 2018 the European Parliament presented a series of amendments, inter alia addressing some of these concerns to varying degrees. At the time of writing, consensus with the European Council and the finalization of the legislative process are pending. However, it is safe to assume that there will be at least some major changes in the way HTA is carried out in the years to come.

6.4 The effectiveness and cost-effectiveness of HTA as a quality strategy

As illustrated in previous sections, HTA is defined as information input to policy and other decision-making in healthcare. As such, its "effectiveness" is primarily evaluated based on its ability to support evidence-informed decisions. In general, the impact of HTA is variable and inconsistently understood. A major influencing factor is the directness of the relationship between an HTA programme, policy-making bodies and healthcare decisions (*see* the procedural framework section, above). HTA reports that are translated directly into policies may have clear and quantifiable impacts, such as the evaluation of new pharmaceuticals for inclusion in the positive list, but the findings of other, often well-carried-out HTA reports, may go unheeded or are not readily adopted into general practice. However, even when the reporting of HTA findings is followed by concrete changes, for example, in policy or use of a technology, it may be difficult to demonstrate the causal effect of the HTA on those changes (NIH, 2017).

Gerhardus & Dintsios (2005) and Gerhardus et al. (2008) proposed a hierarchical model for the impact of HTA reports with six distinguishable steps:

1. Awareness of specific HTA reports

2. Acceptance of the reports and their findings

3. Integration of results in policy processes

4. Formulation of policy decisions which are clearly influenced by HTA results

5. Implementation in (clinical) practice

6. Influence on (health or economic) outcomes

Typically, the key targets of HTA are the third and fourth steps. Steps one and two are prerequisites for implementation and often depend on the perceived legitimacy of the HTA programme, while steps five and six are dependent on implementation and dissemination beyond the original purpose of the HTA report. The additional integration of HTA results into implementation in clinical practice and finally its impact on health outcomes are not to be seen as secondary purposes of HTA, since they are of course the ultimate target for all evaluation activity within healthcare services. However, this part of the utilization is mediated by policy- and decision-making. The mandate of HTA organizations is typically limited to handing over evaluation results to the targeted policy-makers, decision-makers or clinicians. Therefore the ability of HTA to affect practice and outcomes to a large degree depends on the course of policy-making processes, the decisions being made and ultimately their degree of implementation. This illustrates that HTA to a large extent can contribute to other quality strategies within healthcare, such as clinical practice guidelines, standards, clinical pathways and disease management programmes.

Historically, systematic attempts to document the dissemination processes and impacts of HTA programmes have been infrequent, despite recognition that monitoring the impact of individual HTAs and HTA programmes is a key principle for the good practice of HTA (Drummond et al., 2008; NIH, 2017). A systematic review of related evidence carried out in 2008 found a high level of awareness but variable acceptance and perception of influencing power over actual (coverage) decisions. It also highlighted that the vast majority of available evidence pertained to countries with a strong, often institutionalized position for HTA and therefore with limited generalizability to other countries (Gerhardus et al., 2008). In the ensuing decade and at least in part due to efforts at EU level (*see* Boxes 6.1 and 6.2), it is safe to assume that at least for some elements, such as awareness, acceptance and embeddedness in the decision-making process, the impact of HTA will have increased. In fact, many factors can affect the impact of HTA reports beyond their formal integration in decision-making practices and the particular dissemination techniques used (for a comprehensive list, see NIH, 2017). Knowledge about these factors can be used prospectively to improve the impact of HTA (*see* implementation section, below).

Given the lack of clear and general evidence of the effectiveness of HTA, there is of course even less evidence and discussion on cost-effectiveness. An international external evaluation of the now-closed Danish HTA agency DACEHTA in 2003 stated that: "The resources that DACEHTA uses are very limited relative to the total cost of the health service. The use of evidence-based analyses offers a considerable potential for efficiency improvement. The overall assessment, therefore, is that DACEHTA is a cost-effective endeavor" (DHA, 2019). A comprehensive evaluation of the impact of the English HTA programme also concludes that "looking at the economy more broadly, the evidence generated by the HTA programme supports the decisions of NICE and can inform the spending and treatment decisions in the NHS more directly, which should increase the cost-effectiveness of care provided in the NHS" (Guthrie et al., 2015). In countries where the results of evaluation (for example, level of added patient benefit offered by new drugs) directly inform pricing negotiations, such as France and Germany, the impact of HTA can be monetized more directly, but the scope of this is not generalizable (as explained above). Finally, it is also difficult to estimate the cost of producing an HTA report, as scope and therefore comprehensiveness vary both within and across countries. Production costs also depend on the necessity for and extent of primary data collection, meaning that for different research questions but also technology types the overall budget might vary considerably. Further European collaboration and coordination of HTA, as described in the previous section, will probably contribute to more information on the cost of producing HTA and experiences across countries on similar assessments may serve as useful benchmarks for also improving productivity of the HTA processes.

6.5 How can HTA be implemented?

As previously mentioned, the implementation of national HTA strategies (programmes) has been an area of focus for both national and European policy. The EU-funded HTA projects described in Box 6.2 are much more focused on developing systems to support the establishment of sustainable HTA organizations and activities in countries with limited HTA experience and capacity, and analysing institutional development of HTA organizations and requirements for successfully integrating HTA in policy-making (see, for example, EunetHTA, 2008, 2009). They found that, beyond the commitment of politicians, policy-makers and other stakeholders, important factors that co-determine the continuous success of HTA programmes include:

- Human resource development: the process of equipping individuals with the understanding, skills and access to information, knowledge and training that enables them to perform effectively;

- Organizational development: the elaboration of management structures, processes and procedures, not only within organizations but also the management of relationships between the different organizations and sectors: public, private and community; and

- Institutional and legal framework development: making legal and regulatory changes to enable organizations, institutions and agencies at all levels and in all sectors to enhance their capacities) (EUnetHTA, 2009).

When analysing the institutional development of HTA organizations and requirements for successfully integrating HTA in policy-making, it is recognised that there is no single model for success (Banta & Jonsson, 2006). Indeed, as previously illustrated, HTA organizations are part of their own respective health system (Velasco-Garrido, Zentner & Busse, 2008; Velasco-Garrido et al., 2008). Funding mechanisms, target audiences, mandates, types and scope of assessments, and relations to decision-makers vary across HTA organizations (Velasco-Garrido et al., 2008). In fact, despite efforts to align and standardize scientific methodologies in European projects, institutional diversity seems decisive for the way HTA can be used in and integrated into other quality improvement strategies.

Stakeholder involvement is an important part of enabling the establishment and continued usefulness of HTA processes. It can help formulate the overall purpose of HTA reports to make sure that the most relevant issues are addressed, and prepare a smooth utilization process of HTA results by improving the legitimacy in relation to different stakeholder groups (Nielsen et al., 2009). Stakeholder involvement in HTA is system-specific and primarily takes place in a national or regional setting related to specific HTA programmes and reports. However, many have not systematized the framework for including stakeholders in HTA work and those institutions that do have reported that while the practice is fruitful, it is very resource intensive (Pichon-Riviere et al., 2017; Brereton et al., 2017). The development of a permanent European network for HTA requires development of structures for stakeholder involvement at an EU level to ensure the relevance of activities and legitimacy and acceptance of developments in the European HTA field.

Setting up a national HTA mechanism is a complicated and resource-intensive exercise that requires a given timeframe to mature and political commitment to be sustainable and effective (Moharra et al., 2009). Even established HTA systems require a certain degree of flexibility to maintain their usefulness and appropriateness, especially in light of the emergence of new technologies that are increasingly accompanied by high price tags (for example, the Hepatitis C treatment breakthrough in 2014 and the recent approval of CAR-T therapies for oncological indications).

Drummond et al. (2008) formulated a set of key principles for best practice in national HTA programmes (summarized in Fig. 6.4). Follow-up work found

Fig. 6.4 *Key principles for the improved conduct of HTA*

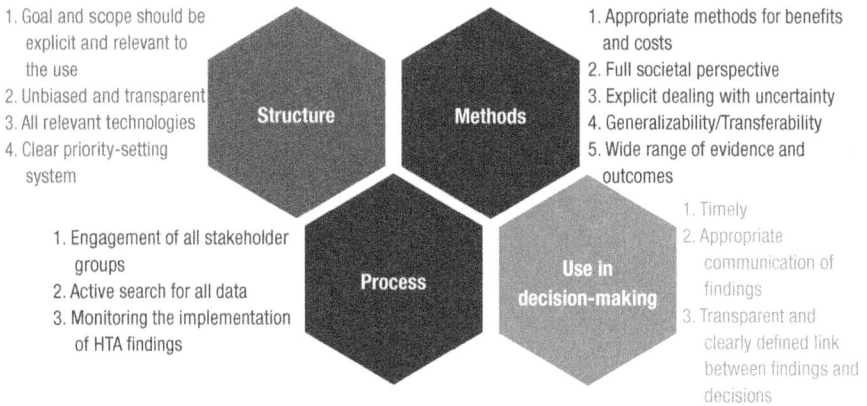

1. Goal and scope should be
   explicit and relevant to
   the use
2. Unbiased and transparent
3. All relevant technologies
4. Clear priority-setting
   system

Structure

Methods

1. Appropriate methods for benefits
   and costs
2. Full societal perspective
3. Explicit dealing with uncertainty
4. Generalizability/Transferability
5. Wide range of evidence and
   outcomes

1. Engagement of all stakeholder
   groups
2. Active search for all data
3. Monitoring the implementation
   of HTA findings

Process

**Use in
decision-making**

1. Timely
2. Appropriate
   communication of
   findings
3. Transparent and
   clearly defined link
   between findings and
   decisions

Source: visualized from Drummond et al., 2008

that these were only partially applied in reality (Neumann et al., 2010; Stephens, Handke & Doshi, 2012). The EUnetHTA Joint Action developed recommendations on overcoming barriers for performing HTA and establishing HTA organizational structures (EUnetHTA, 2011). These are summarized in Box 6.3. Clearly, a number of these principles could apply and are indeed considered in the European Commission's proposal for more formalized collaboration in HTA at the European level; however, additional factors, such as better alignment between evidentiary requirements for marketing approval and HTA as well as the early involvement of stakeholders in this context could play a facilitating role in implementing HTA as a quality assurance strategy.

Indeed, the ISPOR HTA Council Working Group issued a report on Good Practices in HTA in early 2019, pointing out that many good practices have been developed, mostly regarding assessment methodology and certain key aspects of HTA processes, but consensus on good practice is still lacking for many areas, such as defining the organizational aspects of HTA, use of deliberative processes and measuring the impact of HTA (*see* Kristensen et al., 2019, and the discussion above). These findings can help prioritize future work. Many of the areas of priority for further HTA-related research identified by a systematic review in 2011 (Nielsen, Funch & Kristensen, 2011), including disinvestment, evidence development for new technologies, assessing the wider effects of technology use, determining how HTA affects decision-making, and individualized treatments, remain on the table despite the time elapsed.

6.6 Conclusions for policy-makers

HTA's potential to contribute to quality improvement has been clearly demonstrated above. It is not only an important activity that provides the evidence

Box 6.3 *EUnetHTA recommendations for the implementation of HTA at national level (barriers and actions to address them)*

BARRIER: AGREEMENT WITH STAKEHOLDERS

- Identify relevant supporters and opponents regarding organization's place in healthcare system.
- Seek increased assistance of politicians, decision-makers and scientists, establish an ongoing relationship between partners.
- Adjust communication strategy to particular target group.
- Endeavour to regulate uneven data access by legislative initiatives.
- Establish formal processes to disclose conflict of interests.

BARRIER: REACHING POLITICAL INTEREST

- Strengthen trust between scientists and politicians and improve the use of scientific evidence in decision-making through continuous dialogue.
- Define clear position of HTA with regard to the specificity of healthcare system.
- Counteract improper or insufficient use of HTA, which may result in loss of political interest.
- Disseminate HTA products in order to prove their usefulness. Use transparency to make agreement with policy-makers easier to reach. Use different approaches that raise awareness of politicians as beneficiaries of the HTA processes and products.

BARRIER: FUNDING

- Involve HTA in decision-making process to ensure stable funding.
- Prepare an organization-specific business plan that ensures the commitment of relevant parties, helps to minimize risk of failure and facilitate acquirement of funding sources.
- Seek additional sources of funding.
- Use external financial advisers to manage organization's budget.
- Try to precisely determine resources consumed for organization's products. Consider implementation of performance budget or re-negotiations of work-load, regarding organization's stage of development. Avoid competition for funding among institutions by clearly divided responsibilities and seeking cooperation to share work-load.

BARRIER: SHORTAGE OF TRAINED STAFF

- Use various motivating factors to attract people to the organization and protect them from quitting i.e. encouraging salaries, friendly atmosphere at work, stability and prestige, intellectual challenges.
- Create an appropriate sense of mission.
- Invest in people, i.e. ensure appropriate external and internal training.
- Allow flexible hours or part-time working.
- Employ people with experience in other areas and allow them to work part-time.
- Develop new mindsets in the society encouraging building capacity.
- Exchange staff with other institutions, involve external experts, use achievements of others.

base for different levels of decision-making aiming to select safe, effective technologies that provide value for money ("regulating the inputs"), it can also facilitate exchange between various stakeholders and influence processes and – ultimately – outcomes of care.

To achieve good results from an investment in establishing an institutionalized HTA activity, it is necessary to pay close attention to its organization. As described above, an HTA function can be established as a single standing organization or can be integrated into a larger and broader quality improvement organization. Both solutions are viable, but it is decisive to carefully consider the optimal configuration of HTA, depending on the need it aims to meet and the specifics of the system around it. This is preferably achievable by way of a national strategy process since the agreement of all stakeholders and links to policy-making are crucial for impact and thereby return of investment in HTA activities.

In any case, the (re)organization of HTA activities should draw on existing knowledge from the comprehensive experiences with establishing, running and improving the performance of HTA agencies in European countries. Across Europe, different countries have to deal with different challenges, depending on the maturity of their HTA programmes and health system structures. However, it is clear that in the following years, changes at country level will be influenced by European developments. Nevertheless, it is important for national policy-makers to maintain focus on the implementation of HTA findings to the extent that they contribute to quality of care by monitoring and ensuring impact, and likewise to explore potential synergies with other strategies, especially in the realm of evidence synthesis for knowledge translation. Additionally, adapting HTA thinking and methodologies to address the characteristics of new types of technologies, such as digital applications, can be achieved more easily in collaboration. The fundamental principles of HTA and of good governance, including transparency, objectivity, independence of expertise, fairness of procedure and appropriate stakeholder consultations, should not be neglected.

References

Allen N et al. (2013). Development of archetypes for non-ranking classification and comparison of European National Health Technology Assessment systems. *Health Policy*, 113(3):305–12.

Allen N et al. (2017). A Comparison of Reimbursement Recommendations by European HTA Agencies: Is There Opportunity for Further Alignment? *Frontiers in Pharmacology*, 8:384.

Banta HD, Jonsson E (2006). Commentary to: Battista R. Expanding the scientific basis of HTA. *International Journal of Technology Assessment in Health Care*, 22:280–2.

Banta HD, Luce BR (1993). Health Care Technology and its Assessment. Oxford, Oxford Medical Publications (now Oxford University Press).

Banta HD, Kristensen FB, Jonsson E (2009). A history of health technology assessment at the European level. *International Journal of Technology Assessment in Health Care*, 25(Suppl 1):68–73.

Brereton L et al. (2017). Stakeholder involvement throughout health technology assessment: an example from palliative care. *International Journal of Technology Assessment in Health Care*, 33(5):552–61.

Brooks, H (1980). Technology, Evolution, and Purpose. *Daedalus*, 109(1):65–81.

DHA (2019). External evaluation of DACEHTA. Copenhagen: Danish Health Authority. Available at: https://www.sst.dk/en/publications/2003/external-evaluation-of-dacehta#, accessed 14 April 2019.

Drummond MF et al. (2008). Key principles for the improved conduct of health technology assessments for resource allocation decisions. *International Journal of Technology Assessment in Health Care*, 24(3):244–58.

EUnetHTA (2008). EUnetHTA Handbook on Health Technology Assessment Capacity Building. Available at: https://www.eunethta.eu/eunethta-handbook-on-hta-capacity-building/, accessed 14 April 2019.

EUnetHTA (2009). Institutional and performance indicators to assess the level of development of Health Technology Assessment units, programs or agencies. Barcelona: Catalan Agency for Health Technology Assessment and Research.

EUnetHTA (2011). Facilitation of national strategies for continuous development and sustainability of HTA. Available at: https://www.eunethta.eu/ja1-output_facilitation-of-national-strategies-for-continuous-development-and-sustainability-of-hta/, accessed 14 April 2019.

European Commission (2018a). Commission Staff Working Document: Impact Assessment on Strengthening of the EU Cooperation on Health Technology Assessment (HTA), accompanying the document Proposal for a Regulation of the European Parliament and of the Council on health technology assessment and amending Directive 2011/24/EU. Brussels: European Commission.

European Commission (2018b). Proposal for a Regulation of the European Parliament and of the Council on health technology assessment and amending Directive 2011/24/EU. Brussels: European Commission.

Fuchs S et al. (2016). Health Technology Assessment of Medical Devices in Europe: a systematic review of processes, practices and methods in European countries. *International Journal of Technology Assessment in Health Care*, 32(4):1–10.

Gagnon MP et al. (2014). Effects and repercussions of local/hospital-based health technology assessment (HTA): a systematic review. *Systematic Reviews*, 3(129).

Gerhardus A, Dintsios CM (2005). The impact of HTA reports on health policy: a systematic review. *GMS Health Technology Assessment*, 1:Doc02.

Gerhardus A et al. (2008). What are the effects of HTA reports on the health systems? Evidence from the literature. In Velasco-Garrido M et al. (eds.) Health technology assessment and health policy-making in Europe. Current status, challenges and potential. Copenhagen: WHO Regional Office for Europe.

Guthrie S et al. (2015). The impact of the National Institute for Health Research Health Technology Assessment programme, 2003–13: a multimethod evaluation. *Health Technology Assessment*, 19(67):1–291.

INAHTA (2019). INAHTA Members List: Available at: http://www.inahta.org/members/members_list/, accessed 14 April 2019.

Kleijnen S et al. (2015). European collaboration on relative effectiveness assessments: What is needed to be successful? *Health Policy*, 119(5):569–76.

Kristensen FB (2012). Development of European HTA: from Vision to EUnetHTA. *Michael*, 9:147–56.

Kristensen FB et al. (2008). What is health technology assessment? In Velasco-Garrido M et al. (eds.). Health technology assessment and health policy-making in Europe. Current status, challenges and potential. Copenhagen: WHO Regional Office for Europe.

Kristensen FB et al. (2009). European network for Health Technology Assessment, EUnetHTA: Planning, development, and implementation of a sustainable European network for Health Technology Assessment. *International Journal of Technology Assessment in Health Care*, 25(Suppl 2):107–16.

Kristensen FB et al. (2017). The HTA Core Model® – 10 Years of Developing an International Framework to Share Multidimensional Value Assessment. *Value in Health*, 20(2):244–50.

Kristensen FB et al. (2019). Identifying the need for good practices in health technology assessment: summary of the ISPOR HTA Council Working Group report on good Practices in HTA. *Value in Health*, 22(1):13–20.

Lee A, Skött LS, Hansen HP (2009). Organizational and patient-related assessments in HTAs: State of the art. *International Journal of Technology Assessment in Health Care*, 25:530–6.

Luce BR et al. (2010). EBM, HTA, and CER: clearing the confusion. *Milbank Quarterly*, 88(2):256–76.

Moharra M et al. (2009). Systems to support health technology assessment (HTA) in member states of the European Union with limited institutionalization of HTA. *International Journal of Technology Assessment in Health Care*, 25(Suppl 2):75–83.

Neumann P et al. (2010). Are Key Principles for Improved Health Technology Assessment Supported and Used by Health Technology Assessment Organizations? *International Journal of Technology Assessment in Health Care*, 26(1):71–8.

Nielsen CP, Funch TM, Kristensen FB (2011). Health technology assessment: research trends and future priorities in Europe. Journal of Health Services Research and Policy, 16(Suppl 2):6–15.

Nielsen CP et al. (2009). Involving stakeholders and developing a policy for stakeholder involvement in the European Network for Health Technology Assessment, EUnetHTA. *International Journal of Technology Assessment in Health Care*, 25(Suppl 2):84–91.

NIH (2017). HTA 101: IX. MONITOR IMPACT OF HTA. Washington, DC: National Information Center on Health Services Research and Health Care Technology (NICHSR).

O'Donnell JC et al. (2009). Health technology assessment: lessons learned from around the world – an overview. *Value in Health*, 12(Suppl 2):S1–5.

Panteli D, Edwards S (2018). Ensuring access to medicines: how to stimulate innovation to meet patients' needs? Policy brief for the European Observatory on Health Systems and Policies. Copenhagen: WHO Regional Office for Europe.

Panteli D et al. (2015). From market access to patient access: overview of evidence-based approaches for the reimbursement and pricing of pharmaceuticals in 36 European countries. *Health Research Policy and Systems*, 13:39.

Panteli D et al. (2016). Pharmaceutical regulation in 15 European countries: Review. *Health Systems in Transition*, 18(5):1–118.

Pichon-Riviere M et al. (2017). Involvement of relevant stakeholders in health technology assessment development. Background Paper. Edmonton: Health Technology Assessment International.

Sampietro-Colom L, Martin J (eds.) (2016). Hospital-Based Health Technology Assessment. Switzerland: Springer International Publishing.

Stephens JM, Handke B, Doshi J (2012). International survey of methods used in health technology assessment (HTA): does practice meet the principles proposed for good research? *Comparative Effectiveness Research*, 2:29–44.

Velasco-Garrido M, Zentner A, Busse R (2008). Health systems, health policy and health technology assessment. In Velasco-Garrido M et al. (eds.). Health technology assessment and health policy-making in Europe. Current status, challenges and potential. Copenhagen: WHO Regional Office for Europe.

Velasco-Garrido M et al. (2008). Health technology assessment in Europe – overview of the producers. In Velasco-Garrido M et al. (eds.). Health technology assessment and health policy-making in Europe. Current status, challenges and potential. Copenhagen: WHO Regional Office for Europe.

Velasco-Garrido M et al. (2010). Developing Health Technology Assessment to address health care system needs. *Health Policy*, 94:196–202.

WHO (2011). Health Technology Assessment of Medical Devices. WHO Medical Device Technical Series. Geneva: World Health Organization.

Chapter 7

Regulating the input – healthcare facilities

Jonathan Erskine, Grant Mills, Michael Cheng,
Oliver Komma, Dimitra Panteli

Summary

What are the characteristics of the strategy?

The provision of healthcare infrastructure requires agencies to plan and make decisions at different levels. Individual components of the overall infrastructure, which may range from low cost, high volume medical devices to items that require significant investment from capital budgets, are subject to their own requirements and specifications. The arrangement of these components, and of the space within and around a building, is governed by the rules and guidelines contained in regulatory frameworks and embodied in professional expertise. The use of standards and guidelines is recognized as a key component in maintaining and improving quality in healthcare infrastructure. While the term "infrastructure" is often used to encompass all physical, technical and organizational components that are required for the delivery of healthcare services, this chapter focuses on the built environment as a determinant of quality of care. There is a growing body of evidence supporting the notion that the characteristics of the built environment can have a direct impact on quality of care, encompassing the core dimensions of safety, effectiveness and patientcentredness, as well as indirect influence by co-determining staff satisfaction and retention, and cost-effectiveness. The consideration of this evidence in the design of construction or renovation projects has come to be known as "evidence-based design".

What is being done in European countries?

Construction standards in European Union Member States conform to EU-level stipulations for construction products and engineering services: the EN Eurocodes. The Eurocodes apply to the structural design of all public buildings, and refer to geotechnical considerations, fire protection and earthquake protection design, as well as the required properties of common construction materials. However, the planning and design of space within healthcare buildings, and the arrangements made for adjacencies between departments, equipment storage and engineering services, are not amenable to highly prescriptive, European-wide standards. A survey carried out by the European Health Property Network (EuHPN) in 2010 demonstrated that in many countries regulatory systems combine centralized controls (based on non-compliance detection and national benchmarks) and decentralization (based on bottom-up learning, self-adjustment and good practice). Results show that countries range from those that have a central government department role to "arm's-length" national agencies to those countries where healthcare organizations either band together with others to formulate standards or act as independent units, purchasing expert advice as necessary. Some apply a mixed approach, with central government determining standards for some key features of healthcare buildings, but with other, major, design elements left to individual service providers. Germany typifies a different approach, namely that of norms-based best practices rather than rigid top-down standards: healthcare organizations work in close consultation with approved experts and the national institute for standardization to arrive at appropriate standards.

What do we know about the effectiveness and cost-effectiveness of the strategy?

Research has variously demonstrated that the design of healthcare buildings can improve quality in the areas of patient safety (for example, reduction of healthcare-acquired infection rates; patient falls; clinical and medication errors), improved recovery (for example, patient sleep patterns, length of stay), the patient experience (including issues of dignity, privacy, stress levels and overall comfort), and staff satisfaction (for example, recruitment and retention, and absenteeism). The evidence is generally not of high quality and context as well as the patient collective in each case may influence related benefits. Layout design, visibility and accessibility levels are the most cited aspects of design which can affect the level of communication and teamwork in healthcare facilities, impacting patient outcomes and efficiency. Purely structural changes, such as type of airflow and optimizing the auditory and visual environment, is also expected to have some effect on patient outcomes; the evidence is also generally positive but not robust enough for unequivocal conclusions. In light of the expansive evidence base and its inconsistent nature, making the business case for evidence-based design in healthcare is not always straightforward.

How can the strategy be implemented?

It is important to consider both new projects and the upkeep and upgrading of existing infrastructure. Furthermore, the importance of involving users and staff in the planning and design of renovations or new construction has been gaining attention; eliciting opinion in participatory approaches can be facilitated by visual aids. Inclusive, iterative processes for designing the built environment have been developed, for instance to support patient safety. Sustainable and "green" practices should be included in new standard considerations, especially given accumulating findings from the wider research agenda; having said that, balancing sustainability considerations with the primary goal of evidence-based design (for example, safety improvement) needs to be approached with care. The differences in standard development and use described in this chapter mean that homogeneous planning, design and construction cannot be expected across countries; however, it would be helpful to have a common, overarching framework that could be used as a basis to improve the quality, safety, cost-effectiveness and patient-centredness of the healthcare estate. Such a framework would first and foremost necessitate that healthcare providers in all countries have access to agencies that provide information and evidence about different stages in the design process.

Conclusions for policy-makers

In the context of improving the quality of care, addressing the quality of the physical infrastructure of healthcare systems must be a significant concern. Where quality strategies could once be applied separately to the individual elements of healthcare infrastructure, it is now apparent that it should be subject to a more overarching quality management strategy that takes account of the total effect of investment in integrated healthcare infrastructure. This would require that countries have accessible agencies that facilitate the different functions pertinent in each stage, bring together and share resources and facilitate the wider capture and dissemination of evidence between private and public sector institutions and wider stakeholders. Where such expertise is not available at national, regional or local level, policy-makers should consider how best to develop this faculty. Given the general lack of conclusive evidence on different design elements, fostering the creation of a robust evidence base that informs and is informed by new projects seems necessary. The digital transformation currently under way in healthcare provision in most settings can be a contributing factor – as well as a new design attribute – in achieving this goal.

7.1 Introduction: design of healthcare facilities and its contribution to healthcare quality

Across Europe healthcare systems face multiple and familiar challenges: the need to adapt to changing population health needs, the burden of chronic illness, the implications of a long-lasting European financial crisis, increasing costs, and public expectation of more effective and efficient care (see, for example, Busse et al., 2010; Suhrcke et al., 2005). Against this backdrop, policy-makers and healthcare organizations are under pressure to improve the quality of care, and other chapters in this book consider how this can best be achieved across a number of domains. This chapter is concerned with quality in relation to the physical infrastructure of healthcare systems. While the term "infrastructure" is often used to encompass "the total of all physical, technical and organizational components or assets that are prerequisites for the delivery of health care services" (Scholz, Ngoli & Flessa, 2015), this chapter focuses on the built environment as a determinant of quality of care (*see also* WHO, 2009). The regulation of other technical aspects, such as medical equipment, is already partially addressed in Chapters 4 and 6; Box 7.3 at the end of this chapter briefly highlights relevant aspects in relation to medical devices.

Beginning in the 1990s, there is a growing body of evidence supporting the notion that the characteristics of the built environment can have a direct impact on quality of care, encompassing the core dimensions of safety, effectiveness and patient-centredness, as well as indirect influence by co-determining staff satisfaction and retention and cost-effectiveness (AHRQ, 2007). The consideration of this evidence in the design of construction or renovation projects has come to be known as "evidence-based design". According to the US Agency for Health Research and Quality, evidence-based design is "a term used to describe how the physical design of health care environments affects patients and staff" (AHRQ, 2007). It has become an established concept for quality improvement in healthcare architecture (Anåker et al., 2016) and is linked to the concept of the "healing environment" or "healing architecture" (wherein "the interaction between patient and staff produces positive health outcomes within the physical environment"; Huisman et al., 2012).

In the area of safety the most common elements considered in evidence-based design are the prevention of (1) patient falls and their sequelae (for example, by better planning of handrail placement, door opening size and decentralizing nursing stations for faster response); (2) hospital-acquired infections (HAI; for example, by optimizing sink placement and ventilation systems and providing single patient rooms as opposed to wards); and (3) medication errors (for example, by ensuring appropriate lighting and space availability for prescription filling). Furthermore, several design elements have been associated with better patient outcomes and an improved patient experience. Reducing hospital noise reduces stress and can improve and expedite patient recovery. A similar mechanism of action has been attributed to elements such as adequate natural light as well as visual and auditory comfort (for example, by means of artwork or music) towards improving patient outcomes and reducing length of stay (AHRQ, 2007; Huisman et al., 2012; Anåker et al., 2016). Design for easier navigation around the healthcare environment and increased privacy and space for interacting with family and caregivers can also contribute to a better patient experience and facilitate better quality of care (AHRQ, 2007). Finally, the design qualities of the healthcare built environment can be critical for patient safety associated with medical devices (*see also* Cheng et al., 2019a). Box 7.1 highlights attributes of the built environment and their potential for contributing to quality of care and overall performance (*see* Chapter 1 for the distinction between the two concepts).

Essentially, evidence-based design accounts for human and behavioural factors, and their effects on patient care. As an application of systems science, it is an important complement to the medical science underpinning the delivery of care (Clancy, 2013). Given the high public profile of healthcare infrastructure, and the adverse consequences of failing to commission, procure and manage it intelligently, it is important that strategies to improve quality in this area are given the same consideration and status as those concerned with, for example, clinical practice, disease management, workforce development and deployment, or certification, audit and inspection. The provision of healthcare infrastructure requires agencies to plan and make decisions at different levels. Individual components of the overall infrastructure, which may range from low cost, high volume medical devices to items that require significant investment from capital budgets, are subject to their own requirements and specifications. The arrangement of these components, and of the space within and around a building, is governed by the rules and guidelines contained in regulatory frameworks and embodied in professional expertise. The distribution of healthcare infrastructure across a locality, region or country is also influenced by evidence concerning issues of access and equity, safety, current clinical practice and workforce – but this dimension is largely outside the scope of this chapter.

The use of standards and guidelines is recognized as a key component in maintaining and improving quality in healthcare infrastructure, since they provide a baseline for comparison between different options and may variously embody minimum requirements, professionally endorsed rules of thumb, and examples of best practice in relation to safety, the patient experience and cost-effectiveness.

Linking the considerations outlined above to the five-lens framework for quality strategies outlined in Chapter 2 of this book, regulating facilities on the principles of evidence-based design can impact all three core dimensions of

---

Box 7.1 *Aspects of quality and performance and potential influences from the built environment*

Patient-centeredness, including

- using variable-acuity rooms and single-bed rooms
- ensuring sufficient space to accommodate family members
- enabling access to health care information
- having clearly marked signs to navigate the hospital

Safety, including

- applying the design and improving the availability of assistive devices to avert patient falls
- using ventilation and filtration systems to control and prevent the spread of infections
- using surfaces that can be easily decontaminated
- facilitating hand washing with the availability of sinks and alcohol hand rubs
- preventing patient and provider injury
- addressing the sensitivities associated with the interdependencies of care, including work spaces and work processes

Effectiveness, including

- use of lighting to enable visual performance
- use of natural lighting
- controlling the effects of noise

Efficiency, including

- standardizing room layout, location of supplies and medical equipment
- minimizing potential safety threats and improving patient satisfaction by minimizing patient transfers with variable-acuity rooms

Timeliness, by

- ensuring rapid response to patient needs
- eliminating inefficiencies in the processes of care delivery
- facilitating the clinical work of nurses

Equity, by

- ensuring the size, layout, and functions of the structure meet the diverse care needs of patients

Source: Henriksen et al., 2007, as cited in Reiling, Hughes & Murphy, 2008

---

quality (safety, effectiveness and patient-centredness); while it can address all areas of care, the bulk of the literature on healing architecture pertains to acute care ("getting better"). The main activity consists of setting standards (third lens) for the structures of care. Indeed, while this strategy primarily focuses on structures to ultimately improve outcomes of care, it also has the potential to influence processes of care, for example by decentralizing nursing stations or changing from wards to a single-room structure, which also contribute to outcome improvement. This is much in line with Donabedian's understanding of his structure-process-outcome triad (fourth lens). Depending on the set-up of the health system and the project at hand, the targets of the strategy will vary.

The rest of this chapter is structured to first give an overview of the current use of quality standards and guidelines for healthcare infrastructure across Europe and their management and governance. It then looks at the evidence on the effectiveness and cost-effectiveness of evidence-based design and how its principles can be implemented in the construction and renovation of healthcare facilities, primarily in the European context. It wraps up with relevant conclusions for policy-makers.

7.2 What is being done in Europe?

The term "standard" is used across many disciplines, and may variously refer to rules, regulations, specifications, guidance or examples of best practice. The expected degree of compliance, and the relative authority of the standard, largely depends on context and common understanding. Where a standard is referred to in legislation (for example, in relation to public safety) it may have mandatory force, but usually it is a reference point that allows individuals and organizations to have confidence that an object or process is fit-for-purpose. In general, standards are often categorized as being focused on inputs ("how?"), outputs ("what?"), or outcomes ("why?") and these distinctions are important in considering the effect on the quality of healthcare infrastructure.

Standards or guidelines that traditionally specify inputs are sometimes thought to have the advantage of providing sufficient detail to deliver safety through consensus, lower risk and an easier means to check compliance. However, it is also said that this approach may hinder creativity and innovation and, after all, provide less predictability of output/outcome than is claimed. Input standards require considerable maintenance to remain up-to-date and relevant. Furthermore, since they include detailed technical specifications, the risk of the project rests with the commissioning entity entirely. Output standards often focus on performance targets and require a greater level of checking and enforcement during implementation. These standards are less specific in terms of technical detail, and enforcement costs may be higher. The risk for project success partially shifts to the contractor. Finally, standards based on the description of desired outcomes seek to define the positive end goals of regulation. This approach has the advantage of prioritizing patient and end user needs, and may encourage more innovative practice. On the flip side, due to the lack of detailed specifications, both competing bids and the success of the final project are difficult to evaluate. In practice, decisions about healthcare infrastructure will make use of a mix of the above approaches, and stakeholders must consider their use and integration through the lens of diverse infrastructure evidence bases. Box 7.2 provides an example of the three types of standards for clarity.

Construction standards in European Union Member States conform to EU-level stipulations for construction products and engineering services: the EN Eurocodes. The Eurocodes were requested by the European Commission and developed by the European Committee for Standardization. They are a series of 10 European Standards providing a framework for the design of buildings and other civil engineering works and construction products. They are recommended to ensure conformity with the basic requirements of the Construction Products Regulation (Regulation 305/2011 of the European Parliament and of the Council of 9 March 2011, laying down harmonized conditions for the marketing of construction products and repealing Council Directive 89/106/EEC); they are also the pre-ferred reference for technical specifications in public contracts in the European Union. The Eurocodes apply to the structural design of all public buildings, and refer to geotechnical considerations, fire protection and earthquake protection design, as well as the required properties of common construction materials. Fig. 7.1 shows the links between the different Eurocodes.

Box 7.2 *Examples of different types of specifications for building a bridge*

- Input specification: materials to be used and their depth and consistency; volume of asphalt required; applicable standards/regulations for these materials; methods of preparing the surfaces; detailed bill of quantities, plans and schedule.
- Output specification: description of desired outcome – a bridge that has a hard surface, which is 2m wide and has a warranty of workmanship and materials.
- Outcome specification: explanation of the reasons for commissioning the project, e.g. need to provide the shortest and most convenient means of pedestrian access from the main road to the entrance of an office block, which would allow 500 pedestrians to use it simultaneously between the hours of 06:00 to 19:00 on working days.

Source: based on James, 2018

With the exception of some fundamental issues concerning fire and public safety, the planning and design of space within healthcare buildings, and the arrangements made for adjacencies between departments, equipment storage and engineering services, are not amenable to highly prescriptive, European-wide standards. The properties of construction materials and the individual compo-nents of facilities (taps, door handles, roof tiles, flooring materials, etc.) can be closely specified to satisfy regulations on safety and durability, but the higher level features of healthcare facilities – the arrangement of public and staff areas, wards, laboratories, outpatient departments, reception halls and car parks – are influenced by local custom and tradition, financial pressures and the preferences of those who commission, design, build and maintain the infrastructure. Nonetheless, country-specific or regional standards and guidelines are commonly used to orient and direct the commissioners, planners, designers and constructors of healthcare facilities.

Fig. 7.1   *Overview and link between Eurocodes*

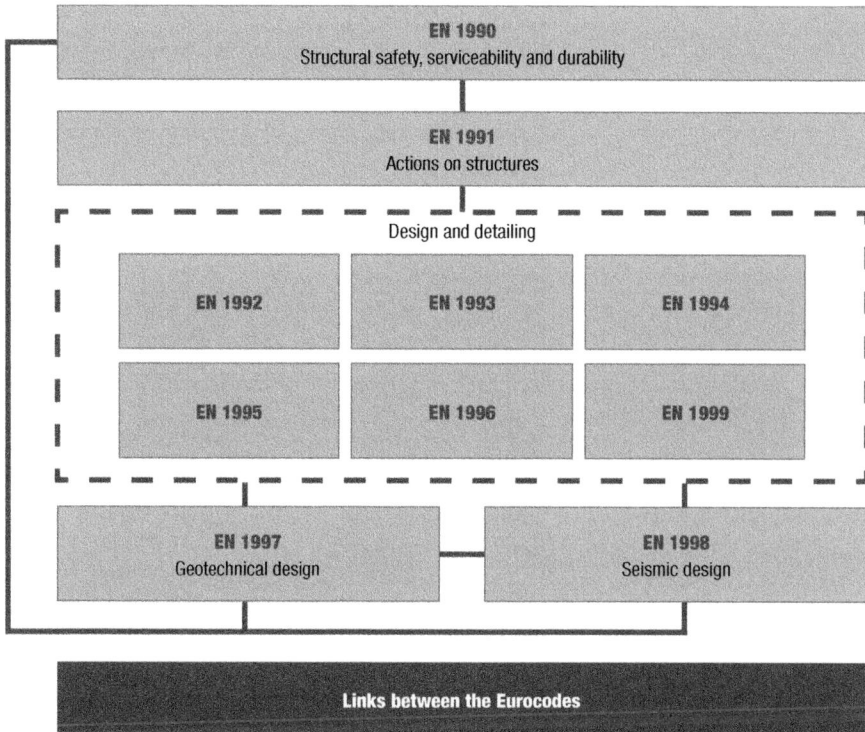

Source: European Commission Joint Research Centre, 2018

Notes: EN 1992 – Concrete; EN 1993 – Steel; EN 1994 – Composite; EN 1995 – Timber; EN 1996 – Masonry; EN 1999 – Aluminium.

It is instructive to compare and contrast the existing differences between European countries in this area to better understand policy options. Following the mandatory transposition of the Eurocodes in 2010, the European Health Property Network (EuHPN) carried out a survey among 11 EU Member States (Finland [FI], Germany [DE], Hungary [HU], Ireland [IE], Italy [IT], Latvia [LV], the Netherlands [NL], Norway [NO], Poland [PL], Romania [RO] and the UK region of Northern Ireland [GBNI]), which included Australia [AU] as an international point of reference (EuHPN, 2011). The survey remains the most comprehensive comparative work today. It reviewed the use of health building standards and guidelines to answer questions about:

- The nature of the standards (incorporating guidelines and indications of best practice) in use for planning and designing healthcare buildings;

- The governance structures that regulate standards and underpin their authority;

- Recent changes to national approaches to standards; and

- The amount of freedom available to individual healthcare organizations when deciding which standards to follow.

The following sections synthesize the survey responses in terms of what they say about the overall nature of infrastructure regulatory systems across Europe.

7.2.1 Regulatory systems for healthcare buildings

The survey demonstrated that in many countries regulatory systems combine centralized controls (based on non-compliance detection and national benchmarks) and decentralization (based on bottom-up learning, self-adjustment and good practice). Systems balance many factors such as: competency, culture, standards development and maintenance, risk, stakeholder power/influence and opportunities for escalation to create smart and responsive assurance frameworks.

Results show that countries range from those that have a central government department role to "arm's-length" national agencies (PL, RO, HU, IE, LV) to those countries where healthcare organizations either band together with others to formulate standards (AU, NL) or act as independent units, purchasing expert advice as necessary (NO). In some cases (for example, FI) there was evidence of a mixed approach, with central government determining standards for some key features of healthcare buildings, but with other, major, design elements left to individual service providers. Fig. 7.2 summarizes the key features of building regulation systems and strategies employed across Europe and sets them against the backdrop of what a learning, responsive system of healthcare infrastructure would entail. There is considerable variability in approach and limited evidence of which system forms the best practice. Mandatory building guidelines often coincided with a National Health Building Quality Assurance and Compliance/Approval organizational structure (GBNI, PL, RO). However, there were occasions where regional or local organizations had devolved responsibilities (FI, DE, IE) and also developed standards and guidance. Different approaches were sometimes apparent (NO) where minimal standards or organizational structures were in place, but were rather guided by professional private expertise and an independent national agency.

7.2.2 Differences in Country Building Standards

Most European countries had mandatory general building standards, with some supporting these with health-specific complete standards sets (for example, UK). Additional clauses, criteria or statements (for example, PL) and private sector supply chain expertise (for example, NO) provided smarter networked regulatory systems. In other countries there was greater cross-sector working to differentiate between health-specific and generic building standards (for example, FI). In the UK hospitals have some flexibility in deciding what proportion of patient accommodation should be in single-bed rooms. However, Northern Ireland has adopted a region-wide mandatory policy of 100% single-bed patient accommodation in new buildings, based on principles of patient dignity and privacy, and infection control.

Some countries apply norms-based best practices rather than rigid top-down standards. Germany typifies this approach, in that healthcare organizations work in close consultation with approved experts and the national institute for standardization (DIN – Deutsches Institut für Normung) to arrive at appropriate standards. For instance, standard DIN 13080 guides the division of hospitals into functional areas and functional sections (DIN, 2016) and rests on the more general standard DIN 277-1 on constructing the areas and volumes of buildings. Other countries put more emphasis on input and output performance specifications, such as energy use, air flow, adaptability of work spaces, levels of natural light, disability access, lifecycle costs and environmental sustainability. Finland reported using a mix of some basic mandatory standards together with performance requirement specifications, managed by stakeholder networks. Countries that operate a market-oriented (or "market-like") healthcare system generally revealed a more flexible, open approach. For example, the Netherlands reported that, apart from requirements that may be imposed by the funder, health estates professionals are free to explore new concepts. The response from Germany was similar – there is freedom in design as long as financial and technical conditions are met.

7.2.3 Changing Regulatory Systems

As health systems change, so, too must the means to ensure that quality of care – including the built environment – is maintained. For instance, Dutch hospitals were largely de-coupled from direct state oversight in tandem with the deregulation of the Dutch healthcare insurance market in 2006 (Kroneman et al., 2016) and this process was matched by the 2010 demise of the National Board for Healthcare Institutions (NBHI), which had been the central authority for setting standards and approving hospital infrastructure projects. Hospitals in the Netherlands now have to source infrastructure capital through banks and the financial markets, and therefore make business cases – including provision for the quality of planning, design and construction, lifecycle costing, etc. – on the basis of return on investment, just as any commercial organization would. In general terms there is a trend towards decentralization of the agencies responsible for setting and overseeing standards for design and planning.

Fig. 7.2 *Overview of regulatory systems for healthcare buildings in European countries*

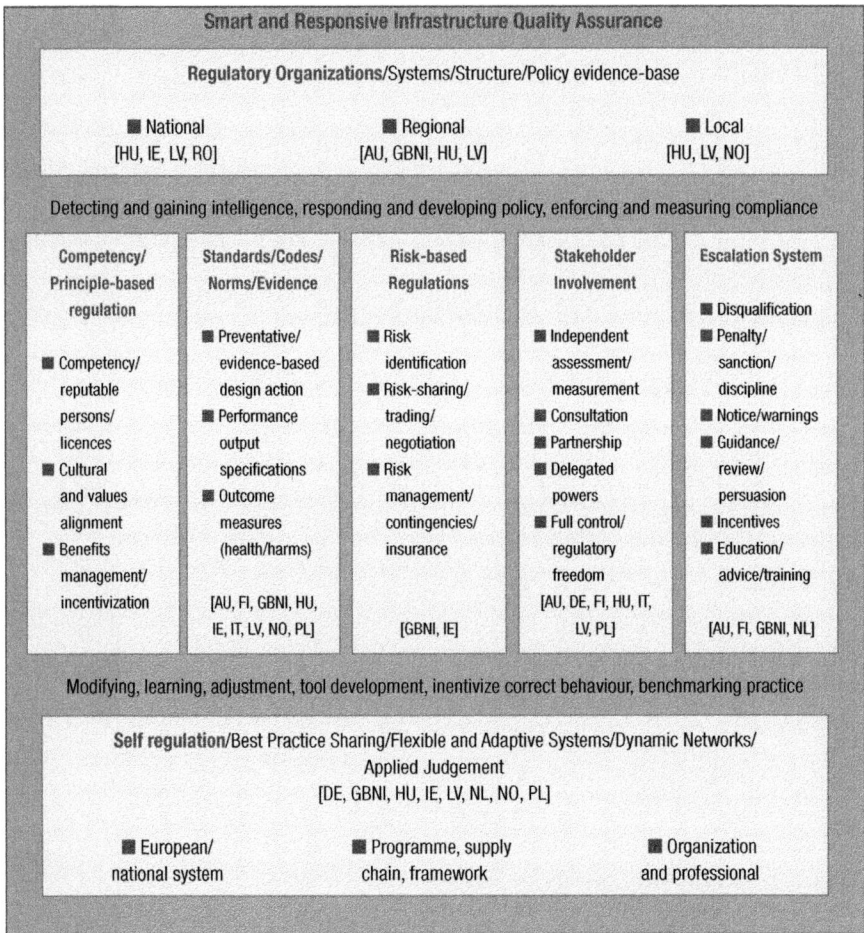

Smart and Responsive Infrastructure Quality Assurance

Regulatory Organizations/Systems/Structure/Policy evidence-base

- National
[HU, IE, LV, RO]
- Regional
[AU, GBNI, HU, LV]
- Local
[HU, LV, NO]

Detecting and gaining intelligence, responding and developing policy, enforcing and measuring compliance

Competency/ Principle-based regulation	Standards/Codes/ Norms/Evidence	Risk-based Regulations	Stakeholder Involvement	Escalation System
■ Competency/ reputable persons/ licences ■ Cultural and values alignment ■ Benefits management/ incentivization	■ Preventative/ evidence-based design action ■ Performance output specifications ■ Outcome measures (health/harms) [AU, FI, GBNI, HU, IE, IT, LV, NO, PL]	■ Risk identification ■ Risk-sharing/ trading/ negotiation ■ Risk management/ contingencies/ insurance [GBNI, IE]	■ Independent assessment/ measurement ■ Consultation ■ Partnership ■ Delegated powers ■ Full control/ regulatory freedom [AU, DE, FI, HU, IT, LV, PL]	■ Disqualification ■ Penalty/ sanction/ discipline ■ Notice/warnings ■ Guidance/ review/ persuasion ■ Incentives ■ Education/ advice/training [AU, FI, GBNI, NL]

Modifying, learning, adjustment, tool development, inentivize correct behaviour, benchmarking practice

Self regulation/Best Practice Sharing/Flexible and Adaptive Systems/Dynamic Networks/
Applied Judgement
[DE, GBNI, HU, IE, LV, NL, NO, PL]

- European/ national system
- Programme, supply chain, framework
- Organization and professional

Finland, for example, reported a process towards more individual and independent decision-making, using a mix of external expert advice and guidance, since the early 1990s. Italy has seen significant devolution of responsibility for healthcare provision to its regions since the late 1990s (Erskine et al., 2009), and this has coincided with development of regional norms and requirements for hospital functionality. Poland and Romania have made little change in the recent past, and little is expected in the near future. In Hungary a number of regulations are intended to specify only requirements, and their associated frameworks, to encourage unencumbered architectural design, based on the joint knowledge of the facility designer and the healthcare facility management. Northern Ireland is undergoing increasing centralized standard setting, as a region small enough to plan centrally.

7.3 The effectiveness and cost-effectiveness of the built environment as a quality strategy

7.3.1 Effectiveness of evidence-based design

As mentioned in the introduction to this chapter, the relationship between health facility design and the effectiveness, safety and patient-centredness of the built environment has been researched extensively, and research outcomes have often influenced the development of regulations, standards and guidelines. Primary research and systematic reviews, mainly in the field of evidence-based design, have variously demonstrated that the design of healthcare buildings can improve quality in the areas of patient safety (for example, reduction of healthcare-acquired infection rates; patient falls; clinical and medication errors), improved recovery (for example, patient sleep patterns, length of stay), the patient experience (including issues of dignity, privacy, stress levels and overall comfort), and staff satisfaction (for example, recruitment and retention, and absenteeism).

Ulrich et al. (2008) compiled a comprehensive overview of design elements and their effects, categorizing outcomes in three categories: patient safety, other patient outcomes and staff outcomes. Their work aimed to guide healthcare design (especially with respect to reducing the frequency of hospital-acquired infections) and identified a number of rigorous studies to support the importance of improving outcomes for a range of design elements, including "single-bed rooms, effective ventilation systems, a good acoustic environment, nature distractions and daylight, appropriate lighting, better ergonomic design, acuity-adaptable rooms, and improved floor layouts and work settings" (Ulrich et al., 2008). Table 7.1 summarizes their findings.

Newer research provides continuous insights into a number of these aspects, although the evidence often remains inconclusive. For example, Taylor, Card & Piatkowski (2018) published a systematic review on single-occupancy patient rooms (SPRs), concluding that "overall, 87% of studies reported advantages

Table 7.1 *Summary of the relationships between design factors and healthcare outcomes*

Design Strategies or Environmental Interventions / Healthcare Outcomes	Single-bed rooms	Access to daylight	Appropriate lighting	Views of nature	Family zone in patient rooms	Carpeting	Noise-reducing finishes	Ceiling lifts	Nursing floor layout	Decentralized supplies	Acuity-adaptable rooms
Reduced hospital-acquired infections	**										
Reduced medical errors	*		*				*				*
Reduced patient falls	*		*		*	*			*		*
Reduced pain		*	*	**			*				
Improved patient sleep	**	*	*				*				
Reduced patient stress	*	*	*	**	*		**				
Reduced depression		**	**	*	*						
Reduced length of stay		*	*	*							*
Improved patient privacy and confidentiality	**				*		*				
Improved communication with patients and family members	**				*		*				
Improved social support	*				*	*					
Increased patient satisfaction	**	*	*	*	*	*	*				
Decreased staff injuries								**			*
Decreased staff stress	*	*	*	*			*				
Increased staff effectiveness	*		*				*		*	*	*
Increased staff satisfaction	*	*	*	*			*				

Source: Ulrich et al., 2008

associated with SPRs (some a combination of advantages and disadvantages or a combination of advantages and neutral results). Outcomes with the best evidence of benefit include communication, infection control, noise reduction/perceived sleep quality, and preference/perception. [Thus], SPRs seem to result in more advantages than disadvantages." They also highlighted that these advantages need to be considered in conjunction with other planning issues, such as necessary workflow modifications, staffing models and inherent trade-offs between privacy and isolation (Taylor, Card & Piatkowski, 2018). This is in line with preceding work, which found that staff perceived worsening of visibility and surveillance, teamwork and remaining close to the patients after changing into a single patient room configuration (Maben et al., 2015a).

For low acuity patients, a different systematic review found that the best quality evidence did not support the use of SPRs for reducing infections, minimizing patient falls, reducing medication errors or improving patient satisfaction (Voigt, Mosier & Darouiche, 2018). Patient acuity refers to a patient's requirements for nursing care, or in other words the number and composition of staff required to ensure good care (Jennings, 2008). Higher acuity necessitates more resources for safe and effective care. So called "acuity-adaptable" patient rooms have been conceptualized as a care model to reduce errors in communication, patient disorientation, dissatisfaction and falls, as a patient is cared for in the same room throughout the care process regardless of their level of acuity. Most of the literature shows a positive impact of the acuity-adaptable patient room on patients (Bonuel & Cesario, 2013) and on the experience of a "healing environment" (Kitchens, Fulton & Maze, 2018). However, the evidence is generally not of high quality, and both context and the patient collective in each case may influence related benefits (Costello et al., 2017).

Other design elements influencing processes of care with the intention of ultimately affecting patient safety outcomes include the positioning of sinks and disinfecting agents for handwashing as well as the decentralization of nursing stations within departments. On the former, recent work has shown that placing of more, easily visible sinks in a surgical transplant unit was associated with improved adherence to handwashing (Zellmer et al., 2015), while increasing distance between the patient zone and the nearest sink was inversely associated with handwashing compliance (Deyneko et al., 2016). Positioning accessible disinfectant dispensers near the patient's bed significantly improved hand hygiene compliance (Stiller et al., 2017). On the latter, while there is no consistent categorization of nurse station typology or standard definition for decentralized nursing stations, there seems to be a positive trend towards patient experience in units with decentralized nurse stations (Fay, Cai & Real, 2018). A survey identified more specific information regarding the effects of nursing floor layout on process outcomes, concluding that "high-performing rooms were generally located a medium distance from the nurse station, with the patient's right side facing the entry door (right-handed), the bed orientation located within the room, and the hand-wash sink facing the patient" (MacAllister, Zimring & Ryherd, 2018). Layout design, visibility and accessibility levels are the most cited aspects of design which can affect the level of communication and teamwork in healthcare facilities, impacting patient outcomes and efficiency (Gharaveis, Hamilton & Pati, 2018; Gharaveis et al., 2018). In fact, a switch to decentralized nurse stations was shown to lead to a perception of decline in nursing teamwork (Fay, Cai & Real, 2018).

All the design elements discussed so far have some component of influencing process of care along with redefining structures. However, purely structural changes are also expected to have some effect on patient outcomes. For instance, determining the best ventilation system for operating rooms can influence the incidence of surgical site infections. A recent systematic review showed no benefit of laminar airflow compared with conventional turbulent ventilation in reducing the risk for infection, and concluded that it should not be considered as a preventive measure (Bischoff et al., 2017). In terms of optimizing the auditory and visual environment for inpatients, the evidence is also generally positive but not robust enough for unequivocal conclusions. A systematic review on noise reduction interventions published in 2018 highlighted this dearth of reliable studies; while concluding that noise reduction interventions are feasible in ward settings and have potential to improve patients' in-hospital sleep experiences, the evidence is insufficient to support the use of such interventions at present (Garside et al., 2018). Work on ICU rooms with windows or natural views found no improvement in outcomes of in-hospital care for general populations of medical and surgical ICU patients (Kohn et al., 2013). At the same time, a systematic review focusing on the effects of environmental design on patient outcomes and satisfaction saw that exposure to particular audio (music and natural sounds) and visual (murals, ornamental plants, sunlight) design interventions contributed to a decrease in patients' anxiety, pain and stress levels (Laursen, Danielsen & Rosenberg, 2014).

7.3.2 Cost-effectiveness of evidence-based design

In light of the expansive evidence base and its inconsistent nature (*see* previous section and Malkin, 2008), making the business case for evidence-based design in healthcare is not always straightforward. Indeed, designing a new or updated facility using the principles described above may add up-front capital costs. However, the prevailing notion is that this investment ultimately decreases medical and financial complications that can result from a poorly designed facility, leading to speedily recouped additional investments (AHRQ, 2007). Sadler, DuBose

& Zimring (2008) point out that, as a result, "central to the business case is the need to balance one-time construction costs against ongoing operating savings and revenue enhancements". They also provide a comprehensive framework for decision-makers to estimate which interventions make sense within their own construction or renovation project and how investment to implement them will be offset by operational gains down the road (Sadler, DuBose & Zimring, 2008).

Individual research projects have focused on balancing efficiency gains with the intended improvement in healthcare outcomes and required investment (see, for instance, Shikder & Price, 2011). For instance, a quasi-experimental before-and-after study of a transformation to 100% single rooms in an acute hospital found that an all single-room hospital can cost 5% more (with higher housekeeping and cleaning costs) but the difference is marginal over time (Maben et al., 2015b). Operational efficiencies improved with SPRs in a maternity ward as well (Voigt, Mosier & Darouiche, 2018), supporting the savings assumption. While ICU rooms with windows or natural views were not found to reduce costs of in-hospital care, they also did not increase them (Kohn et al., 2013). Laursen, Danielsen & Rosenberg (2014) argued that interventions to ameliorate the auditory and visual environment for patients are arguably inexpensive and easily implemented, and therefore feasible in most hospitals. In their framework, Sadler, DuBose & Zimring (2008) differentiate between interventions that all facilities can implement without investing too many resources and those requiring more careful consideration. We reproduce these two clusters in Table 7.2.

7.4 How can facility design be implemented to improve quality of care?

The previous sections already included preliminary considerations about the feasibility of including different elements of evidence-based design into routine construction and/or renovation practices. Indeed, it is important to consider both new projects and the upkeep and upgrading of existing infrastructure. Mills et al. (2015b) highlighted the low rate of new-build replenishment (estimated at less than 4% of the total NHS estate) in the UK, where many existing healthcare buildings suffer from under-investment in maintenance and require significant upgrading (Mills et al., 2015b).

Furthermore, the importance of involving users and staff in the planning and design of renovations or new construction has been gaining attention (Csipke et al., 2016). Involving visual aids to elicit opinion in participatory approaches also merits consideration. Dickerman & Barach described an inclusive, iterative process for designing the built environment to support patient safety, shown in Fig. 7.3 (Dickerman & Barach, 2008). They provide a number of tangible first considerations for organizations and funders to consider, highlighting that

Table 7.2 *Cost-effective interventions by project scope*

Design interventions	Quality and Business-Case Benefits
DESIGN INTERVENTIONS THAT ANY HOSPITAL CAN UNDERTAKE	
1 Install handwashing dispensers at each bedside and in all high-patient-volume areas	Reduced infections
2 Where structurally feasible, install HEPA filters in areas housing immunosuppressed patients	Reduced airborne-caused infections
3 Where feasible, install ceiling-mounted lifts	Reduced staff back injuries
4 Conduct a noise audit and implement a noise-reduction plan	Reduced patient and staff stress; reduced patient sleep deprivation; increased patient satisfaction
5 Install high-performance sound-absorbing ceiling tiles	Reduced patient and staff stress; reduced patient sleep deprivation; increased patient satisfaction
6 Use music as a positive distraction during procedures	Reduced patient stress; reduced patient pain and medication use
7 Use artwork and virtual-reality images to provide positive distractions	Reduced patient stress; reduced patient pain and medication use
8 Improve wayfinding through enhanced signage	Reduced staff time spent giving directions; reduced patient and family stress
DESIGN INTERVENTIONS AS PART OF CONSTRUCTION OR MAJOR RENOVATION	
1 Build single-patient rooms	Reduced infections; increased privacy; increased functional capacity; increased patient satisfaction
2 Provide adequate space for families to stay overnight in patient rooms	Increased patient and family satisfaction; reduced patient and family stress
3 Build acuity-adaptable rooms	Reduced intra-hospital transfers; reduced errors; increased patient satisfaction; reduced unproductive staff time
4 Build larger patient bathrooms with double-door access	Reduced patient falls; reduced staff back injuries
5 Install HEPA filtration throughout patient-care areas	Reduced airborne-caused infections
6 Install handwashing dispenser at each bedside and in all high-patient-volume areas	Reduced infections
7 Install ceiling-mounted lifts in majority of patient rooms	Reduced staff back injuries
8 Meet established noise-level standards throughout the facility	Reduced patient and staff stress; reduced patient sleep deprivation; increased patient satisfaction
9 Use music as a positive distraction during procedures	Reduced patient stress; reduced patient pain and medication use
10 Provide access to natural light in patient and staff areas	Reduced patient anxiety and depression; reduced length of stay; increased staff satisfaction
11 Use artwork and virtual-reality images to provide positive distractions	Reduced patient and staff stress; reduced patient pain and medication use
12 Build decentralized nursing stations	Increased staff time spent on direct patient care
13 Include effective wayfinding systems	Reduced staff time spent on giving instructions; reduced patient and family stress

Source: Sadler, DuBose & Zimring, 2008

large and diverse design teams have the best chance of producing healthcare environments that are conducive to patient safety and function as healing environments. However, managing such teams requires strong leadership – a theme which reappears throughout the literature on evidence-based design (*see also* Anåker et al., 2016).

Fig. 7.3   *Design process model by Dickerman & Barach (2008)*

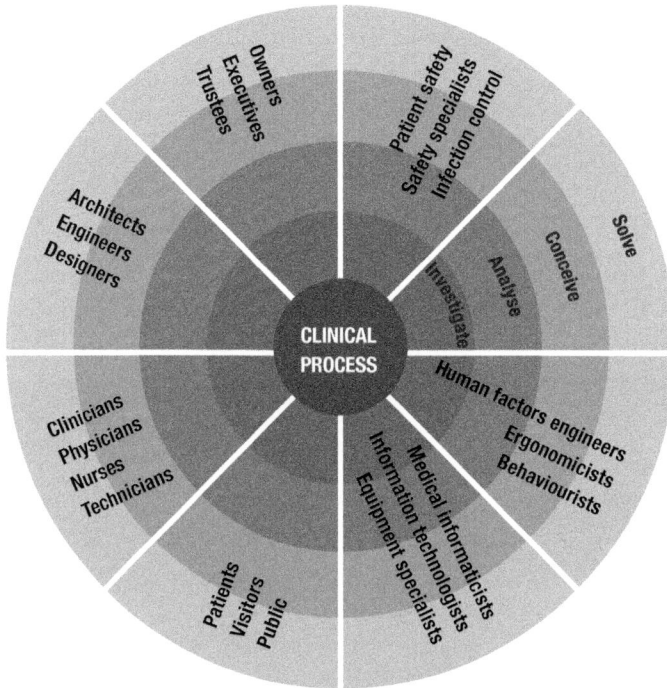

Note: the tenets of this model are: multidisciplinary approach; collaboration essential; patient safety; efficiency and effectiveness; clinical and operational process at the core; good design resonates with the people it serves.

Conceptual work on the meaning of "good quality design" for healthcare facilities found that there were three main themes emerging from the literature regarding perceptions of what the concept can entail: environmental sustainability and ecological values; social and cultural interactions and values; and resilience of engineering and building construction (Anåker et al., 2016). While the latter two elements have been discussed in previous sections, the first theme has not been at the forefront of this chapter's focus. However, it is important to note that sustainable and "green" practices should be included in new standard considerations, especially given accumulating findings from the wider research agenda; having said that, balancing sustainability considerations with the primary goal of evidence-based design (for example, safety improvement) needs to be approached with care (Anåker et al., 2016; Wood et al., 2016).

To support the implementation of evidence-based design, the Center for Health Design in California launched a credentialling programme called Evidence-based Design Assessment and Certification (EDAC) in 2008. The programme aims to ensure that design professionals, healthcare planners and healthcare organization management teams are familiar with how to identify research, create hypotheses, and gather, implement and report the data associated with their projects (Malkin et al., 2008). Key components of EDAC certification include meaningful collaboration with the client/users, recognizing and responding to the unique context of each project, using best available credible evidence from a variety of sources, using critical thinking to interpret the implications of the research on design decisions, understanding the need to protect public safety and health and fostering commitment to share findings with the community (Malkin, 2008). According to the Center for Health Design, EDAC is not reserved for designers, project planners and managers only. It is also useful for researchers and engineering and construction professionals, as well as product manufacturers (CHD, 2018).

Regarding the role of policy-makers at national, regional or local levels in implementing facility standards, it is critical that they understand and play a role in the effect of the built environment on quality of care. The section on existing and changing standards and practice in Europe demonstrated that a one-size-fits-all strategy would probably not be successful given the level of variability. Planning, design and construction practices for healthcare infrastructure vary widely across Europe. Different approaches to the use of standards and guidelines are in place, and there is an uneven distribution of skills and resources for developing and applying quality standards. While local context and history are important in relation to health buildings, and we cannot expect homogeneous planning, design and construction, it would be helpful to have a common, overarching framework that could be used as a basis to improve the quality, safety, cost-effectiveness and patient-centredness of the healthcare estate. Such a framework would first and foremost necessitate that healthcare providers in all countries have access to agencies that provide information and evidence about different stages in the design process. In some countries such agencies may already exist (in national or regional health departments, for example), while in others the same functions may be supplied by a network of Research and Development centres. Where such expertise is not available at national, regional or local level, policy-makers should consider how best to develop this faculty. Such a strategy has echoes in the medical devices sector, where, for example, an updated Clinical Engineering Handbook provided a "systems management framework" which clarified the responsibilities of the stakeholders in choosing, implementing, using and managing the lifecycle of a broad range of medical devices (Cheng et al., 2019b; *see also* Box 7.3).

Box 7.3 *Quality of medical devices as part of healthcare infrastructure*

Medical devices, like drugs, are indispensable for healthcare. But unlike drugs, medical devices span a vast range of different physical forms – from walking sticks and syringes to centrifuges and Magnetic Resonance Imaging (MRI) machines. They also differ from drugs in being even more dependent on user skills to achieve desired outcomes (or to produce undesired effects): the role of the user and engineering support are crucial in ensuring their ultimate safety and performance. Furthermore, many medical devices (for example, imaging and laboratory equipment) represent durable, reusable investments in health facilities.

In Europe the current quality standards of medical devices are provided by the relevant EC Directives, which focus on ensuring product safety and performance (*see also* Chapter 4). Responsibilities are imposed on the manufacturers to comply with regulatory requirements in designing, producing, packaging and labelling their products. The manufacturer is also required to maintain the quality of the device in the delivery process to the consumer as well as conduct post-market surveillance, adverse event reporting, corrective action and preventive action. The effectiveness and safety of medical devices is also increasingly evaluated in the context of Health Technology Assessment (*see* Chapter 6).

Medical device regulations govern manufacturers to ensure *product* safety, but this does not extend to the use of medical devices to ensure *patient* safety. HTA usually evaluates technologies for reimbursement purposes. An overarching framework for the management of medical devices through their lifecycle from the perspective of quality and safety is not formally in place in Europe; Fig. 7.4 highlights important responsibilities to be considered regarding medical device safety in healthcare organizations (*see also* Chapter 11).

Fig. 7.4 *Three-step framework for medical devices – associated patient safety*

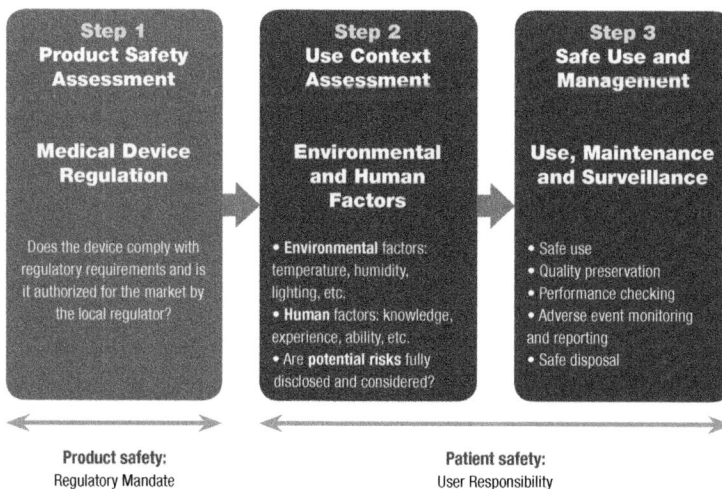

Step 1 Product Safety Assessment	Step 2 Use Context Assessment	Step 3 Safe Use and Management
Medical Device Regulation	Environmental and Human Factors	Use, Maintenance and Surveillance
Does the device comply with regulatory requirements and is it authorized for the market by the local regulator?	• **Environmental** factors: temperature, humidity, lighting, etc. • **Human** factors: knowledge, experience, ability, etc. • Are **potential risks** fully disclosed and considered?	• Safe use • Quality preservation • Performance checking • Adverse event monitoring and reporting • Safe disposal

Product safety:
Regulatory Mandate

Patient safety:
User Responsibility

Source: Cheng et al., 2019a and 2019b

Mills et al. (2015a) explored such an approach for the UK context specifically, especially in light of developments in the country (for example, constrained resources and reorganization of the NHS), which saw a gradual departure from traditional command-and-control arrangements (Mills et al., 2015a). The scenarios explored in this context represent different degrees of devolution of responsibility and are shown in Fig. 7.5. The study further highlighted the need for adaptable, responsive standards to keep up with emerging evidence within a learning system, stating that "there are clear opportunities for meta- and self-regulation regimes and a mix of interventions, tools and networks that will reduce the burden of rewriting standards … and create a wider ownership of building design quality standards throughout the supply chain". For the UK context, the study authors reiterate the importance of leadership (already mentioned above) and conclude that redefining and strengthening successful models of central responsibility in healthcare building design quality improvement strategy, fostering the development and adoption of open and dynamic standards, guidance and tools, and supporting the development of the evidence base to underpin tools for quality improvement are of crucial importance. Despite its context-specific scope, this approach can be adopted in other countries, accounting for system particularities.

Fig. 7.5   *Future national healthcare building design quality improvement scenarios in the UK explored by Mills et al. (2015a)*

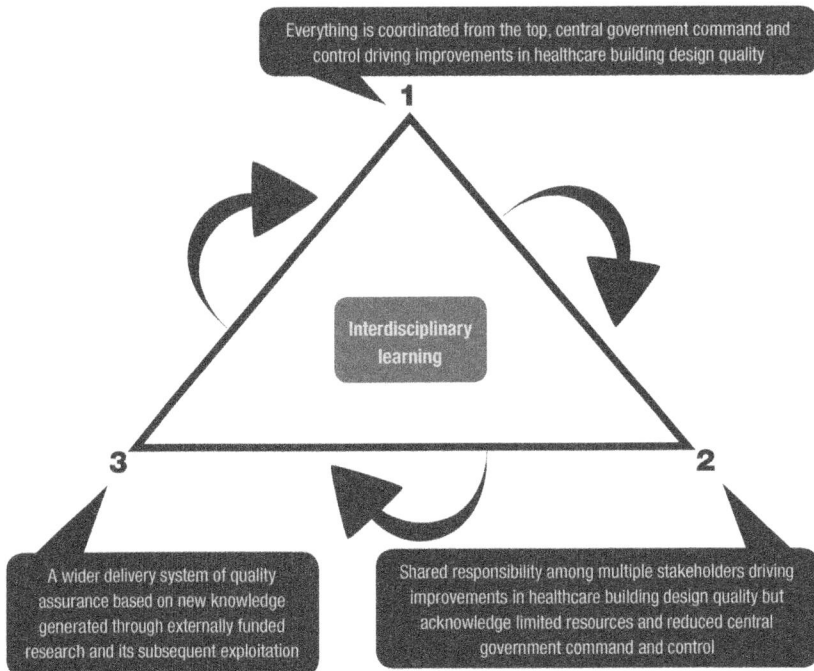

Given the issues discussed in this chapter for the productivity and effectiveness of healthcare infrastructure, it is helpful to know where to find the evidence and research outcomes. Table 7.3 at the end of the chapter contains a listing of selected, web-based information sources in English.

7.5 Conclusions for policy-makers

Policy-makers and healthcare organizations are under pressure to improve the quality of care, and so addressing the quality of the physical infrastructure of healthcare systems must be a significant concern. Healthcare buildings must be integrated and so where quality strategies could once be applied separately to the individual elements of healthcare infrastructure, each with its own processes for planning, commissioning, procurement and maintenance, it is now apparent that healthcare infrastructure should be subject to a more overarching quality management strategy that takes account of the total effect of investment in integrated healthcare infrastructure. This would require that countries have accessible agencies that facilitate the different functions pertinent in each stage, bring together and share resources and facilitate the wider capture and dissemination of evidence between private and public sector institutions and wider stakeholders. Where such expertise is not available at national, regional or local level, policy-makers should consider how best to develop this faculty.

The evidence on the effectiveness and cost-effectiveness of different design elements in the context of quality is expansive but largely inconclusive. Fostering the creation of a robust evidence base that informs and is informed by new projects seems necessary. The digital transformation currently under way in healthcare provision in most settings can be a contributing factor – as well as a new design attribute – in achieving this goal.

Table 7.3   *Selected health facility information resources*

Organization	Website	Areas covered
Centre for Health Design (USA and international)	http://www.healthdesign.org/	Improving patient outcomes through design; better quality healthcare facilities; environments for healthy ageing.
Sykehusbygg (Norway)	http://sykehusbygg.no/	Healthcare planning and physical development of somatic and psychiatric hospitals. Interests in pre- and post-occupancy evaluation, innovation and knowledge transfer.
TNO: the Netherlands' Organization for Applied Scientific Research	https://www.tno.nl/en/	Among other R&D fields, TNO is active in healthcare research and consultancy specializing in health services configuration, strategic demand prognoses, services organization, functional design of health facilities, integrated business case analysis and strategic responses to societal changes posed by demographic change.

Table 7.3   *Selected health facility information resources [continued]*

Organization	Website	Areas covered
THL (National Institute for Health and Welfare; Finland)	http://www.thl.fi/en_US/web/en/home	Interior design of hospitals; the hospital as a healing environment; virtual design tools. Website has a well-populated database of papers and reports on evidence-based design for healthcare infrastructure and ehealth.
European Health Property Network (EuHPN)	http://www.euhpn.eu/	EuHPN is a knowledge-sharing network comprising government health estates departments and other R&D centres with interests in planning, financing and designing healthcare buildings.
Architects for Health (AfH, UK)	https://www.architectsforhealth.com/	AfH is a non-profit organization for those interested in improving health and well-being through healthcare design, underpinned by a membership of design and related professionals.
Centrum för vårdens arkitektur (CVA, Sweden)	https://www.chalmers.se/sv/centrum/cva/Sidor/default.aspx	The Centre for Healthcare Architecture (CVA) is a national arena for the creation, translation, exchange and dissemination of knowledge about healthcare architecture. As an academic centre, CVA conducts research and research training, and contributes with basic and further training in the field. The research focus for CVA is buildings and physical environments as a support and a part of the interaction between healthcare, patients and architecture.
The Bartlett Real Estate Institute, UCL (BREI, UK)	https://www.ucl.ac.uk/bartlett/real-estate/about-us	BREI is part of UCL's faculty of the built environment, focused on interdisciplinary research, education and enterprise – including the design, planning, investment and management of healthcare facilities and projects; sustainable building design and the health and well-being of occupants; and, at the urban scale, public health and the built environment.
Health Facilities Scotland	http://www.hfs.scot.nhs.uk/	Health Facilities Scotland (HFS) plays a key national role in the development and publication of national operational policy, standards, strategy and technical guidance for NHSScotland in relation to non-clinical professional healthcare subjects in the following areas: Property and Capital Planning; Engineering; Environment and Decontamination.
Società Italiana Dell'Architettura e Dell-Ingegneria per la Sanità (Italian Society of Healthcare Architecture and Engineering, SIAIS)	http://www.siais.it/	A non-profit organization which brings together professionals involved in the engineering, architecture and policy considerations relating to all kinds of health and healthcare buildings.
European Healthcare Design Congress, Exhibition and Awards, London, UK	www.europeanhealthcaredesign.eu	Annual international congress, awards and exhibition dedicated to sharing and disseminating global knowledge in the research, practice and policy of designing and planning health systems and services, technology and the built environment, organized by SALUS Global Knowledge Exchange in collaboration with Architects for Health.

Table 7.3   *Selected health facility information resources [continued]*

Organization	Website	Areas covered
SALUS Global Knowledge Exchange	www.salus.global	An online global knowledge community with a vision to improve human and planetary health by design. SALUS publishes an online journal covering news, policy, markets, comment and research, including all the videos of talks and posters from its international events, European Healthcare Design and Healthy City Design. SALUS also features a fully searchable map of over 500 healthcare facility projects from around the world.

References

AHRQ (2007). Transforming Hospitals: Designing for Safety and Quality. AHRQ Publication No. 07-0076-1. Rockville, Maryland, USA: Agency for Healthcare Research and Quality.

Anåker A et al. (2016). Design Quality in the Context of Healthcare Environments: A Scoping Review. *Health Environments Research & Design Journal*, 10(4):136–50.

Bischoff P et al. (2017). Effect of laminar airflow ventilation on surgical site infections: a systematic review and meta-analysis. *Lancet Infectious Diseases*, 17(5):553–61.

Bonuel N, Cesario S (2013). Review of the literature: acuity-adaptable patient room. *Critical Care Nursing Quarterly*, 36(2):251–71.

Busse R et al. (2010). Tackling Chronic Disease in Europe: Strategies, Interventions and Challenges. Brussels: European Observatory on Health Systems and Policies.

CHD (2018). Evidence-Based Design Accreditation and Certification (EDAC). Available at: https://www.healthdesign.org/certification-outreach/edac, accessed on 31 September 2018.

Cheng M et al. (2019a). Medical Device Regulations and Patient Safety. In: Iadanza E (ed.). Clinical Engineering Handbook. Amsterdam: Elsevier.

Cheng M et al. (2019b). A systems management framework for medical device safety and optimal outcomes. In: Iadanza E (ed.). Clinical Engineering Handbook. Amsterdam: Elsevier.

Clancy CM (2013). Creating a healing environment. *Health Environments Research and Design Journal*, J(7):5–7.

Costello JM et al. (2017). Experience with an Acuity Adaptable Care Model for Pediatric Cardiac Surgery. World *Journal for Pediatric and Congenital Heart Surgery*, 8(6):665–71.

Csipke E et al. (2016). Design in mind: eliciting service user and frontline staff perspectives on psychiatric ward design through participatory methods. *Journal of Mental Health*, 25(2):114–21.

Deyneko A et al. (2016). Impact of sink location on hand hygiene compliance after care of patients with Clostridium difficile infection: a cross-sectional study. *BMC Infectious Diseases*, 16:203.

Dickerman KN, Barach P (2008). Designing the Built Environment for a Culture and System of Patient Safety – a Conceptual, New Design Process. In: Henriksen K et al. (eds.). Advances in Patient Safety: New Directions and Alternative Approaches (Vol. 2: Culture and Redesign). Rockville, Maryland, USA: Agency for Healthcare Research and Quality.

DIN (2016). Standard 13080: "Division of hospitals into functional areas and functional sections". Available at: https://www.din.de/en/getting-involved/standards-committees/nabau/standards/wdc-beuth:din21:252635669/toc-2582257/download, accessed on 31 September 2018.

Erskine J et al. (2009). Strategic Asset Planning: an integrated regional health care system, Tuscany, Italy. In: Rechel B et al. (eds.). Capital Investment in Health: Case Studies from Europe. Copenhagen: WHO on behalf of the European Observatory on Health Systems and Policies.

EuHPN (2011). Guidelines and Standards for Healthcare Buildings: a European Health Property Network Survey. Durham: European Health Property Network.

Fay L, Cai H, Real K (2018). A Systematic Literature Review of Empirical Studies on Decentralized Nursing Stations. *Health Environments Research & Design Journal*, doi: 10.1177/1937586718805222 [Epub ahead of print].

Garside J et al. (2018). Are noise reduction interventions effective in adult ward settings? A systematic review and meta analysis. *Applied Nursing Research*, 44:6–17.

Gharaveis A, Hamilton DK, Pati D (2018). The Impact of Environmental Design on Teamwork and Communication in Healthcare Facilities: A Systematic Literature Review. *Health Environments Research & Design Journal*, 11(1):119–37.

Gharaveis A et al. (2018). The Impact of Visibility on Teamwork, Collaborative Communication, and Security in Emergency Departments: An Exploratory Study. *Health Environments Research & Design Journal*, 11(4):37–49.

Henriksen K et al. (2007). The role of the physical environment in crossing the quality chasm. *Joint Commission Journal on Quality and Patient Safety*, 33(11 Suppl):68–80.

Huisman ERCM et al. (2012). Healing environment: a review of the impact of physical environmental factors on users. *Building and Environment*, 58:70–80.

James S (2018). The Smart Way to use Input, Output and Outcome Specifications to get the Most from your Suppliers. Available at: http://www.bestpracticegroup.com/input-output-outcome-specifications/, accessed on 31 October 2018.

Jennings BM (2008). Patient Acuity. In: Hughes RG (ed.). Patient Safety and Quality: An Evidence-Based Handbook for Nurses. Rockville, Maryland, USA: Agency for Healthcare Research and Quality.

Kitchens JL, Fulton JS, Maze L (2018). Patient and family description of receiving care in acuity adaptable care model. *Journal of Nursing Management*, 26(7):874–80.

Kohn R et al. (2013). Do windows or natural views affect outcomes or costs among patients in ICUs? *Critical Care Medicine*, 41(7):1645–55.

Kroneman M et al. (2016). The Netherlands: health system review. *Health Systems in Transition*, 18(2):1–239.

Laursen J, Danielsen A, Rosenberg J (2014). Effects of environmental design on patient outcome: a systematic review. *Health Environments Research & Design Journal*, 7(4):108–19.

Maben J et al. (2015a). Evaluating a major innovation in hospital design: workforce implications and impact on patient and staff experiences of all single room hospital accommodation. Southampton (UK): NIHR Journals Library.

Maben J et al. (2015b). One size fits all? Mixed methods evaluation of the impact of 100% single-room accommodation on staff and patient experience, safety and costs. *BMJ Quality & Safety*, 25(4):241–56.

MacAllister L, Zimring C, Ryherd E (2018). Exploring the Relationships Between Patient Room Layout and Patient Satisfaction. Health Environments Research & Design Journal, doi: 10.1177/1937586718782163 [Epub ahead of print].

Malkin J (2008). A Visual Reference to Evidence-Based Design. Concord, California, USA: The Center for Health Design. ISBN-10: 0974376361.

Mills G et al. (2015a). Rethinking healthcare building design quality: an evidence-based strategy. *Building Research & Information*, 43(4):499–515.

Mills G et al. (2015b). Critical infrastructure risk in healthcare trusts in England: Predicting the impact of trust building portfolio age on the national condition of NHS assets. *International Journal of Strategic Property Management*, 19(2):159–72.

Reiling J, Hughes RG, Murphy MR (2008). The Impact of Facility Design on Patient Safety. In: Hughes RG (ed.), Patient Safety and Quality: An Evidence-Based Handbook for Nurses. Rockville, Maryland, USA: Agency for Healthcare Research and Quality.

Sadler BL, DuBose J, Zimring C (2008). The business case for building better hospitals through evidence-based design. *Health Environments Research & Design Journal*, 1(3):22–39.

Scholz S, Ngoli B, Flessa S (2015). Rapid assessment of infrastructure of primary health care facilities – a relevant instrument for health care systems management. *BMC Health Services Research*, 15:183.

Shikder S, Price A (eds.) (2011). Design and Decision Making to Improve Healthcare Infrastructure. Loughborough: Loughborough University.

Stiller A et al. (2016). Relationship between hospital ward design and healthcare-associated infection rates: a systematic review and meta-analysis. *Antimicrobial Resistance and Infection Control*, 29(5):51.

Suhrcke M et al. (2005). The contribution of health to the economy in the European Union. Brussels: Office for Official Publications of the European Communities.

Taylor E, Card AJ, Piatkowski M (2018). Single-Occupancy Patient Rooms: A Systematic Review of the Literature Since 2006. *Health Environments Research & Design Journal*, 11(1):85–100.

Ulrich RS et al. (2008). A Review of the Research Literature on Evidence-Based Healthcare Design. *Health Environments Research & Design Journal*, 1(3):61–125.

Voigt J, Mosier M, Darouiche R (2018). Private Rooms in Low Acuity Settings: A Systematic Review of the Literature. *Health Environments Research & Design Journal*, 11(1):57–74.

WHO (2009). Guidelines on Hand Hygiene in Health Care: First Global Patient Safety Challenge Clean Care Is Safer Care. Appendix 1, Definitions of health-care settings and other related terms. Geneva: World Health Organization.

Wood L et al. (2016). Green hospital design: integrating quality function deployment and end-user demands. *Journal of Cleaner Production*, 112(1):903–13.

Zellmer C et al. (2015). Impact of sink location on hand hygiene compliance for Clostridium difficile infection. *American Journal of Infection Control*, 43(4):387–9.

Chapter 8

External institutional strategies: accreditation, certification, supervision

Charles Shaw, Oliver Groene, Elke Berger

Summary

What are the characteristics of the strategy?

Accreditation, certification and supervision are quality strategies that intend to encourage the compliance of healthcare organizations with published standards through external assessment. The idea is that healthcare organizations will increase compliance with standards in advance of a planned external inspection. Despite several common characteristics of the three strategies, their origins and initial objectives differ. In general, accreditation refers to the external assessment of an organization by an accreditation organization, leading to the public recognition of the organization's compliance with pre-specified standards. The term certification is usually used in relation to external assessment of compliance with standards published by the International Organization for Standardization (ISO). Supervision means the monitoring of healthcare providers' compliance with minimum standards required for statutory (re)registration, (re-)authorization or (re)licensing.

What is being done in European countries?

External assessment strategies have been widely implemented in Europe. Most countries make use of several strategies, including basic supervision as part of the licensing process for healthcare providers, coupled with certification or accreditation strategies to ensure and improve the quality of care. The scope of these strategies and their regulation differs substantially between countries (and partly between regions of the same country) with regard to the type of standards and assessment, frequency of assessment, level of compliance required or implications of failing to meet standards. There is (still) no register of accredited, certified or licensed healthcare organizations in Europe.

What do we know about the effectiveness and cost-effectiveness of the strategy?

Despite the widespread uptake of external assessment strategies, there is little robust evidence to support their effectiveness and there is a complete absence of evidence on cost-effectiveness. Existing research focuses on healthcare accreditation and little is published on the effects of certification or supervision.

How can the strategy be implemented?

Due to the broad range of external assessments' purposes and given the lack of consensus in the use of terminology, implementation strategies are sparse or missing. However, several facilitators and barriers have been identified that may affect implementation of external assessment strategies in a healthcare organization. These include organizational culture, commercial incentives or staff engagement and communication. Moreover, political, if not financial, support from government is essential, especially in smaller countries.

Conclusions for policy-makers

Policy-makers need to assess the available evidence cautiously. Potentially, external assessment strategies have a positive effect on the organization of professional work and on patient health. However, evidence on the strategies' effectiveness, in whatever form, is not necessarily the determining factor explaining the widespread use of these strategies in Europe. More important might be that external assessments respond to the need of policy-makers, professional associations and potential patients to know that quality in healthcare is under control. In light of the considerable investment in often expensive external assessment strategies, decision-makers should support research into the comparative effectiveness of these strategies, also to better understand the effectiveness of different components of external assessment strategies.

8.1 Introduction: the characteristics of external assessment strategies

Across Europe the interest in external assessment strategies has grown substantially in the last two decades, driven by the requirements and pressures to achieve public accountability, transparency and quality improvement (Shaw, 2001; Alkhenizan & Shaw, 2011; Lam et al., 2018). However, there is wide variation across and sometimes even within countries with regard to the purpose of external assessment, ranging from assessment of compliance with basic regulation (market entry), through assessment of compliance with basic standards (quality assurance) to more comprehensive approaches to improving the quality of care. In addition, there is a lack of consensus in the use of terminology and what might be labelled certification in one context may be called accreditation in another (WHO, 2003).

This chapter focuses on three external assessment strategies: (a) accreditation, (b) certification and (c) supervision. These strategies have at least four common characteristics. First, they usually focus on healthcare provider organizations, not individuals or training programmes. (This chapter ignores the certification of professionals, which is discussed in Chapter 5.) In addition, the focus on organizations distinguishes external assessment strategies from audit and feedback strategies, which usually focus on individual healthcare professionals (*see* Chapter 10). Secondly, all three strategies usually focus on organizational structures and service delivery processes (more than on resource inputs) – an important difference from regulatory strategies (*see* Chapters 5 and 7). Thirdly, they involve assessment against published standards and criteria. And lastly, the aim of all three strategies is to improve safety and quality of care.

Despite these common characteristics, the origin and initial objectives of the three strategies differ considerably. Fig. 8.1 summarizes some of the most important differences between accreditation, certification and supervision, which are related to the origin of the standards against which providers are assessed, the governance of the programme, the assessment bodies, the assessment methods and the output of the assessment. More details are provided in Table 8.1.

In general, *accreditation* refers to the external assessment of an organization by an accreditation body, leading to the public recognition of the organization's compliance with pre-specified standards (WHO, OECD, World Bank, 2018). Accreditation programmes were originally developed and led by healthcare managers and clinicians, and were fully independent of government. Over time, accreditation has become more closely related to governments. In many countries governments have established their own accreditation programmes or are important stakeholders in accreditation bodies. Nevertheless, most healthcare accreditation bodies are usually accountable to an autonomous governing body. Accreditation bodies develop and maintain standards specific to the organization and provision of healthcare – and these standards are fairly consistent worldwide. The improvement process is primarily "bottom-up", based on self-governance, self-assessment, peer review and professional self-regulation. Reports present a

Fig. 8.1 *Key differences between external assessment strategies*

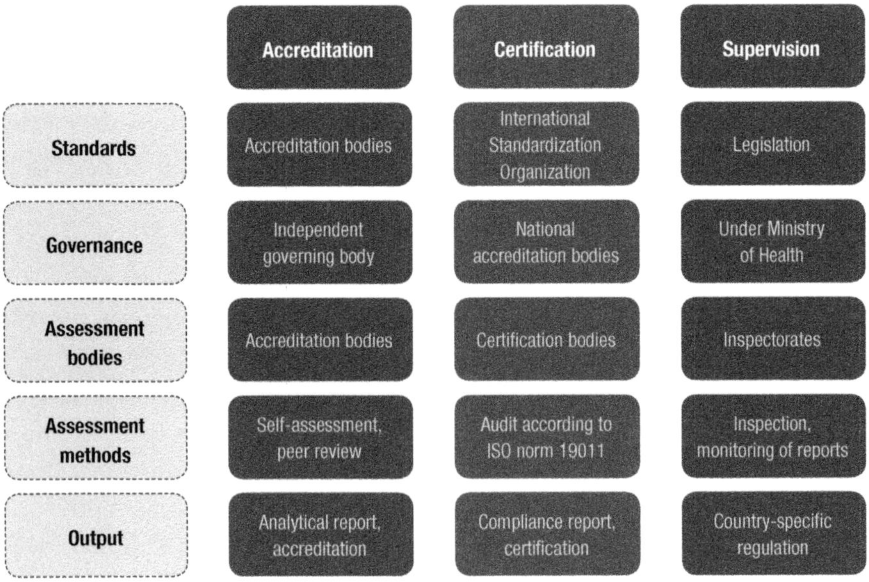

	Accreditation	Certification	Supervision
Standards	Accreditation bodies	International Standardization Organization	Legislation
Governance	Independent governing body	National accreditation bodies	Under Ministry of Health
Assessment bodies	Accreditation bodies	Certification bodies	Inspectorates
Assessment methods	Self-assessment, peer review	Audit according to ISO norm 19011	Inspection, monitoring of reports
Output	Analytical report, accreditation	Compliance report, certification	Country-specific regulation

Source: authors' own compilation

management analysis and recommendations for improvement. Positively assessed healthcare organizations are awarded an accreditation.

The term *certification* is usually used in relation to external assessment of compliance with standards published by the International Organization for Standardization (ISO). Since its commencement in 1946, the ISO provides standards, initially within the European manufacturing industry but now worldwide, and also for quality management in healthcare, against which organizations may be certified. Certification bodies (CBs) are independent of government, but have to be recognized by national accreditation bodies (NABs), which themselves have to be recognized by the national government. Compliance with standards is assessed by accredited auditors through audits that are performed according to ISO 19011 guidelines for auditing of quality management systems. Reports indicate areas of compliance and non-compliance as assessed by the auditor(s), but they do not include recommendations for improvement. A certificate of compliance with ISO 9001 is issued by the CB based on the auditors' report.

The term *supervision* refers to an authoritative monitoring of healthcare providers' compliance with minimum standards required for statutory (re)registration, (re-)authorization or (re)licensing. Standards are set by legislation often with a focus on environmental safety, for example, fire, hygiene, radiation and pharmaceuticals. The purpose is to exclude unsafe providers from the healthcare market. Most supervision programmes also aim for improvement in quality and safety

Table 8.1   *Comparing characteristics of external assessment strategies*

Accreditation	Certification	Supervision
Relation to Health Ministries		
• programmes originated from healthcare managers and clinicians, independent of government • now in Europe one third are governmental, one third independent, and one third hybrids	• certification bodies (CBs) are independent of government • CBs have to be recognized by national accreditation bodies (NABs) • NABs must be recognized by national government, not the Ministry of Health (MoH)	• supervisory bodies and inspectorates are commonly within the MoH, or established as separate regulatory agencies
Governance and stakeholder representation		
• the "average" healthcare accreditation body (AB) is accountable to an autonomous governing body • many stakeholders are included, for example, patients, professionals and insurers	• CBs cover a wide range of products, goods and services; a few focus mainly on healthcare • CBs are regulated by the NABs	• inspectorates are agents of government • supervisory organizations are directly or indirectly under the MoH or the Ministry of Social Affairs
Funding		
• many ABs developed with government funding • later often became self-financing through sales of assessment, training and development services	• CBs are commercial entities • rely on income from services provided	• funded primarily from government • additional income from fees for licensing or registration of providers
Standards, criteria for assessment		
• standards specific to healthcare • developed and maintained by ABs • principles and requirements of standards fairly consistent worldwide • structure, measurement criteria, scoring systems and assessment processes vary • most programmes update standards every two to three years	• standards developed by national standards institutes, the Comité Européen de Normalisation (CEN) and ISO • the ISO 9000 series for quality management is not specific to healthcare • ISO norm 15224, introduced in 2012, is specific for healthcare quality management • all ISO standards are revised every five years	• standards based on legislation at local, regional or national level • may incorporate legislation at European and international level (especially for radiation protection)

systems, such as infection control, medicine management, reporting of adverse events (to an external national body) and comparisons of performance between providers (Eismann, 2011). Supervisory bodies originally focused on periodic inspections of all healthcare facilities, unannounced visits and ad hoc responsive investigation. Many now are using other methods to target attention to priority concerns. In general, methods, assessor competences and duration of licences are subject to country specific regulations (*see* Table 8.1).

Table 8.1   *Comparing characteristics of external assessment strategies [continued]*

Accreditation	Certification	Supervision
Assessment methods		
• originally: internal self-assessment followed by periodic, scheduled on-site visits by peer review teams • now: often also self-reporting of implementation of recommendations and monitoring of key performance indicators • Sometimes: surveys of patients and staff, or evidence that these are regularly done by the institution itself	• audit of compliance by accredited auditors • audits are performed according to ISO 19011 guidelines for auditing quality systems	• originally: periodic inspection of all healthcare facilities, unannounced visits and ad hoc responsive investigation • now: many target attention to priority concerns based on statistical reports, other inspectorates and assessment programmes • sometimes: methods common to accreditation are used, for example, self-assessment, surveys of users and carers, and of staff
Assessors' competences		
• AB surveyors trained to interpret standards, assess compliance on-site, and analyse and report findings	• AB surveyors trained to interpret standards, assess compliance on-site, and analyse and report findings	• country-specific regulations
Duration of award		
• accreditation valid for a fixed term, usually up to four years	• certificates of compliance with ISO 9001 are issued by the CB based directly on the auditors' report	• country-specific regulations • many licenses are issued in perpetuity
Interim and reassessment		
• interim focused surveys, self-reporting and monitoring of performance indicators • reassessment after end of accreditation	• interim annual surveillance visits • reassessment of ISO 9001 after three years • reassessment includes review of past performance	• frequency and depth of regulatory reinspection vary widely between authorities according to the local regulations and the functions concerned • licence renewal often without on-site inspection

Further differences exist between accreditation, certification and supervision with regard to governance, standard development, assessors' competences, funding and supervision (*see* Table 8.1).

In theory, accreditation, certification and supervision could be implemented in any area of healthcare, i.e. preventive, acute, chronic and palliative care. Depending on the individual scheme and strategy, the standards may focus on structures, processes or outcomes in relation to effectiveness, patient-safety and/or patient-centredness. However, most existing external assessment schemes in healthcare use indicators of structure and process rather than outcome and

Table 8.1 *Comparing characteristics of external assessment strategies [continued]*

Accreditation	Certification	Supervision
Supervision of external assessment bodies		
• some ABs in Europe have been independently assessed and accredited by the ISQua (ISQua, 2018a) • some UK programmes are recognized by national regulators as "information providers" under a "concordat" scheme to reduce the burden of inspection on healthcare institutions • ABs in UK may themselves be accredited by the national accreditation body (UKAS) if compliant with the ISO compatible standard PAS 1616	• CBs are assessed by a NAB according to ISO/IEC 17021 as a condition of maintaining their accreditation • NABs themselves are peer reviewed to the standard ISO/IEC 17011 to maintain their status within the European and international mutual recognition arrangements of the European Partnership for Accreditation (EA)	• regulators are subject to government financial audit but have little opportunity for independent rather than political evaluation of their technical performance • many are members of the European Partnership of Supervisory Organisations (EPSO) which is contemplating a system of voluntary peer review • the French *Haute Autorité de Santé* (HAS) is accredited by the ISQua; the Lithuanian State Medical Audit Inspectorate is certified under ISO 9001

Source: authors' own compilation

Notes: AB = Accreditation Body; CB = Certification Body; CEN = Comité Européen de Normalisation; EA = European Partnership for Accreditation; EPSO = European Partnership of Supervisory Organisations; HAS = Haute Autorité de Santé; ISO = International Organization for Standardization; ISQua = International Society for Quality in Health Care; NHS = National Health Service; PAS = Publicly Available Specification

they usually aim to improve quality in terms of effectiveness and patient-safety, although they may also focus on patient-centredness.

External assessment can be linked to economic incentives, for example, as prerequisites for receiving public reimbursement or in so-called pay-for-quality programmes (*see* Chapter 14). Furthermore, accreditation and certification awards are often made publicly available to contribute to informed patient choice (*see* Chapter 13).

This chapter follows the common structure of all chapters in Part 2 of this book. The next section describes the underlying rationale of why accreditation, certification and supervision should contribute to healthcare quality, followed by an overview of what is being done in European countries in respect of the specific quality strategy. This is followed by a description of the available evidence with regard to the effectiveness and cost-effectiveness of the specific strategy, while the next section addresses questions of implementation. Finally, we provide conclusions for policy-makers, bringing together the available evidence and highlighting lessons for implementation of the strategy. The chapter excludes strategies related to specific hospital departments or medical specialities or to accreditation of training, continuing professional development or continuing medical education (*see* Chapter 5). It focuses on generic programmes, omitting the application of accreditation at national or European level of specific departments (for example, of breast cancer centres) and the growing body of specialty-based research (Lerda et al., 2014).

8.2 Why should external assessment strategies contribute to healthcare quality?

The idea of including external assessment strategies is that external verification of organizational compliance with published standards will lead to better, safer healthcare. The underlying rationale is that organizations' managers will carefully review the results of external assessments and implement changes in organizational structures and processes that will ultimately improve quality of care. Similar to other quality improvement strategies (see, for example, Chapters 10 and 2), external assessment strategies are built on the idea of a quality improvement cycle (*see* Fig. 8.2).

The setting of standards by accreditation bodies (accreditation), the International Standards Organization (certification) or government (supervision) is the first step in this cycle. Some may argue that it is the most important step because external assessment will lead to quality improvement only if the standards make requirements for structures or processes that will ultimately lead to improved effectiveness, safety and/or patient-centredness. The second step is the process of external assessment, which will identify areas of adherence and non-adherence with the set of standards. The third step is the improvement process and it includes all actions taken by organizations to implement change. Again, some may argue that this is the most important step because quality will improve only if managers and professionals are motivated to implement changes that will improve quality of care. This motivation is mediated by a combination of pressures on providers as illustrated in Fig. 8.2, including regulations and financial incentives.

The cycle illustrates that there are a number of conditions that need to be fulfilled in order to achieve quality improvement through external assessments: (1) standards need to make requirements that will lead to improved quality of care, (2) external assessments have to be able to reliably detect whether organizations adhere to these standards, (3) managers and professionals have to draw the right conclusions and develop plans of action in response to the assessment, and (4) implementation of the plans has to lead to improvement.

In practice, assessing the link between external assessments and health outcomes empirically is prone to methodological challenges due to the multifaceted nature of the intervention, the scale of the intervention (often at regional or national level) and the timescales from initiation of the intervention to assessment of impact (*see* below).

Fig. 8.2 *Generic framework for external assessment*

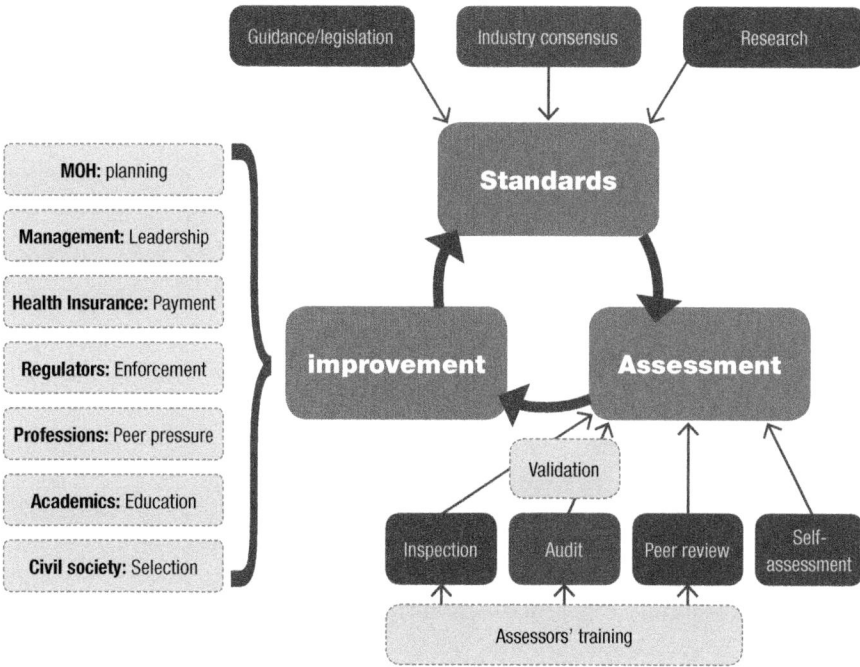

Source: authors' own compilation

Notes: blue = usually related to accreditation; green = usually related to certification; red = usually related to supervision

8.3 What is being done in Europe?

While external assessment strategies have been established for a long time in the US, interest in Europe has grown only in the last two decades. The development has been accompanied by a large number of EU-funded projects that focused on understanding different external assessment strategies and assessing their impact, for example, External Peer Review Techniques (ExPeRT), Deepening our Understanding of Quality improvement in Europe (DUQuE) or Methods of Assessing Response to Quality Improvement Strategies (MARQuIS) (*see also* Chapter 4).

Currently, the EU Joint Research Centre (JRC) is developing a European quality assurance scheme for breast cancer services as part of the European Commission Initiative on Breast Cancer (ECIBC, *see also* Chapter 4). This work is supported by European Accreditation (*see* Box 8.1). Another ongoing EU project, the Partnership for Assessment of Clinical Excellence in European Reference

Networks (PACE-ERN), is developing a manual and toolbox for the assessment of European Reference Networks (ERN) for rare diseases, which may ultimately lead to a system of accreditation for new ERN members.

At the time of writing in 2018, external assessment strategies had been widely implemented in Europe. Most countries make use of several strategies, including basic supervision as part of the licensing process for healthcare providers, coupled with certification or accreditation strategies to ensure and improve the quality of care. The scope of these strategies (type of standards and assessment, frequency of assessment, level of compliance required or implications of failing to meet standards) differs substantially between countries and, partly, between regions of the same country.

There is no register of accredited, certified or licensed healthcare organizations in Europe. This lack of transparency might be related to the fact that strategies for accreditation, certification and supervision themselves differ in the extent to which they are regulated. Accreditation organizations and government inspectorates list publicly those institutions which are recognized but there is no standard system for data reporting or for linkage between websites. Lists of ISO-certified providers are not publicly accessible.

Given the lack of centralized information on the uptake of accreditation, certification and supervision, estimates of activity in Europe presented below are based on annual reports, occasional surveys and health services research.

8.3.1 Accreditation

Table 8.2 presents a list of European countries where accreditation programmes have been introduced over the past thirty years. The table also provides information on the year of introduction and whether programmes are voluntary or mandatory. The table shows that most European countries have voluntary national accreditation programmes. Only Bosnia, Bulgaria, Denmark, France and Romania have mandatory programmes. National uptake of accreditation programmes varies considerably, as does the governance structures of these programmes. According to findings of a survey, about one third of accreditation programmes are run by governments, one third are independent and one third are hybrids (Shaw et al., 2013).

The first national accreditation programme in Europe was introduced in the UK in 1989. Many other countries followed in the 1990s: the Czech Republic, Finland, France, the Netherlands, Poland, Portugal, Spain and Switzerland. Today, national accreditation programmes are thriving in Bulgaria, the Czech Republic, France, Germany, Luxembourg and Poland. In these countries the activity of accreditation programmes has grown considerably and an increasing number of hospitals have been accredited. Subnational programmes, such as in Spain and Italy, are mostly run by regional government. There are relatively few countries in Europe that do not (yet) have a national programme, including Belgium, Estonia, Greece, Latvia, Norway, Slovenia and Sweden. In addition, some 80 hospitals in Europe have been accredited by Joint Commission International (JCI) using published international standards (JCI, 2018), including 16 hospitals in Belgium and one in Greece. In Slovenia five hospitals are accredited by Det Norske Veritas (DNV GL, 2018) and Accreditation Canada (Accreditation Canada, 2018) against their international standards.

The International Society for Quality in Healthcare (ISQua) aims to harmonize accreditation programmes worldwide. ISQua has developed its own Accreditation Programme (IAP). ISQua Accreditation is granted for four years. Across Europe several accreditation programmes or bodies have been accredited according to ISQua standards, for instance in Andalusia (Spain), Denmark, France, the Netherlands, Norway, Romania and the UK (ISQua, 2018a). ISQua has published standards for external assessment organizations, for the development of standards for external assessment, and for the training of external assessors (or "surveyors") (ISQua, 2015).

8.3.2 Certification

In general, ISO standards and certification against those standards have a long history in Europe. There are several EU regulations concerning quality of goods and products (*see* Box 8.1 and Chapter 4).

EN ISO 15224:2012 (updated in 2017) is the first ISO standard that is specific to quality management systems in healthcare. It has a focus on clinical processes and their risk management in order to promote good-quality healthcare. The standard aims to adjust and specify the requirements, as well as the "product" concept and customer perspectives in EN ISO 9001:2008 to the specific conditions of healthcare, where products are mainly services and customers are mainly patients. Before the introduction of the translated version, there was a major variation in the interpretation of key words (for example, product, supplier and design control) such that the standards (and thus any subsequent audit and certification) would not appear to be consistent between countries (Sweeney & Heaton, 2000).

Information on the status of (ISO) certification is even less available than information on accreditation status, partly because this is less directed by national bodies and partly because the level or setting of certification is much more variable, for example, hospital level, service level, laboratory level, diagnostic facility level. There is no clearing house to gather such information in Europe.

Table 8.2   *Selected healthcare accreditation organizations in Europe, 2018*

Country	Agency, organization	Introduced in	Type	Homepage
Europe	Joint Commission International, Europe	1994	voluntary	https://www.jointcommissioninternational.org/
Bulgaria	Accreditation of hospitals and diagnostic-consultative centres	2000	mandatory	n.a.
Croatia	Agency for Quality and Accreditation in Health Care	2007	voluntary	n.a.
Czechia	Spojená akreditační komise	1998	voluntary	www.sakcr.cz
Denmark	The Danish Healthcare Quality Programme (DDKM), IKAS	2006	mandatory	www.ikas.dk
Finland	Social and Health Quality Service (SHQS)	1993	voluntary	www.qualitor.fi
France	Haute Autorité de Santé (HAS)	1996	mandatory	www.has-sante.fr
Germany	Kooperation für Transparenz und Qualität im Gesundheitswesen (KTQ)	2000	voluntary	www.ktq.de
Hungary	Institute for Healthcare Quality Improvement and Hospital Engineering	under discussion	n.a.	www.emki.hu
Ireland	Health Information and Quality Authority	2007	voluntary	www.hiqa.ie
Lithuania	State Health-Care Accreditation Agency (SHCAA)	1999	voluntary	www.vaspvt.gov.lt
Luxembourg	Incitants Qualité (IQ)	2006	voluntary	n.a.
Netherlands	Netherlands Institute for Accreditation in Health Care (NIAZ)	1998	voluntary	www.niaz.nl
Poland	Program Akredytacji	1998	voluntary	www.cmj.org.pl
Portugal	Programa Nacional de Acreditação em Saúde	1999	voluntary	www.dgs.pt
Romania	Autoritatea Nationala De Management Al Calitatii In Sanatate (ANMCS)	2011	mandatory	https://anmcs.gov.ro/web/en
Serbia	Agency for Accreditation of Health Institutions of Serbia (AZUS)	2008	voluntary	www.azus.gov.rs
Slovak Republic	Slovak National Accreditation Service (SNAS)	2002	voluntary	http://www.snas.sk/index.php?l=en
Spain	FADA-JCI	1996	voluntary	www.fada.org
Switzerland	sanaCERT Suisse	1996	voluntary	www.sanacert.ch
UK	CHKS Accreditation; previously Health Quality Service	1989	voluntary	www.chks.co.uk

Sources: Legido-Quigley et al., 2008; Walcque et al., 2008; Shaw et al., 2010a; European Observatory on Health Systems and Policies, 2018; programmes' homepages

Note: n.a. = not applicable

Box 8.1   *EU Regulations on certification of medical products*

The regulation EC 765/2008 defines requirements for accreditation and market surveillance relating to the marketing of (medical) products. It aims to reduce variation between countries and to establish uniform national bodies responsible for conformity assessment. When conformity assessment bodies (CABs) are accredited by their national accreditation body (NAB) and a mutual recognition agreement exists between the NABs, their certification is recognized across national borders. The European Cooperation for Accreditation (EA) supervises national systems to evaluate the competence of CABs throughout Europe, including peer evaluation among NABs. EA has been formally appointed by the European Commission under Regulation (EC) 765/2008 to develop and maintain a multilateral agreement of mutual recognition based on a harmonized accreditation infrastructure.

The Comité Européen de Normalisation (CEN) is the competent body of the European Union (EU) and European Free Trade Area (EFTA) to develop and publish European standards, either on request by business entities (bottom-up), or mandated by the European Commission (top-down). Certification of management systems (such as compliant with ISO 9001) is by bodies which are themselves accredited according to IEC ISO 17021 by the national accreditation body, which is in turn accredited by the European Cooperation for Accreditation.

Searchable lists of ISO certificated healthcare organizations are not freely available at national or European level. However, an annual survey from ISO itself provides an overview of awarded health and social care organizations in accordance with 9001 norm series (*see* Fig. 8.3). However, information on the newer norm 15224 is not available.

Fig. 8.3   *Number of ISO-certificates in health and social care, 1998–2017*

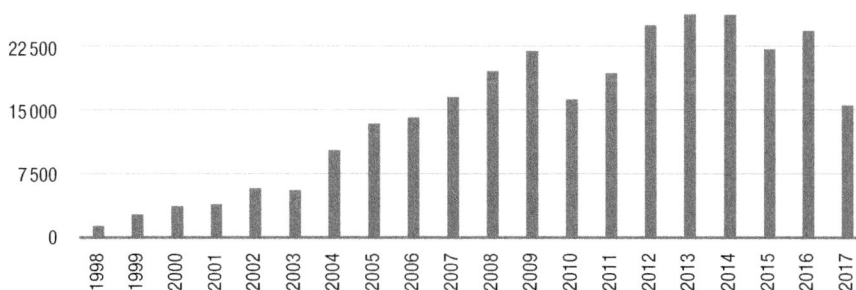

Source: authors' graph based on ISO, 2018

The Healthcare in Transition (HiT) profiles published by the WHO European Observatory on Health Systems and Policies provides further information on ISO certification status of healthcare organizations in European countries. Although ISO standards are mentioned in several HiT profiles, detailed information on

ISO certification is often not available. Countries where at least some hospitals (or departments) have been ISO-certified include Bulgaria, Cyprus, Denmark, Germany, Greece, Hungary, Poland, Slovenia and the UK. In Poland certified (and accredited) hospitals receive higher reimbursements. In other countries, for example, the Czech Republic, Ireland, Lithuania, Spain and the Netherlands either ISO-based certification schemes were developed or it was mentioned that some healthcare organizations in general (not explicitly hospitals) are ISO-certified.

8.3.3 Supervision

Many countries have several forms of supervision. Apart from basic supervision as part of the licensing or authorization process that allows organizations to act as healthcare providers, there is often additional supervision and licensing related to fire safety, pharmacy and environmental health. Many of these supervision and licensing functions are commonly delegated to separate agencies of national or local government. Thus the law may be national but the supervision and licensing may be regional or local.

No systematic overview is available of supervision arrangements in different European countries. However, the European Partnership for Supervisory Organisations (EPSO), an informal group of government-related organizations enforcing or supervising health services in EU and EFTA countries, provides a list of national member bodies (*see* Table 8.3). EPSO aims to support the exchange of information and experiences in healthcare supervision and control of medical and pharmaceutical products, instruments and devices.

However, the presence of a national supervisory organization does not necessarily mean that there is a system of regular supervision and (re)licensing in a country. In a survey of the European Accreditation Network (EAN) half of the responding 14 countries reported either no requirement for hospital licensing or the issue of a licence in perpetuity. The remainder reissue licences periodically, with or without re-inspection (Shaw et al., 2010a).

In many countries the relationship between accreditation, regulation and ISO quality systems is unclear. One notable exception is England, where an alliance of professional associations was established in 2013 to harmonize clinical service accreditation between the specialties in order to minimize administrative burden and to support the regulatory function of the healthcare regulator, the Care Quality Commission (CQC). The Alliance worked with the British Standards Institution (BSI) to reconcile the various requirements of the CQC, the ISO accreditation body (UKAS) and professionally led clinical review schemes. This could be a transferable model for legally based collaboration between the healthcare regulator, ISO certification and professional peer review in other European

Table 8.3   *National supervisory organizations members of European Partnership for Supervisory Organisations (EPSO), 2018*

Country	Organization	Website
Belgium (Flanders)	The Flemish Care Inspectorate (Zorginspectie)	www.zorginspectie.be
Bulgaria	Executive Agency for Medical Audit (EAMA)	www.eama.bg
Denmark	National Board of Health (NBH)	www.sst.dk
	The Danish Patient Safety Authority	www.stps.dk/en
Estonia	Estonian Health Board	www.terviseamet.ee/
Finland	Valvira	www.valvira.fi
France	Haute Autorité de Santé (HAS)	www.has-sante.fr
Iceland	Directorate of Health (DoH)	www.landlaeknir.is/
Ireland	Health Information and Quality Authority (HIQA)	www.hiqa.ie
Italy	The National Agency for Health Services	www.agenas.it/
Kosovo	Ministry of Health (MoH)	www.msh-ks.org/
Latvia	Health Inspectorate of Latvia	www.vi.gov.lv/en
Lithuania	State Medical Audit Inspectorate	www.vmai.lt
Malta	Department for Social Welfare Standards (DSWS)	www.dsws.gov.mt
	Medical Council Malta	www.ehealth.gov.mt
Netherlands	Health Care Inspectorate (IGZ)	www.igz.nl
	Inspectorate for Youth Care	www.inspectiejeugdzorg.nl/
Norway	Norwegian Board of Health Supervision	www.helsetilsynet.no
Portugal	Portuguese Health Regulation Authority (ERS)	www.ers.pt
Slovenia	Health Inspectorate of the Republic of Slovenia (HIRS)	www.mz.gov.si/en/.
Sweden	Health and Social Care Inspectorate (IVO)	www.ivo.se
UK England	Care Quality Commission (CQC)	www.cqc.org.uk
UK N Ireland	Regulation and Quality Improvement Authority (RQIA)	www.rqia.org.uk/
UK Scotland	Healthcare Improvement Scotland	www.healthcareimprovementscotland.org
	Care Inspectorate (CI)	www.careinspectorate.com
UK Wales	Health Inspectorate Wales (HIW)	www.hiw.org.uk

Source: EPSO, 2018

countries. One result of the collaboration is Publicly Available Specification (PAS) 1616, which describes the required characteristics of the content and structure of standards used for generic clinical service assessment (BSI, 2016). These represent a fusion of ISQua principles for external assessment standards and elements of ISO standards for quality and risk management.

8.4 The effectiveness and cost-effectiveness of external assessment strategies

Given the large amount of money spent on external assessment, purchasers, managers, clinicians, patients and the public at large demand evidence that the money is well spent. In response, a research agenda on external assessment, mostly hospital accreditation, has developed over the last decade (ISQua, 2018b). For this chapter, we performed a rapid review to provide an overview on key findings published in the scientific literature (*see* Box 8.2) (Khangura et al., 2012).

Box 8.2   *Rapid review of the scientific literature*

In order to identify studies on the effectiveness of external assessment strategies we conducted a SCOPUS search, which includes MEDLINE, the Cochrane Library, EMBASE and several other relevant databases. As a first step we searched only for review articles using the search terms "accreditation (MeSH, 1966+)", "Joint Commission on accreditation of Healthcare", "certification", "licensing", "external assessment", "ISO", "International Standards Organization", combined with "Hospitals (MeSH, 1991+)". After screening of titles and abstracts we identified nine relevant systematic reviews (Alkhenizan & Shaw, 2011; Brubbak et al., 2015; Flodgren, Gonçalves-Bradley & Pomey, 2016; Flodgren et al., 2011; Greenfield & Braithwaite, 2008; Mumford et al., 2013; NOKC, 2006; NOKC, 2009; Yousefinezhadi et al., 2015) (*see* Table 8.4 for accreditation). In addition, one Cochrane review concerning supervision was identified via handsearch (Wiysonge et al., 2016). As a second step, we expanded our search to other original research articles to identify studies not included in existing reviews. This search retrieved 1815 potentially relevant titles. After assessing titles and abstracts and via snowballing, we identified nine further large-scale and experimental studies (*see* Table 8.5) not included in the systematic reviews mentioned above.

8.4.1 Accreditation

Eight systematic reviews were identified, which included between 2 and 66 original studies. These had been conducted mostly in the US or other non-European countries, for example, Australia, Canada, Japan and South Africa, thus limiting the transferability of findings to the European context. In addition, interpretation of results is complicated by the heterogeneity of accreditation schemes in different countries.

In general, evidence on the effectiveness, let alone cost-effectiveness, of hospital accreditation to improve quality of care is limited (*see* Table 8.4). Part of the problem is that there are very few controlled studies to evaluate such effects. It seems that accreditation has effects on the extent to which hospitals prepare for accreditation, which in turn may have a positive effect on team culture and generic service organization. However, whether this translates into better process measures and improved clinical outcomes is not clearly established.

The only systematic review that aimed to assess costs and cost-effectiveness identified six studies conducted in non-European countries. The findings give an indication of accreditation's costs (including preparation), ranging from 0.2 to 1.7% of total hospital expenditures per annum averaged over the accreditation cycle of usually three years. However, the number of studies was small and none of them carried out a formal economic evaluation. Thus, no reliable conclusions on the cost-effectiveness of accreditation can be drawn (Mumford et al., 2013).

In addition, nine relatively recent large-scale studies, which were not included in the systematic reviews presented above, have assessed either the effectiveness or costs of accreditation programmes (*see* Table 8.5).

Seven studies assessed the effectiveness of accreditation programmes, and they generally reported mixed results. Two studies evaluating the effects on mortality of a German (Pross et al., 2018) and a US accreditation programme (Lam et al., 2018) found no association between hospital accreditation and mortality. However, a third study of a Danish accreditation programme (Falstie-Jensen, Bogh & Johnsen, 2018) did find an association between low compliance with accreditation standards and high 30-day mortality. Findings on the effects of accreditation on readmission rates in the same three studies are also inconclusive.

Another study conducted in Australia reported a significant reduction of Staphylococcus aureus bacteraemia (SAB) rates, which were nearly halved in accredited hospitals compared to non-accredited hospitals (Mumford et al., 2015b). The findings of Bogh et al. (2017) suggest that the impact of accreditation varies across conditions: heart failure and breast cancer care improved less than other areas and improvements in diagnostic processes were smaller than improvements in other types of processes. Moreover, the studies of Shaw et al. (2010b, 2014) reported a positive effect of accreditation (and certification) for three out of four clinical services (*see* the section on certification for a more detailed description of both studies).

Two of the nine identified studies focused on the costs of accreditation. In an Australian mixed-methods study including six hospitals the costs ranged from 0.03 to 0.60% of total expenditures per annum averaged on the accreditation cycle of four years. The authors extrapolated the costs to national level, which would accumulate to $A37 million – 0.1% of total expenditures for acute public hospitals (Mumford et al., 2015a). The other study did not assess costs directly, but evaluated the value of accreditation from the hospital's perspective. The study found that most hospitals increased expenditures in staff training, consultants' costs and infrastructure maintenance, and that almost one third of

Table 8.4 *Evidence on effectiveness and cost-effectiveness of accreditation from systematic reviews*

Author (year)	Period covered	Number of studies included	Country coverage	Main findings
Flodgren, Gonçalves & Pomey (2016)	up to 2015	update of Flodgren et al. (2011), no further study met inclusion criteria		
Brubakk et al. (2015)	1980–2010	4 (3 SRs, 1 RCT)	RCT from ZA (1)	• the RCT showed inconclusive results (*see* details in Flodgren et al., 2011) • findings from the reviews included were mixed and therefore no conclusions could be reached to support effectiveness of hospital accreditation
Mumford et al. (2013)	up to 2011	Effectiveness		
		15	AU (2), DE (1), Europe (1), JP (1), SAU (1), US (8), ZA (1)	• studies on effectiveness were inconclusive in terms of showing clear evidence of effects on patient safety and quality of care
		Costs and cost-effectiveness		
		6	"AU (1), US (4), ZM (1)	• no formal economic evaluation has been carried out to date • incremental costs ranged from 0.2 to 1.7% of total expenditures per annum
Alkhenizan & Shaw (2011)	1983–2009	26	AU (1), CA (1), DK (1), EG (1), JP (1), KR (1), PH (1), SG (1), ZA (1), US (16), ZM (1)	• overall there was a positive association between accreditation and processes of care • associations are potentially overestimated as they stem mostly from uncontrolled studies

the responding hospitals considered accreditation a worthy investment (Saleh et al., 2013). However, due to the lack of formal economic evaluations it remains unclear whether accreditation is cost-effective or not.

In summary, the available evidence from several systematic reviews (Flodgren et al., 2011; Greenfield & Braithwaite, 2008) and individual studies (Saleh et al., 2013; Shaw et al., 2014) suggests that accreditation may have a positive impact at the professional and/or organizational level, for example, in terms of clinical leadership, clinical organization, nurses' perception of clinical quality, participation and teamwork, and professional development. However, it remains unclear whether hospital accreditation is effective at improving quality of care at the patient level. In addition, cost-effectiveness remains uncertain as formal economic evaluations of accreditation are not available. However, given the heterogeneity

Table 8.4 *Evidence on effectiveness and cost-effectiveness of accreditation from systematic reviews [continued]*

Author (year)	Period covered	Number of studies included	Country coverage	Main findings
Flodgren et al. (2011)	up to 2011	2 (cluster-RCT, ITS)	England (1), ZA (1)	• positive effects of hospital accreditation on compliance with accreditation standards were shown in the cluster-RCT; effects on quality indicators were mixed: only one out of eight indicators improved ("nurses perception of clinical quality, participation and teamwork") • the ITS showed a statistically non-significant effect of accreditation on hospital infections
NOKC (2009)	up to 2009	update of NOKC (2006), no further study met inclusion criteria		
Greenfield & Braithwaite (2007)	1983–2006	66	not reported	• findings suggest association between accreditation and promoting change and professional development • inconsistent associations between accreditation and professionals' attitudes to accreditation, organizational and financial impact, quality measures and programme assessment • evidence for an association between accreditation and consumer views or patient satisfaction is inconclusive
NOKC (2006)	1966–2006	2 (cohort-study, before-after study)	AU (1), DE (1)	• results suggest that accreditation might positively influence nurse's working conditions, and the frequency of safety routines • regarding certification the authors concluded that it might result in cost reduction and an increase of satisfaction among cooperating cardiologists

Notes: ITS = interrupted time series; RCT = randomized controlled trial; SR = systematic review

Country abbreviations: AU = Australia; CA = Canada; DK = Denmark; EG = Egypt; JP = Japan; KR = Korea; PH = Philippines; SAU = Saudi Arabia; SG = Singapore; ZA = South Africa; US = United States of America; ZM = Zambia.

of accreditation schemes, both within and across countries, findings from the literature have to be interpreted with care and generalizability is limited.

8.4.2 Certification

There is little published research or descriptive evidence for the effectiveness of certification in healthcare. A review conducted by NOKC (2006) covered both accreditation and certification but only two of the references retrieved from the literature review complied with the inclusion criteria, of which one study was related to accreditation and one study to certification. The latter suggests that a quality system according to ISO 9001 might result in cost reduction of

Table 8.5 *Recent large-scale and experimental research on effectiveness and costs of healthcare accreditation*

Study	Design	Country	Aim	Hospitals (patients)	Key findings
Pross et al., 2018	secondary data analysis	DE	to assess the impact of hospital accreditation on 30-day mortality of stroke patients	n = 1100–1300 per year, from 2006 to 2014	• no effects of hospital accreditation on 30-day stroke mortality were shown
Lam et al., 2018	secondary data analysis	US	to assess the association between accreditation and mortality	n = 4.400 (> 4 mio.)	• hospital accreditation was not associated with lower mortality, and was only slightly associated with reduced readmission rates for the 15 common medical conditions selected in this study
Falstie-Jensen, Bogh & Johnsen, 2018	nationwide population-based study from 2012 to 2015	DK	to examine the association between compliance with hospital accreditation and 30-day mortality	n = 25 (> 170.000)	• persistent low compliance with the DDKM (in Danish: Den Danske Kvalitetsmodel) accreditation was associated with higher 30-day mortality and longer length of stay compared to high compliance • no difference was seen for acute readmission
Bogh et al., 2017	multilevel, longitudinal, stepped-wedge study	DK	to analyse the effectiveness of hospital accreditation on process indicators	n = 25	• the impact of accreditation varied across conditions: heart failure and breast cancer improved less than other disease areas and diagnostic processes were less enhanced than other types of processes • hospital characteristics were no reliable predictors for assessing the effects of accreditation
Mumford et al., 2015a	mixed method study	AU	to evaluate the costs of hospital accreditation	n = 6	• the average costs through the four-year accreditation cycle ranged from 0.03% to 0.60% of total hospital operating costs per year • extrapolated to national level that would accumulate to $A36.83 mio. (0.1% of acute public hospital expenditure) • limitation is the small sample size (n = 6) of hospitals

Study	Design	Country	Aim	Hospitals (patients)	Key findings
Mumford et al., 2015b	retrospective cohort study	AU	to analyse the impact of accreditation scores on SAB rates in hospitals	n = 77	• significantly reduced SAB rates (1.34 per 100 000 bed days to 0.77 per 100 000 bed days) • although the authors support using SAB rates to measure the impact of infection control programmes, there is less evidence whether accreditation scores reflect the implementation status of infection control standards
Saleh et al., 2013	observational cross-sectional designed survey	LBN	to assess the hospital's view on accreditation as a worthy or not worthy investment	n = 110	• most hospitals had increased expenditure in training of staff (95.8%), consultants' costs (80%) and infrastructure maintenance (77.1%) • nearly two thirds (64.3%) of all responding hospitals considered accreditation as a worthy investment • most common arguments were that accreditation has positive effects on quality and safety
Shaw et al., 2014	mixed method multilevel cross-sectional design	CZ, DE, ES, FR, PL, PRT, TUR	to assess the effect of certification and accreditation on quality management in four clinical services	n = 73	• accreditation and certification are positively associated with clinical leadership, systems for patient safety and clinical review, but not with clinical practice • both systems promote structures and processes, which support patient safety and clinical organization but have limited effect on the delivery of evidence-based patient care
Shaw et al., 2010b	cross-sectional study	BE, CZ, ES, FR, IRL, PL, UK	to assess the association between type of external assessment and a composite score of hospital quality	n = 71	• quality and safety structures and procedures were more evident in hospitals with either type of external assessment • overall composite score was highest for accredited hospitals, followed by hospitals with ISO **certification**

Note: SAB = Staphylococcus aureus bacteraemia.

Country abbreviations: AU = Australia; CZ = Czechia; DE = Germany; ES = Spain; FR = France; LBN = Lebanon; PL = Poland; PRT = Portugal; TUR = Turkey; UK = United Kingdom; US = United States

medical expenses (–6.1%) and total laboratory costs (–35.2%) and an increase of satisfaction among cooperating cardiologists. However, the study was of low quality and conducted in a pre-and-post design without a control group. An update of the review in 2009 could not identify further studies for inclusion (NOKC, 2009) (*see* Table 8.4).

Another review that specifically aimed to assess the effects of ISO 9001 certification and the European Foundation for Quality Management (EFQM) excellence model on improving hospital performance included a total of seven studies (Yousefinezhadi et al., 2015). Four of them related to ISO certification, reporting the results of four quasi-experimental studies from Germany, Israel, Spain and the Netherlands. Implementation of ISO 9001 was found to increase the degree of patient satisfaction, patient safety and cost-effectiveness. Moreover, the hospital admissions process was improved and the percentage of unscheduled returns to the hospital decreased. However, the review authors conclude that there is a lack of robust evidence regarding the effectiveness of ISO 9001 (and EFQM) because most results stem from observational studies.

Two of the original studies identified in our literature search assessed the impact of accreditation **and** certification on hospital performance (*see* Table 8.5). The study conducted by Shaw et al. (2014), covering 73 hospitals in seven European countries, showed that ISO certification (and accreditation) is positively associated with clinical leadership, systems for patient safety and clinical review. Moreover, ISO certification (and accreditation) was found to promote structures and processes, which support patient safety and clinical organization. However, no or limited effects were found with regard to clinical practices, such as the delivery of evidence-based patient care. The second study, covering 71 hospitals in seven countries, also assessed the effect of both accreditation and certification. It suggested that accredited hospitals showed better adherence to quality management standards than certified hospitals, but that compliance in both was better than in non-certified hospitals (Shaw et al., 2010b).

In addition, several descriptive single-centre studies discuss motivations, processes and experiences of certification (Staines, 2000). While these studies are relevant to inform managers, their contribution to answering the question as to whether certification is effective is limited. The authors of two reviews that address more broadly the lessons learned from the evaluations of ISO certification acknowledge that the majority of studies on ISO certification in healthcare are supported by descriptive statistics and surveys only, thus not allowing causal inference on the impact of certification on organizational performance and other outcomes (Sampaio et al., 2009; Sampaio, Saraiva & Monteiro, 2012).

8.4.3 Supervision

There is little published research on the effectiveness of supervision in healthcare. Results of one review (Sutherland & Leatherman, 2006), covering three studies conducted in England and the US, suggest that the prospect of inspection catalyzes organizational efforts to measure and improve performance. Although inspections rarely uncover issues that are unknown to managers, they are able to focus attention and motivate actors to address problems. However, the review authors concluded that evidence is drawn from a small number of observational studies and therefore the links between regulation and improvements in quality are primarily associative rather than causal.

No further studies on the effectiveness and/or cost-effectiveness of supervision were identified. Thus, where evidence on accreditation and certification is inconsistent or lacks experimental data, evidence on the effects of supervision is almost non-existent.

8.5 Implementing external assessment strategies: what are the organizational and institutional requirements?

Important challenges for the implementation of accreditation programmes include unstable business (for example, limited market, low uptake) and unstable politics. In particular, voluntary programmes in small countries are hard to sustain financially because the market for accreditation is not sufficiently large. In order to ensure high rates of participation among healthcare providers, strong ethical, political or financial incentives are needed.

In general, programmes in small countries face particular challenges. Often external assessments lack credibility because the country is too small for peer-reviewers to be considered objective. Small countries are likely to benefit significantly from international collaboration in the area of healthcare accreditation. In addition, strong political (and financial) support from government is particularly important in small countries.

A recent review of 26 research papers (Ng et al., 2013) identified a number of facilitators and barriers for implementation of hospital accreditation programmes (*see* Table 8.6). The results are in line with a study (Fortes et al., 2011) not included in the review that examined implementation issues with accreditation standards according to the Joint Commission on Accreditation of Healthcare Organizations (JCAHO).

The review highlights that organizations should support multidisciplinary team building and collaboration and should choose a participative approach involving healthcare professionals in order to prevent reluctance and an organizational

Table 8.6 *Facilitators and barriers for implementation of accreditation and certification*

	Facilitators	Barriers
Organizational factors	• staff engagement and communication • multidisciplinary team-building and collaboration • change in organizational culture • enhanced leadership and staff training • integration and utilization of information • increased resources dedicated to CQI	• organizational culture of resistance to change • increased staff workload • lack of awareness about CQI • insufficient staff training and support for CQI • lack of applicable standards for local use • lack of performance measures
System-wide factors	• additional funding • public recognition • advantage in market competition • development of suitable accreditation standards for local use	• Hawthorne effects and opportunistic behaviours • resource and funding cuts • lack of incentives for participation • a regulatory approach for mandatory participation • high costs for sustaining the programmes

Source: based on Ng et al., 2013

Note: CQI = continuous quality improvement

culture of resistance to change. To do so, enhanced leadership and staff training is necessary and also useful to prevent a lack of awareness about the idea of continuous quality improvement. Moreover, organizations should be aware of an increased demand on (personnel) resources when implementing a continuous quality improvement model. Furthermore, effects of a certification or accreditation scheme on performance should be measurable. Finally, the success of an external assessment strategy depends on the standards used and that they are applicable and adapted to the context of a healthcare organization.

At the system level accreditation programmes benefit if additional funding is available and if the public recognizes the relevance of accreditation, which may lead to advantages in market competition. Furthermore, the development of accreditation standards that are perceived to be applicable to the local situation is essential in order for the standards to be perceived as relevant and acceptable by organizations. A regulatory approach, mandating participation in accreditation programmes, has advantages and disadvantages. While mandatory participation may ensure financial viability of the accreditation bodies, it may also create resistance on the side of the provider organizations. In addition, the costs of the accreditation programme need to be adjusted to the potential market for accreditation, which does not necessarily have to be confined within the national borders of a particular country.

Findings from a systematic review conducted by Sutherland & Leatherman (2006) suggest that factors facilitating supervision are different, possibly related to its regulatory character. Important aspects for the successful implementation of supervision strategies are inspectors' competences, and the existence of clear goals both for inspection regimes and for inspected organizations. In addition, a balance needs to be struck between checking compliance with national standards and allowing sufficient local flexibility to set meaningful improvement priorities. Furthermore, costs should not be excessive, for example, there does not need to be detailed annual assessment of high-performing organizations. Finally, the review identified a number of aspects that hinder effective supervision, including resistance, ritualistic compliance, regulatory capture, performance ambiguity and data problems.

8.6 Conclusions for policy-makers

Almost all countries in Europe have implemented external assessment strategies. However, in some countries uptake of accreditation and certification has been relatively limited. In view of the widespread uptake of external assessment strategies, there is surprisingly little robust evidence to support the effectiveness of these strategies. Despite the amount of money invested in the implementation of accreditation programmes, evidence on cost-effectiveness is almost nonexistent. Existing research focuses on healthcare accreditation and little is published on the effects of certification or supervision. The findings of existing studies require careful interpretation and the lack of statistical significance may not mean that there is no effect on the quality of care. In light of the substantial investments in external assessment strategies, decision-makers should further support research into the comparative effectiveness of external assessment, also to better understand the key components of effective programmes.

The available (limited) evidence needs to be assessed cautiously, taking into account the effects of accreditation on a range of outcomes, including patient-related outcomes, but also outcomes related to professions or organizations. However, it needs to be acknowledged that evidence takes different forms and not all relevant evidence needed by decision-makers fits the paradigm of evidence-based medicine. Likewise, evidence, in whatever form, is only one of the factors influencing policies of external assessment, and not necessarily the determining one.

When planning the implementation of an external assessment programme, several aspects have to be taken into account. First, the involvement of relevant stakeholders, for example, the public or purchasers, in establishing standards and setting policies for external assessment strategies has been highlighted as an important aspect for a successful and sustainable programme. In particular, stakeholder involvement can contribute to preventing resistance among professionals and it can support the development of applicable and useful standards (Ng et al., 2013).

Second, strong ethical, political or financial incentives to participate in external assessment are required to ensure high rates of participation among healthcare providers (giving a critical mass for health system impact). Thus, linking external assessment to funding mechanisms was identified as one of the main drivers for hospitals to participate in accreditation programmes. In light of high costs for implementation and sustainability of accreditation programmes, a lack of incentives may act as hindering factor (Ng et al., 2013).

Closely related to the question of financial incentives is the question whether a mandatory or a voluntary approach to external assessment should be chosen. Mandatory accreditation or certification programmes with a mandatory nature may be perceived as a measure of governmental control and distrust which could create resistance among healthcare professionals (Ng et al., 2013). However, voluntary programmes in small countries are hard to sustain financially and lack credibility as independent assessments. Beside funding mechanisms, incentives could also include prestige/marketing, intrinsic motivation for quality improvement and becoming consistent with legal requirements and government policy.

Third, the relationship between governments and organizations responsible for external assessment has to be clearly defined. The decision as to whether accreditation/certification/supervisory bodies should be related to the government or not should be taken in light of the programme's purpose. If the purpose is quality assurance and accountability, the programme should be managed and funded by the government. However, if the purpose is quality improvement, the programme can be independent and voluntary – but this means that high-quality hospitals are usually more likely to participate.

Finally, it is clear that strong political, if not financial, support from government is essential for the successful implementation of external assessment strategies, which should always be designed in consideration of an individual health system's characteristics (Fortes et al., 2011).

References

Accreditation Canada (2018). Find an Internationally Accredited Service Provider. Available at: https://accreditation.ca/intl-en/find-intl-accredited-service-provider/, accessed 28 November 2018.

Alkhenizan A, Shaw C (2011). Impact of accreditation on the quality of healthcare services: a systematic review of the literature. *Annals of Saudi Medicine*, 31(4):407–16.

Bogh SB et al. (2017). Predictors of the effectiveness of accreditation on hospital performance: a nationwide stepped-wedge study. *International Journal for Quality in Health Care*, 29(4):477–83.

BSI (2016). Publicly Available Specification (PAS) 1616:2016 Healthcare – Provision of clinical services – Specification. British Standards Institution. Available at: https://shop.bsigroup.com/ProductDetail/?pid=000000000030324182, accessed 21 March 2019.

Brubakk K et al. (2015). A systematic review of hospital accreditation: the challenges of measuring complex intervention effects. *BMC Health Services Research*, 15:280. doi: 10.1186/s12913-015-0933-x.

DNV GL (2018). Accredited hospitals. Available at: https://www.dnvgl.com/assurance/healthcare/accredited-hospitals.html, accessed 28 November 2018.

Eismann S (2011). "European Supervisory Bodies and Patient Safety". Survey of 15 respondents (Belgium, Denmark, England, Estonia, Finland, France, Germany, Ireland, Lithuania, Netherlands, Northern Ireland, Norway, Scotland, Slovenia, Sweden). CQC.

EPSO (2018). EPSO member countries and partners (including not active). Available at: http://www.epsonet.eu/members-2.html, accessed 28 November 2018.

European Observatory on Health Systems and Policies (2018). Health Systems in Transitions Series. Available at: http://www.euro.who.int/en/who-we-are/partners/observatory/health-systems-in-transition-hit-series/countries, accessed 29 November 2018.

Falstie-Jensen AM, Bogh SB, Johnsen SP (2018). Consecutive cycles of hospital accreditation: Persistent low compliance associated with higher mortality and longer length of stay. *International Journal for Quality in Health Care*, 30(5):382–9. doi: 10.1093/intqhc/mzy037.

Flodgren G, Gonçalves-Bradley DC, Pomey MP (2016). External inspection of compliance with standards for improved healthcare outcomes. *Cochrane Database of Systematic Reviews*, 12: CD008992. doi: 10.1002/14651858.CD008992.pub3.

Flodgren G et al. (2011). Effectiveness of external inspection of compliance with standards in improving healthcare organisation behaviour, healthcare professional behaviour or patient outcomes. *Cochrane Database of Systematic Reviews*: 11: CD008992. doi: 10.1002/14651858.CD008992.pub2.

Fortes MT et al. (2011). Accreditation or accreditations? A comparative study about accreditation in France, United Kingdom and Cataluña. *Revista da Associação Médica Brasileira (English Edition)*, 57(2):234–41. doi: 10.1016/S2255-4823(11)70050-9.

Greenfield D, Braithwaite J (2008). Health sector accreditation research: a systematic review. *International Journal for Quality in Health Care*, 20(3):172–83.

ISO (2018). 9. ISO Survey of certifications to management system standards. Full results. Available at: https://isotc.iso.org/livelink/livelink?func=ll&objId=18808772&objAction=browse&viewType=1, accessed 26 November 2018.

ISQua (2015). Guidelines and Principles for the Development of Health and Social Care standards. Available at: http://www.isqua.org/reference materials.hrm, accessed 28 November 2018.

ISQua (2018a). ISQua's International Accreditation Programme. Current Awards. Available at: https://www.isqua.org/accreditation.html, accessed 28 November 2018.

ISQua (2018b). ISQua Research. Available at: https://www.isqua.org/research.html, accessed 29 November 2018.

JCI (2018). JCI – Accredited Organizations. Available at: https://www.jointcommissioninternational.org/about-jci/jci-accredited-organizations/, accessed 28 November 2018.

Khangura S et al. (2012). Evidence summaries: the evolution of a rapid review approach. *Systematic Reviews* 1(10). doi: 10.1186/2046-4053-1-10.

Lam MB et al. (2018). Association between patient outcomes and accreditation in US hospitals: observational study. BMJ *(Clinical research edition)*, 363, k4011. doi: 10.1136/bmj.k4011.

Legido-Quigley H et al. (2008). Assuring the quality of health care in the European Union: a case for action. Copenhagen: WHO Regional Office for Europe.

Lerda D et al. (2014). Report of a European survey on the organization of breast cancer care services. European Commission. Joint Research Centre. Institute for Health and Consumer Protection. Luxembourg (JRC Science and Policy Reports).

Mumford V et al. (2013). Health services accreditation: what is the evidence that the benefits justify the costs? *International Journal for Quality in Health Care*, 25(5):606–20. doi: 10.1093/intqhc/mzt059.

Mumford V et al. (2015a). Counting the costs of accreditation in acute care: an activity-based costing approach. *BMJ Open*, 5(9).

Mumford V et al. (2015b). Is accreditation linked to hospital infection rates? A 4-year, data linkage study of Staphylococcus aureus rates and accreditation scores in 77 Australian Hospitals? *International Journal for Quality in Health Care*, 27(6):479–85.

Ng, GKB et al. (2013). Factors affecting implementation of accreditation programmes and the impact of the accreditation process on quality improvement in hospitals: a SWOT analysis. *Hong Kong medical journal = Xianggang yi xue za zhi*, 19(5):434–46. doi: 10.12809/hkmj134063.

NOKC (2006). Effect of certification and accreditation on hospitals. Rapport fra Kunnskapssenterat: nr 27-2006. Oslo: Norwegian Knowledge Centre for the Health Services. Available at: https://www.fhi.no/globalassets/dokumenterfiler/rapporter/2009-og-eldre/rapport_0627_isosertifisering_akkreditering_ver1.pdf, accessed 1 April 2019.

NOKC (2009). Effect of certification and accreditation on hospitals. Rapport fra Kunnskapssenterat: nr 30-2009. Oslo: Norwegian Knowledge Centre for the Health Services. Available at: https://www.fhi.no/globalassets/dokumenterfiler/rapporter/2009-og-eldre/rapport_0930_sertifisering_akkreditering_sykehus.pdf, accessed 1 April 2019.

Pross C et al. (2018). Stroke units, certification, and Outcomes in German hospitals: a longitudinal study of patient-based 30-day mortality for 2006–2014. *BMC Health Services Research*, 18(1):880. doi: 10.1186/s12913-018-3664-y.

Saleh SS et al. (2013). Accreditation of hospitals in Lebanon: is it a worthy investment? *International Journal for Quality in Health Care*, 25(3):284–90.

Sampaio P, Saraiva P, Monteiro A (2012). ISO 9001 Certification pay-off: myth versus reality. *International Journal of Quality and Reliability Management*, 29(8):891–914.

Sampaio P et al. (2009). ISO 9001 certification research: questions, answers and approaches. *International Journal of Quality and Reliability Management*, 26:36–58.

Shaw CD (2001). External assessment of health care. *BMJ*, 322(72990):851–4.

Shaw CD et al. (2010a). Sustainable Healthcare Accreditation: messages from Europe in 2009. *International Journal for Quality in Health Care*, 22:341–50.

Shaw CD et al. (2010b). Accreditation and ISO certification: Do they explain differences in quality management in European hospitals? *International Journal for Quality in Health Care*, 22:445–51.

Shaw CD et al. (2013). Profiling health-care accreditation organizations: an international survey. International Journal for Quality in Health Care, 25(3):222–31.

Shaw CD et al. (2014). The effect of certification and accreditation on quality management in 4 clinical services in 73 European hospitals. *International Journal for Quality in Health Care*, 26(S1):100–6.

Staines A (2000). Benefits of an ISO 9001 certification – the case of a Swiss regional hospital. *International Journal of Health Care Quality Assurance Incorporating Leadership in Health Services*, 13:27–33.

Sutherland K, Leatherman S (2006). Regulation and quality improvement. A review of the evidence. The Health Foundation.

Sweeney J, Heaton C (2000). Interpretations and variations of ISO 9000 in acute health care. *International Journal for Quality in Health Care*, 12:203–9.

Walcque CDE et al. (2008). Comparative study of hospital accreditation programs in Europe. KCE (KCE reports, 70C). Available at: https://kce.fgov.be/sites/default/files/atoms/files/d20081027303.pdf, accessed 29 November 2018.

WHO (2003). Quality and accreditation in health care services: A global review. Geneva: World Health Organization. Available at: http://www.who.int/hrh/documents/en/quality_accreditation.pdf, accessed 3 December 2018.

WHO, OECD, World Bank (2018). Delivering quality health services: a global imperative for universal health coverage. Geneva. (CC BY-NC-SA 3.0 IGO).

Wiysonge CS et al. (2016). Public stewardship of private for-profit healthcare providers in low- and middle-income countries (Review). *Cochrane Database Systematic Reviews*, 8(CD009855).

Yousefinezhadi T et al. (2015). The Effect of ISO 9001 and the EFQM Model on Improving Hospital Performance: A Systematic Review. *Iranian Red Crescent Medical Journal*, 17(12):1–5.

Chapter 9

Clinical Practice Guidelines as a quality strategy

Dimitra Panteli, Helena Legido-Quigley, Christoph Reichebner,
Günter Ollenschläger, Corinna Schäfer, Reinhard Busse

Summary

What are the characteristics of the strategy?

Clinical guidelines (or "clinical practice guidelines") are "statements that include recommendations intended to optimize patient care that are informed by a systematic review of evidence and an assessment of the benefits and harms of alternative care options". They have the potential to reduce unwarranted practice variation, enhance translation of research into practice, and improve healthcare quality and safety, if developed and implemented according to international standards. They can be used to provide best practice recommendations for the treatment and care of people by health professionals, to develop standards to assess the clinical practice of individual health professionals and healthcare organizations, to help educate and train health professionals and to help patients make informed decisions. A valid guideline has the potential of influencing care outcomes, but for that it needs to be effectively disseminated and implemented (informing processes of care).

What is being done in European countries?

Less than half of European countries surveyed in 2011 reported having an official basis for guidelines, although implementation still mostly took place on a voluntary basis. Across countries guidelines can be developed at national, regional and/or local level; in most cases professional associations are involved in the endeavour. About one third of countries have a central agency developing clinical guidelines in collaboration with professional associations; several countries reported having multiple levels of clinical guideline development, with regional and local bodies as well as several professional organizations contributing to the centrally coordinated process; finally, fewer countries had no central coordination of the guideline development process at all: professional associations or providers often step in to fill the void. Countries with "well established" activities and wide experience in guideline development and implementation include Belgium, England, France, Germany and the Netherlands; many others have introduced some form of guideline production. There is no newer systematically collected evidence along these lines, but varying degrees of progress can be expected among countries depending on recent reform activity.

What do we know about the effectiveness and cost-effectiveness of the strategy?

A systematic review carried out in 2011 found that while significant effects on outcomes have been measured in some studies, others show no or unclear effects of treatment according to guideline recommendations. Newer studies also show mixed results regarding the effect of guidelines on outcomes, but a clear link with implementation modalities. Regarding cost-effectiveness, the scope of evidence is even more limited. Most of the relevant studies only partially accounted for costs incurred in the process of guideline production. Given the vastly differing practices in guideline production across countries and contexts, an overall conclusion on whether the strategy as a whole is cost-effective or not is very difficult to draw.

How can the strategy be implemented?

There is increasing consensus that incorporating implementation considerations already in the guideline development process can have a substantial influence on implementability, and a number of tools have been developed for that purpose. The uptake of clinical guidelines is influenced by factors that fall under two broad aims: the creation of content and the communication of that content. Education for professionals or patients and print material are the most commonly employed strategies for translating guidelines to practice, but practices vary considerably and gaps have been identified both in the scope and follow-up of interventions. Despite the general recognition of the importance of implementation tools, most guidelines have been found to not be accompanied by such applications. One of the most prominent developments in the area of guideline implementation in recent years has been the increased utilization of information technologies to facilitate guideline adherence, such as decision support software, and the use of guidelines at the bedside, such as mobile guideline apps. Guideline formats that support shared decision-making have been gaining focus in recent years, as has the importance of editorial independence and declaration of conflicts of interest.

Conclusions for policy-makers

The overview of country-specific practices presented in this chapter clearly demonstrates how divergent guideline practices can be, especially when viewed as national strategies for quality improvement. The fact that in several countries practitioners "borrow" recommendations produced abroad combined with existing international initiatives points to a considerable potential for more active knowledge exchange in the future. However, the context-specific nature of produced guidelines must always be taken into account. A lot has already been undertaken in the context of guideline adaptability but earlier, more intensive collaboration might be fruitful, especially on issues such as optimizing guideline development and implementation in the age of multimorbidity. There is currently no discussion about centralizing the dissemination (let alone the development) of guidelines at EU level, but perhaps it is time to consider such a mechanism, especially given the recent suspension of the USA-based clearinghouse that served internationally as a frequently used resource.

9.1 Introduction: the characteristics of clinical practice guidelines

Clinical practice guidelines (in this chapter simply "clinical guidelines") have been defined by the US Institute of Medicine (IOM, 2011) as "statements that include recommendations intended to optimize patient care that are informed by a systematic review of evidence and an assessment of the benefits and harms of alternative care options". They can be used to: inform individual clinical decision-making, provide best practice recommendations for the treatment and care of people by health professionals, develop standards to guide and assess the clinical practice of individual health professionals and healthcare organizations, help educate and train health professionals, and help patients make informed decisions (ESF, 2011).

As per their definition, clinical guidelines are part of the armamentarium of evidence-based medicine (EBM). The term "evidence-based" in relation to healthcare practices found its first use in the early 1990s as one of the possible bases for the development of clinical guidelines (Eddy, 2005). It subsequently became increasingly well-established in the context of evidence-based medicine, which came to be widely understood as "the conscientious, explicit, and judicious use of current best evidence in making decisions about the care of individual patients" (Sackett et al., 1996). The main idea behind this definition, namely relying on scientific evidence with low risk of bias to inform decision-making, increasingly permeated practices beyond the individual patient level, not only in the aforementioned field of clinical guidance development but also in the context of coverage decision-making (Eddy, 2005), mainly through the use of Health Technology Assessment (HTA; *see* Chapter 6).

Both clinical guidelines and HTA are based on the same foundation, that is the synthesis of available clinical evidence in a manner that is useful to their intended users, particularly in light of the ever-increasing volume of primary research. As such, they are both knowledge translation tools. However, HTA focuses on a particular intervention and mainly addresses policy-makers' needs and questions whilst clinical guidelines are primarily focused not on a narrow clinical question but on broader and more complex topics (i.e. disease management), as well as on supporting clinical practice. As such, they are part and parcel of structuring the knowledge base underpinning the work of healthcare professionals. However, given their common scientific rationale, clinical guidelines and HTA may inform each other's development (*see* Table 9.1).

Table 9.1   *Evidence-based medicine, clinical guidelines and HTA in context*

	Evidence-based medicine	Clinical guidelines	Health Technology Assessment
Target group/ Users	Clinicians	Healthcare professionals Managers	Decision-makers
Target population	Individual patients	Patient groups (also applied to individual clinical decision-making)	Population, population groups
Context of application	Clinical decision-making	Clinical decision-making (inter alia to address unjustified practice variation)	Coverage decisions, Investments, Regulation
Methods	Systematic reviews Meta-analyses Decision analyses	Systematic reviews Meta-analyses Decision analyses	Systematic reviews Meta-analyses Clinical trials Economic evaluations Ethical, sociocultural, organizational, legal analyses
Challenges	Lack of specific methodology Requires user training Potentially hampered by reality of service provision	Lack of specific methodology Requires user training Potentially hampered by reality of service provision	Lack of evidence Impact difficult to measure Frequently only considers medical and economic aspects

Source: adapted from Perleth et al., 2013

For clinical guidelines, another important distinction to make is that from clinical pathways. Despite the fact that the definition of a clinical pathway varies (*see* Chapter 12), they generally aim to operationalize translated knowledge and transform it into everyday care processes; they tend to focus on the care of patients within one provider institution and ensure flow of information throughout the treatment process. Where guidelines tend to focus on specific physician-patient decisions (what should be done), pathways tend to focus more on the operational and logistical aspects (who should do what, when and where). A similar distinction can be made between clinical practice guidelines and clinical protocols or bundles (*see* JCI, 2016). The development of clinical pathways and other operationalization tools can be informed by clinical guidelines (*see* also Kredo et al., 2016).

To reiterate, clinical guidelines focus on how to approach patients with defined healthcare problems either throughout the entire care process or in specific clinical situations. As such they can be considered as a tool to inform healthcare delivery, with a specific focus on the clinical components, considering the practice of medicine as an applied science. However, it is important to understand the difference in terminology used in international literature regarding the different components of transforming evidence-based clinical practice at the provider level. Box 9.1 provides such a disambiguation of relevant terms (Wiles et al., 2017). The aim of this chapter is to provide an insight on the role clinical guidelines can and do play as healthcare quality improvement tools in the European context and highlight potential open questions for future research.

9.2 Why should clinical guidelines contribute to healthcare quality?

Clinical guidelines have the potential to reduce unwarranted practice variation and enhance translation of research into practice. In the context of Donabedian's triad (the fourth lens of the five-lens quality framework presented in Chapter 2), the overall hypothesis is that a well developed guideline which is also well implemented will help improve patient outcomes by optimizing the process of care (IOM, 2011; Qaseem et al., 2012; *see* Fig. 9.1). However, cross-fertilization with other knowledge translation tools, such as HTA, could in theory extend their influence to structural elements as well.

Fig. 9.1   *Influence of clinical guidelines on process and outcomes of care*

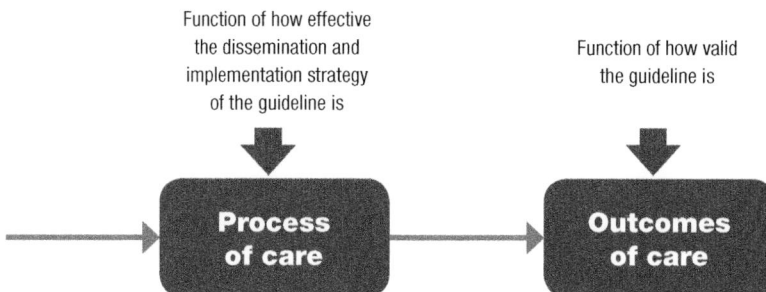

Source: Grimshaw et al., 2012

Box 9.1 *Terminology around clinical guidelines*

Clinical practice guidelines are:

- "statements that include recommendations intended to optimize patient care that are informed by a systematic review of evidence and an assessment of the benefits and harms of alternative care."

A clinical standard:

- is an integrated process that should be undertaken or an outcome that should be achieved for a particular circumstance, symptom, sign or diagnosis (or a defined combination of these); and
- should be evidence-based, specific, feasible to apply, easy and unambiguous to measure, and produce a clinical benefit and/or improve the safety and/or quality of care at least at the population level.

If a standard cannot or should not be complied with, the reason/s should be briefly stated.

A clinical indicator:

- describes a measurable component of the standard, with explicit criteria for inclusion, exclusion, timeframe and setting.

A clinical tool:

- should implicitly or explicitly incorporate a standard or component of a standard;
- should constitute a guide to care that facilitates compliance with the standard;
- should be easy to audit, preferably electronically, to provide feedback; and
- should be able to be incorporated into workflows and medical records.

Source: Wiles et al., 2017

For clinical guidelines to have an actual impact on processes and ultimately outcomes of care, they need to be well developed and based on scientific evidence. Efforts to identify the attributes of high-quality clinical guidelines prompted extensive debates on which criteria are most important. Desirable attributes of clinical guidelines were defined by the IOM in 1990 (Box 9.2). The Council of Europe (2001) endorsed both the use of guidelines themselves and the importance of developing them based on a sound methodology and reliable scientific evidence so as to support best practice. With the increasing interest in the implications of guideline use, methodologies for their development, critical assessment, dissemination and implementation, as well as their adaptation and updating, have been developed and several studies on their appropriateness and usefulness have been carried out (*see* below).

Regarding guideline development, a number of guidebooks in different formats are available from different actors in different contexts ("guidelines for

Box 9.2	*Desirable attributes of clinical guidelines*
Validity	Will the guideline produce intended healthcare outcomes?
Reliability and reproducibility	Would another group of experts derive similar guidelines given the same evidence and methodology? Would different caregivers interpret and apply the guideline similarly in identical clinical circumstances?
Clinical applicability	Does the document describe the clinical settings and the population to which the guideline applies?
Clinical flexibility	Are the recommendations sufficiently flexible depending on the clinical circumstances? Are the alternatives and exceptions explicitly stated?
Clarity	Are the guidelines stated in unambiguous and precise terms?
Multidisciplinary process	Were stakeholders included at various stages of guideline development allowing their comment and participation?
Scheduled review	Is a schedule for update and revision provided?
Documentation	Is the method used for developing guidelines explicitly stated?

Source: Heffner, 1998, based on IOM, 1990

guidelines"; *see*, for example, Shekelle et al., 1999; Woolf et al., 2012; and Schünemann et al., 2014). Increasingly since its inception in 2003, guideline development tools include the GRADE approach (Guyatt et al., 2011; Neumann et al., 2016; Khodambashi & Nytrø, 2017). The Grading of Recommendations Assessment, Development and Evaluation (GRADE) approach was created by the synonymous working group,[1] which is a collaborative consisting mainly of methodologists and clinicians. It provides a framework for assessing the quality (or "certainty") of the evidence supporting, inter alia, guideline recommendations and therefore their resulting strength (GRADE Working Group, 2004). Essentially, GRADE classifies recommendations as strong when a recommended intervention or management strategy would presumably be chosen by a majority of patients, clinicians or policy-makers in all care scenarios, and as weak when different choices could be made (reflecting limited evidence quality, uncertain benefit-harm ratios, uncertainty regarding treatment effects, questionable cost-effectiveness, or variability in values and preferences (*see*, for example, Vandvik et al., 2013)). The GRADE evidence-to-decision framework further helps guideline developers in structuring their process and evaluation of available evidence (Neumann et al., 2016).

On the user side, several tools to evaluate ("appraise") the methodological quality of clinical guidelines exist (for example, Lohr, 1994; Vlayen et al.,

---

1   www.gradeworkinggroup.org

2005, Siering et al., 2013; Semlitsch et al., 2015). The most commonly used instrument to assess the quality of a guideline is that developed by the AGREE (Appraisal of Guidelines for Research and Evaluation) Collaboration, initially funded through an EU research grant. The instrument comprises 23 criteria grouped in the following six domains of guideline development addressed by the AGREE instrument in its second iteration (AGREE II): scope and purpose; stakeholder involvement; rigour of development; clarity and presentation; applicability; and editorial independence (Brouwers et al., 2010). To facilitate the consideration of AGREE II elements already in the guideline development process, a reporting checklist was created in 2016 (Brouwers et al., 2016). There have been calls for more content-focused guideline appraisal tools, as existing options were considered by some to be mainly looking at the documentation of the guideline development process (Eikermann et al., 2014). At the same time, there is recognition that the development of good clinical guidelines often requires trade-offs between methodological rigour and pragmatism (Browman et al., 2015; Richter Sundberg, Garvare & Nyström, 2017). Several studies have evaluated the overall quality of guidelines produced in certain contexts, invariably demonstrating that there is considerable variation in how guidelines score on the various AGREE domains (for example, Knai et al., 2012). However, there seems to be an overall improvement in quality over time (Armstrong et al., 2017). Research shows that while guideline appraisals often use arbitrarily set AGREE cut-off scores to categorize guidelines as being of good or bad quality (Hoffmann-Eßer et al., 2018b), the scoring of specific criteria, such as rigour of development and editorial independence, seems to be the major influencer of final scores (Hoffman-Eßer et al., 2018a).

Beyond the methodological quality of the guideline itself, however, the issue of applicability is also of great importance (*see also* Box 9.2). Heffner noted that as guidelines were rarely tested in patient care settings prior to publication (as would a drug before being approved), the quality of clinical guidelines is defined narrowly by an analysis of how closely recommendations are linked to scientific and clinical evidence (Heffner, 1998). This concern remains today, though it is now more explicitly addressed (*see*, for example, Steel et al., 2014; Li et al., 2018), raising the question of whether guidelines should be systematically pilot-tested in care delivery settings before being finalized. Furthermore, local contextual considerations often influence how guideline recommendations can be used. The science of guideline adaptation aims to balance the need for tailored recommendations with the inefficiency of replicating work already carried out elsewhere. Here as well, a number of frameworks have been developed to guide adaptation efforts (Wang, Norris & Bero, 2018).

Finally, considering the speed with which medical knowledge progresses and the pace of knowledge production at primary research level, it is to be expected that guideline recommendations need to be kept up-to-date. A comprehensive review on the issue concluded that one in five recommendations is outdated three years post-launch of the guideline and concluded that longer updating intervals are potentially too long (Martínez García et al., 2014). In light of the considerable resources required for both the development and the updating of clinical guidelines, approaches for efficient, potentially "real time" updating of (individual) guideline recommendations as new evidence emerges are being discussed ("living guidelines" – *see* Akl et al., 2017, as well as Elliott et al., 2014, for the concept of "living" systematic reviews; *see also* Vernooij, 2014; Martínez García et al., 2015). However, their usefulness needs to be balanced against the potential of updating recommendations too soon, i.e. without a sufficiently mature evidence base, and running the risk of encouraging the use of as-yet-unproven options in the delivery of care. Furthermore, continuous updating is in itself resource-intensive.

For clinical guidelines to have an actual impact on processes and ultimately outcomes of care they need to be not only well developed and based on scientific evidence but also disseminated and implemented in ways that ensure they are actually used by clinicians. So-called guideline clearinghouses, such as the one operated by the US Agency for Healthcare Research and Quality,[2] which was defunded in the summer of 2018, as well as online repositories hosted by large guideline-producing institutions (such as the National Institute for Health and Care Excellence in the UK) or professional associations and/or their umbrella organizations serve as passive dissemination tools. The work of the Guidelines International Network[3] further promotes the dissemination of guideline-related content and provides an exchange platform for guideline developers and users. Tools to assist with the implementation of guideline recommendations (such as point-of-care mobile applications or checklists for clinicians, patient self-management tools and evaluation tools for managers) have progressed along with other developments around clinical practice guidelines in recent years. However, it seems that there is still considerable variation in the availability of such tools by condition, country and the organization responsible for issuing the guidelines (Gagliardi & Brouwers, 2015; Liang et al., 2017).

We discuss the above issues in more detail later in the chapter. At this juncture it is important to note that the points raised so far implicitly focus on improving the effectiveness and safety of patient care. However, as discussed in Chapter 2, the dimension of patient-centredness – i.e. the importance of considering patients' needs and preferences, as well as those of their caregivers – is important not only for the delivery of care but also for its outcomes (Hewitt-Taylor, 2006;

---

2 www.guideline.gov
3 http://www.g-i-n.net/

May, Montori & Mair, 2009; Gupta, 2011). This issue constitutes a more recent focus of discussion around guideline development and utilization processes, with guidelines ideally not only facilitating patient education but also endorsing engagement and fostering shared decision-making, thus assuring that individual patient values are balanced against the "desired" outcomes embedded in the trials that form the basis of the recommendations in the guidelines (see, for example, van der Weijden et al., 2013). Ideally, guidelines should help in determining the treatment plan and individual treatment goals before each intervention, particularly for chronic patients. Different modalities of patient involvement exist in different contexts: patient group representatives are sometimes included in the guideline development process and guideline documents are increasingly produced in different formats for practitioners and patients (*see*, for example, G-I-N, 2015; as well as Elwyn et al., 2015; Fearns et al., 2016; Schipper et al., 2016; Zhang et al., 2017; Cronin et al, 2018).

In summary, clinical guidelines have the potential to influence mainly processes and ultimately outcomes of care, targeting primarily professionals and dealing with the effectiveness, safety and increasingly also patient-centredness of care. To fulfill this potential, they need to be:

- based on the best available scientific evidence;

- developed by a balanced, multidisciplinary panel following formal, robust consensus techniques;

- well disseminated, and implemented in a context and user-specific manner; and

- kept up-to-date.

The following sections look at how these aspects are addressed in European countries, and how the potential contribution of clinical guidelines to quality of care can be understood and optimized.

9.3 What is being done in Europe?

9.3.1 Extent of formalization of guidelines

There is no recent comprehensive comparison of practices around the development and use of clinical guidelines in European countries. The most systematic effort to approach this issue remains the survey carried out by Legido-Quigley et al. in 2011. The survey included 80 respondents from 29 European countries and looked at a number of issues including the regulatory basis underpinning guidelines in each health system, the guideline development process, mechanisms of quality control, implementation modalities, and evaluation of produced recommendations (Legido-Quigley et al., 2012).

Overall, the study identified three broad categories of engagement in clinical guideline development among participating European countries:

- The first category included those with "well established" activities and wide experience in guideline development and implementation. This category comprised the leaders in guideline development (Belgium, England, France, Germany and the Netherlands) and other countries that had, and have, well established programmes (Denmark, Finland, Italy, Norway and Sweden).

- The second category comprised countries that had introduced some form of guideline production and were therefore "making progress" towards having adequate systems in place (for example, Luxembourg).

- The third category involved cases where clinical guidelines had either been "recently adopted" or were "in the planning stage" at the time of investigation.

The majority of countries had no legal basis for the development and implementation of clinical guidelines. Only 13 reported having an officially established basis for guidelines, although implementation still mostly took place on a voluntary basis. Such examples are the French Health Authority (*Haute Authorité de Santé*, HAS) and the National Disease Management Guidelines Programme in Germany (*Programm für Nationale Versorgungsleitlinien*, NVL), which develop clinical guidelines, disseminate them and evaluate their implementation within their respective healthcare system. In France, while clinical guidelines are established by national regulations, their use by practitioners is not mandatory and an initial phase of financial penalties for non-compliance was soon abandoned. In Germany, the NVL programme is run by the highest authorities in the self-governance of physicians, the German Medical Association (*Bundesärztekammer*), the National Association of Statutory Health Insurance Physicians (*Kassenärztliche Bundesvereinigung*), and the Association of the Scientific Medical Societies in Germany (*Arbeitsgemeinschaft der Wissenschaftlichen Medizinischen Fachgesellschaften*, AWMF). NVL guidelines follow a defined methodology (Bundesärztekammer, 2017) and usually inform the content of national disease management programmes (DMPs). Physicians who are voluntarily enrolled in these programmes sign an obligation to rely on the DMP standards and to document their (non)-compliance (*see also* Stock et al., 2011); however, the mission statement of the NVL programme clearly highlights that guidelines are recommendations and practitioners "can – and sometimes must" deviate from them in justified cases.

9.3.2 Systems and structures of guideline development

The same survey showed that across countries guidelines can be developed at national, regional and/or local level; in most cases professional associations are involved in the endeavour. Three main modalities could be discerned:

- about one third of countries had a central agency developing clinical guidelines in collaboration with professional associations;

- several countries reported having multiple levels of clinical guideline development, with regional and local bodies as well as several professional organizations contributing to a centrally coordinated process; and

- finally, fewer countries had no central coordination of the guideline development process at all: professional associations or providers often stepped in to fill the void following personal initiative.

An example of a national agency entirely in charge of a top-down endorsement of recommendations is the National Institute for Health and Care Excellence (NICE) in England, a government-funded organization responsible for providing national guidance and setting quality standards on the promotion of good health and the prevention and treatment of ill-health. Although NICE guidance is developed for the context of England and Wales, it is often used by institutions and health professionals in other countries (*see* below). The Scottish Intercollegiate Guidelines Network (SIGN) is part of the Evidence Directorate of Healthcare Improvement Scotland, a public body within the Scottish National Health Service. It develops and disseminates national clinical guidelines containing recommendations for effective practice based on current evidence and has established itself as one of the go-to instances for guideline best practice in Europe. In Norway the development of official national guidelines falls under the responsibility of the Directorate of Health, although professional associations produce their own guidance in parallel (central and decentralized development). In Belgium several institutions have emerged and are involved in the production and dissemination of clinical guidelines, such as the Colleges of Physicians, the Belgian Health Care Knowledge Centre (KCE), the Belgian Centre for Evidence-Based Medicine (CEBAM), the EBPracticeNet and the Federal Council for the Quality of Nursing. In Germany the AWMF – the umbrella organization of more than 160 scientific medical associations – is responsible for maintaining an online guideline repository and determining the methodology for guideline development across medical societies (AWMF, 2012); the methodology for the previously described NVL programme is defined separately. The inclusion of all developed guidelines in the online repository of the AWMF necessitates certain minimum standards and guidelines are categorized according to their evidence base and mode of development (*see* Fig. 9.2).

Fig. 9.2   *AWMF criteria for guideline categorization*

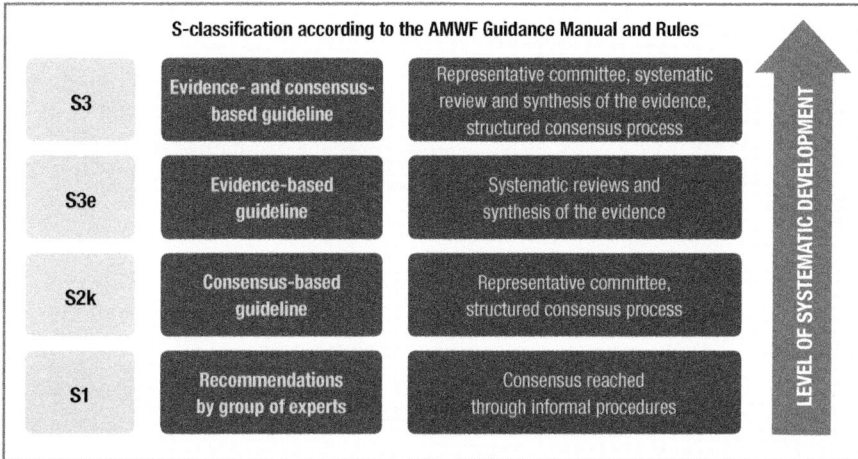

Source: Nothacker et al., 2016

At the other end of the spectrum in the study by Legido-Quigley et al. (2012), practitioners in countries such as Greece and Slovenia had to rely on their own efforts to obtain evidence usually produced abroad; at the time of investigation, professional associations had begun to show interest in the field and both countries have made progress since then (Albreht et al., 2016; Economou & Panteli, 2019).

9.3.3 Use of quality appraisal tools

Legido-Quigley et al. (2012) confirmed that the general acceptance and use of the AGREE II instrument (*see* above) applies to practices in European countries as well: nine countries reported that the instrument was widely used and three more reported not having a formal quality appraisal requirement but working with AGREE if guideline quality was assessed. Some countries employed either adapted versions of the AGREE II instruments or their own appraisal tools. Respondents from twelve countries indicated that no processes to appraise the quality of guidelines were in place. For example, the NICE *Guidelines Manual* explicitly states that its provisions are based on AGREE II (NICE, 2014). In Germany guidelines in the AWMF system are checked for quality before being listed, using the German Instrument for Methodological Guideline Appraisal (*Deutsches Instrument zur Bewertung der methodischen Leitlinienqualität*, DELBI) checklist, which is based on the AGREE I instrument and adapted to the German context (*see* Semlitsch et al., 2015).

9.3.4 Formal pathways for guideline implementation and stimulation of their usage

Ascertaining the extent to which guidelines are actually being implemented – and used – is difficult in most cases; in general there is only very limited systematic data collection of this type of information (we return to this issue in the section on optimizing implementation, below). However, Legido-Quigley et al. (2012) did investigate if underlying conditions for guideline implementation were enforced in European countries, including mandatory nature of utilization, official dissemination practices and financial incentives.

Implementation of clinical guidelines was found generally to not be mandatory. Only Hungary, Lithuania, the Netherlands and Sweden reported some type of general legal requirement but no penalties for non-compliance seemed to be in place. For instance, in the Netherlands clinical guidelines use was mandatory only in certain cases, such as in end-of-life care. Respondents from Hungary indicated that guidelines formulated by single providers (for example, hospitals) were binding within the establishment in question.

In Germany National Disease Management Guidelines are used as a basis to define mandatory standards for disease management programmes. Furthermore, the German Guideline Programme in Oncology, launched in 2008 to foster the development, implementation and evaluation of evidence-based clinical practice guidelines in oncology, regularly derives quality indicators during the guideline development process (*see* Chapter 3 for more information on quality indicators in general). These then flow directly into the certification of oncology centres, which are the cornerstone of healthcare delivery for cancer in Germany. Data on the indicators are collected and fed back to the guideline developers to aid with the updating process.

In some countries and contexts clinical guidelines were not mandatory but clinicians were expected to follow them. For example, in the English NHS healthcare professionals are expected to take NICE clinical guidelines fully into account when exercising their clinical judgement and they are required to record their reasons for not following guideline recommendations. In Germany whether or not treatment was carried out according to official guidelines has been used as an argument during malpractice cases (Legido-Quigley et al., 2012).

In terms of dissemination practices, in most countries guidelines were published on the websites of the agencies responsible for producing and disseminating them and are thus made accessible to a wide audience, albeit in a passive manner. In

Germany guidelines are collected and made available by the German guideline repository (see above and Figure 9.2).[4] Among the countries surveyed by Legido-Quigley et al. (2012) a number of more proactive approaches to dissemination could be observed, including tailored versions for different target groups and newsletters. In Sweden, for example, updated clinical guidelines were sent to each registered practitioner and a short version was compiled for the lay public. Regarding implementation support tools, some countries reported concrete measures, including checklists and how-to guides accompanying new guidelines, as well as IT tools (websites, apps, etc., see below).

Most notably, NICE has a team of implementation consultants that work nationally to encourage a supportive environment and locally to share knowledge and support education and training; additionally, it has developed generic implementation tools (for example, an overall "how-to" guide) and specific tools for every guideline (for example, a costing template and a PowerPoint presentation for use within institutions). Interestingly, NICE's smartphone app, which allowed users to download guidance and use it offline during practice was retired at the end of 2018 and users are now encouraged to use the revamped NICE website. This decision reflects developments in IT infrastructures, personal mobile connectivity (i.e. data) limits and NICE's recognition of the importance of ensuring clinicians' access to up-to-date recommendations (NICE, 2018).

In the Netherlands the use of clinical guidelines is promoted through electronic web pages, some developed with interactive learning. A national website contains a series of implementation tools[5] and certain guideline content is integrated in electronic patient record systems. The latter was reported as being the cornerstone of guideline implementation in Finland as well: guidelines are integrated with the Evidence-Based Medicine electronic Decision Support (EBMeDS) system, allowing clinicians to open them from within the electronic patient record. Moreover, summaries, patient versions, PowerPoint slide series and online courses are developed. In Germany indicator-based approaches are used to monitor and endorse implementation (*see* below), while additional tools include IT-applications in hospitals and the use of guideline-based clinical pathways. At the time of Legido-Quigley et al.'s investigation in 2011, smartphone applications to further simplify guideline implementation had also started to appear (for example, García-Lehuz, Munoz Guajarado & Arguis Molina, 2012). In the intervening years many developers have produced implementation apps (ranging from content repositories to interactive operationalization tools) and guideline repositories have their own app-based platforms for guideline-based decision support (we return to this in the section on good implementation practice, below).

---

4   www.awmf.org
5   http://www.ha-ring.nl/

Financial incentives seem not to be a particularly frequently used tool to encourage the use of clinical guidelines. Legido-Quigley et al. (2012) found that Romanian health units which developed and implemented treatment protocols based on national clinical guidelines received additional funding. In Portugal financial incentives for doctors, nurses and staff were given, based on their score in the annual audit of family physician performance, which also includes clinical guidelines. In the Netherlands some insurers provided financial incentives to support clinical guidelines implementation but largely as a secondary mechanism.

9.3.5 Systematic evaluation of guideline programmes

Overall, there are few examples of systematic formal evaluation of the development, quality, implementation and use of clinical guidelines. NICE produces implementation reports which measure the uptake of specific recommendations taken from selected pieces of guidance by means of routine data analysis. Researchers assess the uptake and effectiveness of guidance on an ad hoc basis. In Sweden the development, quality control, implementation and use of guidelines are regularly evaluated by the National Board of Health and Welfare as well as by county councils or universities on request. Finally, in Germany the development and quality of guidelines are regularly evaluated by AWMF; the quality of the National Guideline Programme is surveyed and closely controlled by the Medical Centre for Quality in Health Care (*Ärztliches Zentrum für Qualität in der Medizin*, ÄZQ) and the AWMF, while the Institute for Quality and Efficiency in Health Care (*Institut für Qualität und Wirtschaftlichkeit im Gesundheitswesen*, IQWiG) is responsible for systematically researching and evaluating current guidelines (German and international) to determine necessity for updating DMP standards (Legido-Quigley et al., 2012).

9.4 The effectiveness and cost-effectiveness of clinical guidelines as a quality strategy

As mentioned earlier in this chapter, the main components of evaluating the usefulness of clinical guidelines as a quality strategy target their implementation and validity: do they reach their target (are clinicians and patients aware of them) and affect the way clinicians treat their patients (influence on process of care) and do they actually support better healthcare (if implemented, do health outcomes actually improve)? (*See also* Fig. 9.1.)

Seminal work by Grimshaw & Russel (1993) looked into the influence of clinical guidelines on medical practice in the early nineties and found that although interest in guidelines was increasing, their utilization and effectiveness remained unclear. It is known that important barriers for guideline implementation rest with lack of awareness (Cabana et al., 1999) and the reluctance of physicians to change their approach to the management of disease (Michie & Johnston, 2004). A public survey on NICE guidelines discovered that awareness of a guideline did not necessarily imply that respondents understood or knew how to use it (McFarlane et al., 2012). A related study carried out in the German primary care context found awareness of clinical guidelines to be relatively low and the inclination to treat according to guidelines not to be higher – and occasionally even lower – in those practitioners who were aware of their existence compared to those who were not (Karbach et al., 2011). Similarly, a study in the French primary care context concluded that, while a favourable disposition towards guidelines in general meant a higher likelihood of awareness of specific guidelines, it did not have a significant effect on the actual application of guideline recommendations in practice (Clerc et al., 2011). Cook et al. (2018) showed that while clinicians believed practice variation should be reduced, they were less certain that this can be achieved. In the Swiss context, despite a generally favourable disposition towards guidelines, barriers to adherence comprised lack of guideline awareness and familiarity, applicability of existing guidelines to multimorbid patients, unfavourable guideline factors and lack of time, as well as inertia towards changing previous practice (Birrenbach et al., 2016). In a scoping review capturing evidence published up to the end of 2015, Fischer et al. (2016) found that barriers to guideline implementation can be differentiated into personal factors, guideline-related factors and external factors, and that structured implementation can improve guideline adherence.

Regarding drivers towards guideline awareness and utilization, Francke et al. (2008) showed that the simpler a guideline is to follow, the more likely it is to be accepted by practitioners. Work by Brusamento et al. (2012) supports the conclusions already drawn by Grimshaw et al. (2004) that the effect of different implementation strategies on care processes varies but spans from non-existence to moderate, with no clear advantage of multifaceted or single interventions. The latter finding was confirmed by a review of reviews in 2014 (Squires et al., 2014), as well as for specific areas of care (for example, Suman et al., 2016). Looking at the issue of guideline adherence over time, recent work found that it decreased about half of the time after more than one year following implementation interventions but the evidence was generally too heterogeneous for really robust conclusions (Ament et al., 2015). A number of studies have tackled the concept of guideline "implementability" in the past few years and are discussed more closely in the next section.

Early work investigating the effects of guidelines on outcomes in primary care found little evidence of effect, citing methodological limitations of the evidence body (Worral, Chaulk & Freake, 1997). Evidence from the Netherlands also suggests that while clinical guidelines can be effective in improving the process and structure of care, their effects on patient health outcomes were studied far less and data are less convincing (Lugtenberg, Burgers & Westert, 2009). This was substantiated by further work in the area (Grimshaw et al., 2012). The systematic review by Brusamento et al. (2012) confirmed the lack of conclusive evidence: while significant effects had been measured, for example regarding the percentage of patients who achieved strict hypertension control through guideline compliant treatment, other studies showed no or unclear effects of guideline-concordant treatment. Newer studies also show mixed results regarding the effect of guidelines on outcomes, but a clear link with implementation modalities (Roberts et al., 2016; Cook et al., 2018; Kovacs et al., 2018; Shanbhag et al., 2018).

Regarding cost-effectiveness, the scope of evidence is even more limited. A comprehensive analysis should include the costs of the development phase, the dissemination/implementation and the change determined in the health service by putting the guideline into practice. However, in practice data on the cost of guideline development are scarce and – given the vast variability of settings and practices – likely not generalizable (Köpp et al., 2012; Jensen et al., 2016). A systematic review by Vale et al. (2007) pointed out that among 200 studies on guideline implementation strategies (only 11 from Europe), only 27% had some data on cost and only four provided data on development and implementation. Most of the relevant studies only partially accounted for costs incurred in the process of guideline production. Having said that, NICE has developed methods to assess the resource impact of its guidelines; for a subset of cost-saving guidelines, savings ranged from £31 500 to £690 per 100 000 population. An investigation of one component of guideline use, namely that of active implementation in comparison to general dissemination practices, found that while the former requires a substantial upfront investment, results regarding optimized processes of care and improved patient outcomes may not be sufficient to render it cost-effective (Mortimer et al., 2013). A related but separate issue is the use of cost-effectiveness analyses *in* clinical guidelines; challenges and opportunities have been identified in the international literature (Drummond, 2016; Garrison, 2016).

9.5 How can clinical guidelines be implemented to improve quality of care?

The previous section touched on the variability of evidence (both in terms of demonstrated effect and strength) regarding the success of different guideline implementation strategies. In this section we look at recent insights on how the implementation of clinical guidelines can be optimized to further facilitate their contribution to good-quality care. This timeframe also reflects the recent increased attention to implementation science in healthcare in general.

There is increasing consensus that incorporating implementation considerations already in the guideline development process can have a substantial influence on implementability. This is reflected in the checklist for implementation planning developed by Gagliardi et al. (2015), which provides a set of concrete actionable items, based on the premise that "implementation should be considered at the beginning, and throughout the guideline development process" (Gagliardi et al., 2015; *see also* Richter-Sundberg et al., 2015 for an example from Sweden). A tool to assist guideline developers with ensuring context-specific implementability elements throughout the guideline process has also been developed (GUIDE-M; *see* Brouwers et al., 2015). Other work into good implementation practice for clinical guidelines has identified specific implementability domains that influence the uptake of clinical guidelines, differentiating between components that fall under two broad aims: the creation of content and the communication of that content (Kastner et al., 2015; Box 9.3).

Box 9.3   *Dimensions of guideline implementability*

Creation of content: The four interrelated domains of content creation are (i) stakeholder involvement (including credibility of the developers and disclosure of conflicts of interest); (ii) evidence synthesis (specifying what evidence is needed and how and when it is synthesized); (iii) considered judgement (including clinical applicability and values); and (iv) feasibility (local applicability, resource constraints and novelty). These domains may be considered non-sequentially and iteratively.

Communication of content: Communication of guidelines entails fine-tuning both the message of the recommendations (through use of simple, clear and persuasive language) and their format (through representation in multiple versions, inclusion of specific components and effective layout and structure).

Source: Kastner et al., 2015

An investigation into trends in guideline implementation found that education for professionals or patients and print material were the most commonly employed strategies for translating guidelines into practice, but practices vary considerably and gaps have been identified both in the scope and follow-up of interventions (Gagliardi & Alhabib, 2015). In fact, despite the general recognition that implementation tools are important for ensuring guideline recommendations reach their intended goal, most guidelines were found not to be accompanied by such applications (Gagliardi & Brouwers, 2015; Liang et al., 2017).

What is more, conclusive evidence supporting the superiority of certain implementation modalities is generally lacking. Fischer et al. (2016) found that the following aspects are central elements of successful implementation approaches:

target-oriented dissemination, education and training, social interaction, decision support systems and standing orders; and tailoring implementation strategies to settings and target groups. At the same time, a comprehensive review of dissemination and implementation practices commissioned by the German Federal Ministry of Health (Althaus et al., 2016) investigated the effects of a number of approaches (distribution of educational materials; educational meetings; educational outreach visits; influence of local opinion leaders; audit and feedback; reminder systems; interventions tailored to local circumstances; organizational interventions; and ensuring continuity of care by means of guideline-based clinical pathways) and found that the systematically collected evidence base was inconclusive for all of them. Against this backdrop, the report recommended a number of steps for strengthening guideline implementation in the German context. Next to endorsing further work into developing appropriate and effective implementation approaches, it supported the creation of legal requirements for guidelines and highlighted the importance of developing guidelines of high methodological quality and relevance to practice (in line with internationally acknowledged criteria of guideline good practice: see introduction).

A different systematic review conducted by the National Heart, Lung, and Blood Institute (NHLBI) in the United States a year later, aiming to synthesize evidence from published implementation science literature to identify effective or promising strategies for the adoption and implementation of clinical guidelines, found that audit and feedback as well as educational outreach visits were generally effective in improving both process of care and clinical outcomes, while the respective effectiveness of provider incentives was mixed. Reminders only sometimes improved process of care and were generally ineffective for clinical outcomes. The study also identified barriers and facilitators for clinician adoption or adherence to guidelines. Barriers included time constraints, limited staffing resources, clinician scepticism, clinician knowledge of guidelines and higher age of the clinician. Guideline characteristics, such as format, resources and end-user involvement were identified as facilitators, along with stakeholder involvement, leadership support, organizational culture (for example, multidisciplinary teams) and electronic guidelines systems. The review confirmed the substantial gaps in the evidence on effectiveness of implementation interventions, especially regarding clinical outcomes, cost-effectiveness and contributory contextual issues (Chan et al., 2017).

One of the most prominent developments in the area of guideline implementation in recent years has been the increased utilization of information technologies to facilitate (a) push mechanisms for guideline adherence, such as decision support components integrated into clinical management software (for example, alerts, reminders or standing orders; *see*, for example, Wright et al., 2010); (b) the use of guidelines at the bedside (for example, mobile guideline apps); and (c) the faster, potentially "real time" updating of (individual) guideline recommendations as new evidence emerges (for example, with "living guidelines"; *see*, Akl et al., 2017 and Thomas et al., 2017, and caveat on this issue earlier in this chapter).

The MAGIC ("Making GRADE the Irresistible Choice") project was established to facilitate the "authoring, dissemination, and dynamic updating of trustworthy guidelines" (Vandvik et al., 2013) and combines the use of all these aspects. It draws on the GRADE principles (*see* introduction to this chapter) as well as the work of the DECIDE project, which aims to optimize communication modalities for evidence-based recommendations targeting healthcare professionals and providers, patients and citizens, and policy-makers.[6] Its approach to solving identified issues with traditional guideline practices is shown in Table 9.2. As mentioned in the introduction, these new approaches still need to be evaluated to ensure that the right balance between benefit and potential harm and/or loss of resources is achieved.

Table 9.2   *Challenges in guideline practice and MAGIC solutions*

What is the problem?	Possible solution
1. Lacking trustworthiness of guidelines	Guideline-authoring platform that facilitates adherence to standards for trustworthy guidelines and use of the GRADE system
2. Inefficient guideline authoring, adaptation and dynamic updating	Online guideline-authoring and publication platform
3. Inefficient guideline dissemination to clinicians at point of care	Structured and tagged content created in an online authoring and publication platform to allow dissemination in a wide range of devices: web platforms, application for tablets and smartphones, and integration in EMRs
4. Suboptimal presentation formats of guideline content	Multilayered guideline content in presentation formats that meet clinicians' information needs at point of care
5. Inconsistent and underdeveloped systems for integration of trustworthy guidelines in EMRs	CDSSs customized to current standards for trustworthy guidelines (for example, both strong and weak recommendations)
6. Limited support for shared decision-making at point of care	Electronic DAs linked to recommendations in guidelines, for use by clinicians and patients in consultations

Notes: CDSS = clinical decision support system; DA = decision aid; EMR = electronic medical records; GRADE = Grading of Recommendations Assessment, Development and Evaluation

Source: Vandvik et al., 2013

The need for rapid responses in emergency situations (for example, epidemics) has prompted research into so-called "rapid guidelines", which approach the balance between expedience of process, methodological rigour and implementability in a systematic manner (Florez et al., 2018; Kowalski et al., 2018; Morgan et al., 2018). Another consideration in this direction is the potential of observational

---

6   https://www.decide-collaboration.eu/

data for updating guideline recommendations. The "living guideline" concept relies on the quick identification of clinical trial results, but there are examples of registry data flowing into the development or updating of clinical practice guidelines (OECD, 2015). Observational data is necessary to describe current health provision (and its quality), pinpoint potential patient groups that are adequately covered by guideline recommendations, and identify gaps and issues to be resolved by clinical research. They are also vital for identifying late onset treatment harms and drug safety issues. However, they are not first choice when deciding about the benefits of treatment recommendations. A review of NICE guidance found that the uptake of such data in guidelines was slow (Oyinlola, Campbell & Kousoulis, 2016).

Performance measurement is another area that lends itself to synergy between clinical guidelines and healthcare data. More and more guideline groups develop quality indicators along with the recommendation sets (Blozik et al., 2012). While these are usually primarily intended as general performance measures (i.e. the guideline, as a summary of best knowledge, informs the choice of indicator), a closer look at measurement results can provide insights on the extent to which practice reflects guideline recommendations (i.e. the indicators inform guideline adherence surveillance). Few countries use guideline-based quality indicators for nationwide quality assurance, such as the hospital benchmarking system in Germany (Szecsenyi et al., 2012) and the German Guideline Programme in Oncology described earlier in the chapter. In the UK a guidelines-based indicator framework was recently developed to monitor primary care practice (Willis et al., 2017). The Guidelines International Network provides reporting guidance for guideline-based performance measurement tools (Nothacker et al., 2016).

While traditionally the development and implementation of clinical guidelines (and other summaries of evidence) has been geared towards meeting the needs of clinicians, formats that support shared decision-making have been gaining focus in recent years (Agoritsas et al., 2015; Härter et al. 2017). Guideline-based decision support tools to facilitate clinician-patient interactions and shared decision-making are a standard accompaniment of the German NVL programme (*see* above), and are among the activities in MAGIC (*see also* Table 9.2 and the SHARE IT project).

Finally, an issue that has been garnering attention in the past few years is that of editorial independence in clinical guideline development. Implementing guideline recommendations that have been created under unclear influence conditions is not only ethically questionable but may also endanger quality of care, as the content may not actually reflect best available evidence. An international survey of 29 institutions involved in clinical guideline development found variability in the content and accessibility of conflict of interest policies; some institutions did not have publicly available policies and of the available policies several did not clearly report critical steps in obtaining, managing and communicating disclosure of relationships of interest (Morciano et al., 2016). Recent work from Germany indicates that while financial conflicts of interest seem to be adequately disclosed in the most rigorously developed guidelines, active management of existing conflicts of interest is lagging behind (Napierala et al., 2018); this is also reflected in work from Canada, which discovered frequent relations between guideline producing institutions and, for example, the pharmaceutical industry and no clear management strategy (Campsall et al., 2016; Shnier et al., 2016). This type of issue was also identified in Australia, with one in four guideline authors without disclosed ties to pharmaceutical companies showing potential for undisclosed relevant ties (Moynihan et al., 2019). To foster trust and implementation, it is clear that institutions involved in guideline development should invest resources in explicitly collecting all relevant information and establish clear management criteria; the structure of disclosure formats also has a role to play here (Lu et al., 2017).

Box 9.4 shows the conflicts of interest management principles defined by the Guidelines International Network (Schünemann et al., 2015). In Germany the website Leitlinienwatch.de ("guideline watch") uses an explicit evaluation matrix to appraise how new German guidelines address the issue of financial conflicts of interest. Beyond measures for direct financial conflicts of interest, the management of indirect conflicts of interest (for example, issues related to academic advancement, clinical revenue streams, community standing and engagement in academic activities that foster an attachment to a specific point of view, *cf.* Schünemann et al., 2015) is also important in guideline development. Ensuring that guidelines are developed based on robust consensus processes by a multidisciplinary panel can contribute to mitigating the effect of such conflicts (*see*, for instance, Ioannidis, 2018).

9.6 Conclusions for policy-makers

Systematically developed, evidence-based clinical guidelines are being used in many countries as a quality strategy. Their usefulness in knowledge translation, particularly in the context of ever-growing volumes of primary research, is not contested. However, their rigour of development, mode of implementation and evaluation of impact can be improved in many settings to enable their goal of achieving "best practice" in healthcare. One of the most important knowledge gaps in this direction is the extent to which guidelines affect patient outcomes and how this effect can be enhanced to ensure better care. For that purpose, both quantitatively measured parameters and service user experience should be taken into account. The latter is already attempted to varying degrees by means

---

Box 9.4 *G-I-N principles for dealing with conflicts of interests in guideline development*

- Principle 1: Guideline developers should make all possible efforts to not include members with direct financial or relevant indirect conflicts of interest.
- Principle 2: The definition of conflict of interest and its management applies to all members of a guideline development group, regardless of the discipline or stakeholders they represent, and this should be determined before a panel is constituted.
- Principle 3: A guideline development group should use standardized forms for disclosure of interests.
- Principle 4: A guideline development group should disclose interests publicly, including all direct financial and indirect conflicts of interest, and these should be easily accessible for users of the guideline.
- Principle 5: All members of a guideline development group should declare and update any changes in interests at each meeting of the group and at regular intervals (for example, annually for standing guideline development groups).
- Principle 6: Chairs of guideline development groups should have no direct financial or relevant indirect conflicts of interest. When direct or indirect conflicts of interest of a chair are unavoidable, a co-chair with no conflicts of interest who leads the guideline panel should be appointed.
- Principle 7: Experts with relevant conflicts of interest and specific knowledge or expertise may be permitted to participate in discussion of individual topics, but there should be an appropriate balance of opinion among those sought to provide input.
- Principle 8: No member of the guideline development group deciding about the direction or strength of a recommendation should have a direct financial conflict of interest.
- Principle 9: An oversight committee should be responsible for developing and implementing rules related to conflicts of interest.

---

of stakeholder involvement, but the practice should be enhanced and expanded to ensure representative and acceptable results. New developments that aim to ensure that guideline recommendations are based on best available evidence, are easily accessible to clinicians and patients, and stay up-to-date should be further explored and evaluated.

The overview of country-specific practices presented in this chapter clearly demonstrates how divergent guideline practices can be, especially when viewed as national strategies for quality improvement. The fact that in several countries practitioners "borrow" recommendations produced abroad combined with existing international initiatives point to a considerable potential for more active knowledge exchange in the future. However, the context-specific nature of produced guidelines must always be taken into account. A lot has already been undertaken in the context of guideline adaptability but earlier, more intensive collaboration might be fruitful, especially on issues such as optimizing guideline development and implementation in the age of multimorbidity. Indeed, this chapter did not focus on the issue of guideline applicability in light of ageing and multimorbidity; implementing guideline recommendations based on evidence derived from young(er) populations without comorbidities does not reflect best practice and can endanger good quality of care for older, multimorbid patients.

In contrast to Health Technology Assessment (HTA; *see* Chapter 6), there is currently no discussion about centralizing the dissemination (let alone the development) of guidelines at EU level, although umbrella organizations of different professional associations produce European guidelines for their specialties. Perhaps it is time to consider such a mechanism, especially given the recent suspension of the USA-based clearinghouse that served internationally as a frequently used resource.

References

Agoritsas T et al. (2015). Decision aids that really promote shared decision making: the pace quickens. *BMJ*, 350:g7624.

Akl EA et al. (2017). Living systematic reviews: 4. Living guideline recommendations. *Journal of Clinical Epidemiology*, 91:47–53. doi: 10.1016/j.jclinepi.2017.08.009.

Albreht T et al. (2016). Slovenia: Health system review. *Health Systems in Transition*, 18(3):1–207.

Althaus A et al. (2016). Implementation of guidelines – obstructive and beneficial factors. Cologne: Institute for Quality and Efficiency in Health Care.

Ament SM et al. (2015). Sustainability of professionals' adherence to clinical practice guidelines in medical care: a systematic review. *BMJ Open*, 5(12):e008073. doi: 10.1136/bmjopen-2015-008073.

Armstrong JJ et al. (2017). Improvement evident but still necessary in clinical practice guideline quality: a systematic review. *Journal of Clinical Epidemiology*, 81:13–21.

AWMF (2012). Ständige Kommission Leitlinien. AWMF-Regelwerk "Leitlinien". Available at: http://www.awmf.org/leitlinien/awmf-regelwerk.html, accessed 14 April 2019.

Birrenbach T et al. (2016). Physicians' attitudes toward, use of, and perceived barriers to clinical guidelines: a survey among Swiss physicians. *Advances in Medical Education and Practice*, 7:673–80. doi: 10.2147/AMEP.S115149.

Blozik E et al. (2012). Simultaneous development of guidelines and quality indicators – how do guideline groups act? A worldwide survey. *International Journal of Health Care Quality Assurance*, 25(8):712–29.

Brouwers M et al. (2010). AGREE II: Advancing guideline development, reporting and evaluation in healthcare. *Canadian Medical Association Journal*, 182:E839–842.

Brouwers MC et al. (2015). The Guideline Implementability Decision Excellence Model (GUIDE-M): a mixed methods approach to create an international resource to advance the practice guideline field. *Implementation Science*, 10:36. doi: 10.1186/s13012-015-0225-1.

Brouwers MC et al. (2016). The AGREE Reporting Checklist: a tool to improve reporting of clinical practice guidelines. *BMJ*, 352:i1152. doi 10.1136/bmj.i1152.

Browman GP et al. (2015). When is good, good enough? Methodological pragmatism for sustainable guideline development. *Implementation Science*, 10:28. doi: 10.1186/s13012-015-0222-4.

Brusamento S et al. (2012). Assessing the effectiveness of strategies to implement clinical guidelines for the management of chronic diseases at primary care level in EU Member States: a systematic review. *Health Policy*, 107(2–3):168–83.

Bundesärztekammer (2017). Programm für Nationale Versorgungsleitlinien – Methodenreport. 5. Auflage 2017. doi: 10.6101/AZQ/000169.

Cabana MD et al. (1999). Why don't physicians follow clinical practice guidelines? A framework for improvement. *Journal of the American Medical Association*, 282(15):1458–65.

Campsall P et al. (2016). Financial Relationships between Organizations that Produce Clinical Practice Guidelines and the Biomedical Industry: a Cross-Sectional Study. *PLoS Medicine*, 13(5):e1002029.

Chan WV et al. (2017). ACC/AHA Special Report: Clinical Practice Guideline Implementation Strategies: a Summary of Systematic Reviews by the NHLBI Implementation Science Work Group: a Report of the American College of Cardiology/American Heart Association Task Force on Clinical Practice Guidelines. *Journal of the American College of Cardiology*, 69(8):1076–92.

Clerc I et al. (2011). General practitioners and clinical practice guidelines: a reexamination. *Medical Care Research and Review*, 68(4):504–18.

Cook DA et al. (2018). Practice variation and practice guidelines: attitudes of generalist and specialist physicians, nurse practitioners, and physician assistants. *PloS One*, 13(1):e0191943.

Council of Europe (2001). Recommendation of the Committee of Ministers to Member States on developing a methodology for drawing up guidelines on best medical practices. Available at: https://search.coe.int/cm/Pages/result_details.aspx?ObjectID=09000016804f8e51, accessed 14 April 2019.

Cronin RM et al. (2018). Adapting medical guidelines to be patient-centered using a patient-driven process for individuals with sickle cell disease and their caregivers. *BMC Hematology*, 18:12. doi: 10.1186/s12878-018-0106-3.

Drummond M (2016). Clinical Guidelines: a NICE Way to Introduce Cost-Effectiveness Considerations? *Value in Health*, 19(5):525–30. doi: 10.1016/j.jval.2016.04.020.

Economou C, Panteli D (2019). Assesment report monitoring and documenting systemic and health effects of health reforms in Greece. WHO Regional Office for Europe.

Eddy DM (2005). Evidence-based medicine: a unified approach. *Health Affairs (Millwood)*, 24(1):9–17.

Eikermann M et al. (2014). Tools for assessing the content of guidelines are needed to enable their effective use – a systematic comparison. *BMC Research Notes*, 7:853. doi: 10.1186/1756-0500-7-853.

Elliott JH et al. (2014). Living systematic reviews: an emerging opportunity to narrow the evidence-practice gap. *PLoS Medicine*, 11(2):e1001603. doi: 10.1371/journal.pmed.1001603.

Elwyn G et al. (2015). Trustworthy guidelines – excellent; customized care tools – even better. *BMC Medicine*, 13:199. doi: 10.1186/s12916-015-0436-y.

ESF (2011). Implementation of Medical Research in Clinical Practice. European Science Foundation. Available at: http://archives.esf.org/fileadmin/Public_documents/Publications/Implem_MedReseach_ClinPractice.pdf, accessed 14 April 2019.

Fearns N et al. (2016). What do patients and the public know about clinical practice guidelines and what do they want from them? A qualitative study. *BMC Health Services Research*, 16:74. doi: 10.1186/s12913-016-1319-4.

Fischer F et al. (2016). Barriers and Strategies in Guideline Implementation – a Scoping Review. *Healthcare (Basel, Switzerland)*, 4(3):36. doi: 10.3390/healthcare4030036.

Florez ID et al. (2018). Development of rapid guidelines: 2. A qualitative study with WHO guideline developers. *Health Research Policy and Systems*, 16(1):62. doi: 10.1186/s12961-018-0329-6.

Francke AL et al. (2008). Factors influencing the implementation of clinical guidelines for health care professionals: a systematic meta-review. *BMC Medical Informatics and Decision Making*, 8:38.

Gagliardi AR, Brouwers MC (2015). Do guidelines offer implementation advice to target users? A systematic review of guideline applicability. *BMJ Open*, 5(2):e007047. doi: 10.1136/bmjopen-2014-007047.

Gagliardi AR, Alhabib S, members of Guidelines International Network Implementation Working Group (2015). Trends in guideline implementation: a scoping systematic review. *Implementation Science*, 10:54. doi: 10.1186/s13012-015-0247-8.

Gagliardi AR et al. (2015). Developing a checklist for guideline implementation planning: review and synthesis of guideline development and implementation advice. *Implementation Science*, 10:19. doi: 10.1186/s13012-015-0205-5.

Garcia-Lehuz JM, Munoz Guajardo I, Arguis Molina S (2012). Mobile application to facilitate use of clinical practice guidelines in the Spanish National Health Service. Poster presentation, G-I-N International Conference, Berlin 22–25 August 2012.

Garrison LP (2016). Cost-Effectiveness and Clinical Practice Guidelines: Have We Reached a Tipping Point? An Overview. *Value in Health*, 19(5):512–15. doi: 10.1016/j.jval.2016.04.018.

G-I-N (2015). G-I-N Public Toolkit: patient and Public Involvement in Guidelines. Pitlochry: Guidelines International Network.

GRADE Working Group (2004). Grading quality of evidence and strength of recommendations. *BMJ*, 328(7454):1490–4.

Grimshaw JM, Russell IT (1993). Effect of clinical guidelines on medical practice: a systematic review of rigorous evaluations. *Lancet*, 342(8883):1317–22.

Grimshaw JM et al. (2004). Effectiveness and efficiency of guideline dissemination and implementation strategies. *Health Technology Assessment*, 8(6):iii–iv, 1–72.

Grimshaw JM et al. (2012). Knowledge translation of research findings. *BMC Implementation Science*, 7:50.

Gupta M (2011). Improved health or improved decision making? The ethical goals of EBM. *Journal of Evaluation in Clinical Practice*, 17(5):957–63.

Guyatt GH et al. (2011). GRADE guidelines: a new series of articles in the Journal of Clinical Epidemiology. *Journal of Clinical Epidemiology*, 64(4):380–2. doi: 10.1016/j.jclinepi.2010.09.011.

Härter M et al. (2017). Shared decision making in 2017: International accomplishments in policy, research and implementation. *Zeitschrift für Evidenz, Fortbildung und Qualität im Gesundheitswesen*, 123–124:1–5.

Heffner JE (1998). Does evidence-based medicine help the development of clinical practice guidelines? *Chest*, 113(3 Suppl):172S–8S.

Hewitt-Taylor J (2006). Evidence-based practice, clinical guidelines and care protocols. In: Hewitt-Taylor J (ed.). Clinical guidelines and care protocols. Chichester: John Wiley & Sons, pp. 1–16.

Hoffmann-Eßer W et al. (2018a). Guideline appraisal with AGREE II: online survey of the potential influence of AGREE II items on overall assessment of guideline quality and recommendation for use. *BMC Health Services Research*, 18(1):143. doi: 10.1186/s12913-018-2954-8.

Hoffmann-Eßer W et al. (2018b). Systematic review of current guideline appraisals performed with the Appraisal of Guidelines for Research & Evaluation II instrument – a third of AGREE II users apply a cut-off for guideline quality. *Journal of Clinical Epidemiology*, 95:120–7. doi: 10.1016/j.jclinepi.2017.12.009.

Ioannidis JPA (2018). Professional Societies Should Abstain From Authorship of Guidelines and Disease Definition Statements. *Circulation: Cardiovascular Quality and Outcomes*, 11(10):e004889. doi: 10.1161/CIRCOUTCOMES.118.004889.

IOM (2011). Clinical Practice Guidelines We Can Trust (Consensus Report). Washington DC: National Academies Press.

JCI (2016). Clinical Practice Guidelines: Closing the gap between theory and practice. A White Paper by the Joint Commission International. Oak Brook (USA): Joint Commission International.

Jensen CE et al. (2016). Systematic review of the cost-effectiveness of implementing guidelines on low back pain management in primary care: is transferability to other countries possible? *BMJ Open*, 6(6):e011042. doi: 10.1136/bmjopen-2016-011042.

Karbach UI et al. (2011). Physicians' knowledge of and compliance with guidelines: an exploratory study in cardiovascular diseases. Deutsches Arzteblatt International, 108(5):61–9.

Kastner M et al. (2015). Guideline uptake is influenced by six implementability domains for creating and communicating guidelines: a realist review. *Journal of Clinical Epidemiology*, 68:498–509. doi: 10.1016/j.jclinepi.2014.12.013.

Khodambashi S, Nytrø Ø (2017). Reviewing clinical guideline development tools: features and characteristics. *BMC Medical Informatics and Decision Making*, 17(1):132. doi: 10.1186/s12911-017-0530-5.

Knai C et al. (2012). Systematic review of the methodological quality of clinical guideline development for the management of chronic disease in Europe. *Health Policy*, 107(2–3):157–67.

Köpp J et al. (2012). Financing of Clinical Practice Guidelines (CPG) – what do we really know? Poster presentation, G-I-N International Conference, Berlin 22–25 August 2012.

Kovacs E et al. (2018). Systematic Review and Meta-analysis of the Effectiveness of Implementation Strategies for Non-communicable Disease Guidelines in Primary Health Care. *Journal of General Internal Medicine*, 33(7):1142–54. doi: 10.1007/s11606-018-4435-5.

Kowalski SC et al. (2018). Development of rapid guidelines: 1. Systematic survey of current practices and methods. *Health Research Policy and Systems*, 16(1):61. doi: 10.1186/s12961-018-0327-8.

Kredo T et al. (2016). Guide to clinical practice guidelines: the current state of play. *International Journal for Quality in Health Care*, 28(1):122–8.

Legido-Quigley H et al. (2012). Clinical guidelines in the European Union: Mapping the regulatory basis, development, quality control, implementation and evaluation across Member States. *Health Policy*, 107(2–3):146–56.

Li H et al. (2018). A new scale for the evaluation of clinical practice guidelines applicability: development and appraisal. *Implementation Science*, 13(1):61. doi: 10.1186/s13012-018-0746-5.

Liang L et al. (2017). Number and type of guideline implementation tools varies by guideline, clinical condition, country of origin, and type of developer organization: content analysis of guidelines. *Implementation Science*, 12(1):136. doi: 10.1186/s13012-017-0668-7.

Lohr KN (1994). Guidelines for clinical practice: applications for primary care. *International Journal for Quality in Health Care*, 6(1):17–25.

Lu Y et al. (2017). Transparency ethics in practice: revisiting financial conflicts of interest disclosure forms in clinical practice guidelines. *PloS One*, 12(8):e0182856. doi: 10.1371/journal.pone.0182856.

Lugtenberg M, Burgers JS, Westert GP (2009). Effects of evidence-based clinical practice guidelines on quality of care: a systematic review. *Quality and Safety in Health Care*, 18(5):385–92. doi: 10.1136/qshc.2008.028043.

McFarlane E et al. (2012). DECIDE: survey on awareness of NICE guidelines and their implementation. Poster presentation, G-I-N International Conference, Berlin 22–25 August 2012.

Martínez García L et al. (2014). The validity of recommendations from clinical guidelines: a survival analysis. *Canadian Medical Association Journal*, 186(16):1211–19.

Martínez García L et al. (2015). Efficiency of pragmatic search strategies to update clinical guidelines recommendations. *BMC Medical Research Methodology*, 15:57. doi: 10.1186/s12874-015-0058-2.

May C, Montori VM, Mair FS (2009). We need minimally disruptive medicine. *BMJ*, 339:b2803. doi: 10.1136/bmj.b2803.

Michie S, Johnston M (2004). Changing clinical behaviour by making guidelines specific. *BMJ*, 328(7435):343–5.

Morciano C et al. (2016). Policies on Conflicts of Interest in Health Care Guideline Development: a Cross-Sectional Analysis. *PloS One*, 11(11):e0166485. doi: 10.1371/journal.pone.0166485.

Morgan RL et al. (2018). Development of rapid guidelines: 3. GIN-McMaster Guideline Development Checklist extension for rapid recommendations. *Health Research Policy and Systems*, 16(1):63. doi: 10.1186/s12961-018-0330-0.

Mortimer D et al. (2013). Economic evaluation of active implementation versus guideline dissemination for evidence-based care of acute low-back pain in a general practice setting. *PloS One*, 8(10):e75647. doi: 10.1371/journal.pone.0075647.

Moynihan R et al. (2019). Undisclosed financial ties between guideline writers and pharmaceutical companies: a cross-sectional study across 10 disease categories. *BMJ Open*, 9:e025864. doi: 10.1136/bmjopen-2018-025864.

Napierala H et al. (2018). Management of financial conflicts of interests in clinical practice guidelines in Germany: results from the public database GuidelineWatch. *BMC Medical Ethics*, 19(1):65. doi: 10.1186/s12910-018-0309-y.

Neumann I et al. (2016). The GRADE evidence-to-decision framework: a report of its testing and application in 15 international guideline panels. *Implementation Science*, 11:93. doi: 10.1186/s13012-016-0462-y.

NICE (2014). Developing NICE guidelines: the manual. Process and methods guides. London: National Institute for Health and Care Excellence.

NICE (2018). NICE to retire Guidance app. Available at: https://www.nice.org.uk/news/article/nice-to-retire-guidance-app, accessed 13 April 2019.

Nothacker M et al. (2016). Reporting standards for guideline-based performance measures. *Implementation Science*, 11:6. doi: 10.1186/s13012-015-0369-z.

OECD (2015). Health Data Governance: Privacy, Monitoring and Research. Paris: OECD. Available at: http://www.oecd.org/health/health-systems/health-data-governance-9789264244566-en.htm.

Oyinlola, JO, Campbell J, Kousoulis AA (2016). Is real world evidence influencing practice? A systematic review of CPRD research in NICE guidances. *BMC Health Services Research*, 16:299. doi: 10.1186/s12913-016-1562-8.

Perleth M et al. (2013). Health Technology Assessment: Konzepte, Methoden, Praxis für Wissenschaft und Entscheidungsfindung. MWV Medizinisch Wissenschaftliche Verlagsgesellschaft.

Qaseem A et al. (2012). Guidelines International Network: Toward International Standards for Clinical Practice Guidelines. *Annals of Internal Medicine*, 156:525–31.

Richter Sundberg L, Garvare R, Nyström ME (2017). Reaching beyond the review of research evidence: a qualitative study of decision making during the development of clinical practice guidelines for disease prevention in healthcare. *BMC Health Services Research*, 17(1):344. doi: 10.1186/s12913-017-2277-1.

Richter-Sundberg L et al. (2015). Addressing implementation challenges during guideline development – a case study of Swedish national guidelines for methods of preventing disease. *BMC Health Services Research*, 15:19. doi: 10.1186/s12913-014-0672-4.

Roberts ET et al. (2016). Evaluating Clinical Practice Guidelines Based on Their Association with Return to Work in Administrative Claims Data. *Health Services Research*, 51(3):953–80. doi: 10.1111/1475-6773.12360.

Sackett DL et al. (1996). Evidence based medicine: what it is and what it isn't. *BMJ*, 312(7023):71–2.

Schipper K et al. (2016). Strategies for disseminating recommendations or guidelines to patients: a systematic review. *Implementation Science*, 11(1):82. doi: 10.1186/s13012-016-0447-x.

Schünemann HJ et al. (2014). Guidelines 2.0: systematic development of a comprehensive checklist for a successful guideline enterprise. *Canadian Medical Association Journal*, 186(3):E123–42. doi: 10.1503/cmaj.131237.

Schünemann HJ et al. (2015). Guidelines International Network: Principles for Disclosure of Interests and Management of Conflicts in Guidelines. *Annals of Internal Medicine*, 163(7):548–53. doi: 10.7326/M14-1885.

Semlitsch T et al. (2015). Evaluating Guidelines: A Review of Key Quality Criteria. *Deutsches Arzteblatt International*, 112(27–28):471–8.

Shanbhag D et al. (2018). Effectiveness of implementation interventions in improving physician adherence to guideline recommendations in heart failure: a systematic review. *BMJ Open*, 8(3):e017765. doi: 10.1136/bmjopen-2017-017765.

Shekelle PG et al. (1999). Clinical guidelines: developing guidelines. *BMJ*, 318(7183):593–6.

Shnier A et al. (2016). Reporting of financial conflicts of interest in clinical practice guidelines: a case study analysis of guidelines from the Canadian Medical Association Infobase. *BMC Health Services Research*, 16:383. doi: 10.1186/s12913-016-1646-5.

Siering U et al. (2013). Appraisal tools for clinical practice guidelines: a systematic review. *PLoS One*, 8(12):e82915. doi: 10.1371/journal.pone.0082915.

Squires JE et al. (2014). Are multifaceted interventions more effective than single-component interventions in changing health-care professionals' behaviours? An overview of systematic reviews. *Implementation Science*, 9:152. doi: 10.1186/s13012-014-0152-6.

Steel N et al. (2014). A review of clinical practice guidelines found that they were often based on evidence of uncertain relevance to primary care patients. *Journal of Clinical Epidemiology*, 67(11):1251–7.

Stock S et al. (2011). Disease-management programs can improve quality of care for the chronically ill, even in a weak primary care system: a case study from Germany. The Commonwealth Fund, 24 (1560).

Suman A et al. (2016). Effectiveness of multifaceted implementation strategies for the implementation of back and neck pain guidelines in health care: a systematic review. *Implementation Science*, 11(1):126. doi: 10.1186/s13012-016-0482-7.

Szecsenyi J et al. (2012). Tearing down walls: opening the border between hospital and ambulatory care for quality improvement in Germany. *International Journal for Quality in Health Care*, 24(2):101–4. doi: 10.1093/intqhc/mzr086.

Thomas J et al. (2017). Living systematic reviews: 2. Combining human and machine effort. *Journal of Clinical Epidemiology*, 91:31–7. doi: 10.1016/j.jclinepi.2017.08.011.

Vale L et al. (2007). Systematic review of economic evaluations and cost analyses of guideline implementation strategies. *European Journal of Health Economics*, 8(2):111–21.

van der Weijden T et al. (2013). How can clinical practice guidelines be adapted to facilitate shared decision making? A qualitative key-informant study. *BMJ Quality and Safety*, 22(10):855–63. doi: 10.1136/bmjqs-2012-001502. Epub 2013 Jun 7.

Vandvik PO et al. (2013). Creating clinical practice guidelines we can trust, use, and share: a new era is imminent. *Chest*, 144(2):381–9. doi: 10.1378/chest.13-0746.

Vernooij RW (2014). Guidance for updating clinical practice guidelines: a systematic review of methodological handbooks. *Implementation Science*, 9:3. doi: 10.1186/1748-5908-9-3.

Vlayen J et al. (2005). A systematic review of appraisal tools for clinical practice guidelines: multiple similarities and one common deficit. *International Journal for Quality in Health Care*, 17(3):235–42.

Wang Z, Norris SL, Bero L (2018). The advantages and limitations of guideline adaptation frameworks. *Implementation Science*, 13(1):72. doi: 10.1186/s13012-018-0763-4.

Wiles LK et al. (2017). STANDING Collaboration: a study protocol for developing clinical standards. *BMJ Open*, 7(10):e014048. doi: 10.1136/bmjopen-2016-014048.

Willis TA et al. (2017). Variations in achievement of evidence-based, high-impact quality indicators in general practice: an observational study. *PloS One*, 12(7):e0177949. doi: 10.1371/journal.pone.0177949.

Woolf S et al. (2012). Developing clinical practice guidelines: types of evidence and outcomes; values and economics, synthesis, grading, and presentation and deriving recommendations. *Implementation Science*, 7:61. doi: 10.1186/1748-5908-7-61.

Worrall G, Chaulk P, Freake D (1997). The effects of clinical practice guidelines on patient outcomes in primary care: a systematic review. *Canadian Medical Association Journal*, 156(12):1705–12.

Wright A et al. (2010). Best Practices in Clinical Decision Support: the Case of Preventive Care Reminders. *Applied Clinical Informatics*, 1(3):331–45.

Zhang Y et al. (2017). Using patient values and preferences to inform the importance of health outcomes in practice guideline development following the GRADE approach. *Health and Quality of Life Outcomes*, 15(1):52. doi: 10.1186/s12955-017-0621-0.

Chapter 10

Audit and Feedback as a Quality Strategy

Gro Jamtvedt, Signe Flottorp, Noah Ivers

Summary

What are the characteristics of the strategy?

Audit and feedback is a strategy that intends to encourage professionals to change their clinical practice. An audit is a systematic review of professional performance based on explicit criteria or standards. This information is subsequently fed back to professionals in a structured manner. The underlying assumption for audit and feedback is that highly motivated health professionals who receive information showing that their clinical practice is inconsistent with desired practice, as described in evidence-based guidelines, and/or in comparison to peers, will shift their attention to focus on areas where improvements are needed. Most audit processes measure adherence to recommendations and may include measures of structures, processes and/or outcomes of care; any or all three domains of quality may be assessed: effectiveness, safety and/or patient-centredness.

What is being done in European countries?

The UK and the Netherlands are the countries in Europe that have the longest history of audit and feedback but other countries have become increasingly active since the late 1990s and early 2000s. Audit and feedback initiatives are conducted at local, regional and national levels. They have usually focused on indicators in the effectiveness and/or safety domains, as these are usually easiest to measure using administrative databases and/or electronic medical records. In some regions patient surveys are used to add indicators of patient-centredness to measurement systems. Feedback reports are provided to providers and/or professionals, and feedback is often combined with other quality initiatives such as accreditation, financial incentives or quality circles.

What do we know about the effectiveness and cost-effectiveness of the strategy?

More than 140 randomized trials involving audit and feedback interventions were included in a 2012 review by the Cochrane Collaboration. Studies show a small to moderate effect of audit and feedback on professional compliance with desired clinical practice. The available evidence on effects on patient outcomes is less clear, although several studies indicate positive results. Cost-effectiveness of audit and feedback in comparison with usual care has not been evaluated in systematic reviews. However, cost-effectiveness will likely depend on the clinical topic. It remains unclear whether audit and feedback is more effective than other quality improvement interventions, such as reminders, educational outreach activities, opinion leaders, etc., and whether it is more effective when combined with any of these interventions.

How can the strategy be implemented?

The clinical topic of audit and feedback needs to be carefully selected. Audit and feedback is more effective when focusing on providers with poor performance at baseline. Schemes should always include clear targets and an action plan specifying necessary steps to achieve the targets. The feedback should provide a clear message that directs the professionals' attention to actionable, achievable tasks that will improve patient care. Organizational commitment to a constructive (i.e. non-punitive) approach to continuous quality improvement is essential, with iterative cycles of multimodal feedback provided from a credible source. Local conditions, such as the availability of reliable, routinely collected data that are perceived as valid, have an important impact on the costs of an intervention.

Conclusions for policy-makers

Audit and feedback can contribute to improved quality of care, and can be implemented with minimal cost when data are available. However, it is not the ideal strategy for all clinical problems and the design features of audit and feedback interventions have an important impact on its effectiveness.

10.1 Introduction: the characteristics of audit and feedback

Audit and feedback is a strategy that is widely used in European countries in various ways. The spectrum ranges from mandatory schemes run by government bodies to voluntary, smaller-scale initiatives led by professionals. Some audit and feedback initiatives aim to improve accountability (for example, towards the public, the payer, etc.), while others aim at continuous quality improvement and professional development. In some countries audit and feedback strategies are described as clinical audits, underlining their focus on clinical practice (in contrast to, for example, financial audits). All audit and feedback initiatives have in common the intention to encourage professionals to change their clinical practice when needed by showing them how they perform compared to descriptive or normative benchmarks or targets.

An audit is a review of professional performance based on explicit criteria or standards, preferably developed on the basis of evidence-based clinical guidelines or pathways (*see* Chapters 9 and 12). Performance information is subsequently fed back to professionals, showing how they perform in relation to their peers, standards or targets. In addition, there should be a formal process to identify possible actions in order to change current practice and to improve performance.

Audit and feedback can be used for any area of healthcare, i.e. preventive, acute, chronic and palliative care. Audits can attempt to assess individual health professionals' performance or that of teams, departments, hospitals or regions. The audit may focus on various indicators of quality measured in terms of structures, processes or outcomes of care (*see also* Chapter 3). Audits could also focus on any of the three domains of healthcare quality (effectiveness, safety, patient-centredness), as well as on many other aspects of performance, such as timeliness, efficiency and equity. However, in practice most audits focus on processes of care and/or patient outcomes that are strongly correlated with processes of care, and the focus of most initiatives has been on effectiveness and patient safety.

Audits can be based on routinely available information, such as administrative databases, electronic patient records or medical registries, or they may be based on purposefully collected data from medical records or direct observations. Audit and feedback initiatives can be internal (conducted by individual or local groups of practitioners for their own practice), or external (conducted by professional bodies, research groups or government structures). In either case the indicators measured can be determined by outside sources (i.e. top-down) or by the recipients of the feedback (i.e. bottom-up) or by a combination of both (Foy et al., 2002). Ultimately, the approach taken depends on the underlying purpose (for example, accountability versus quality improvement or knowledge translation/implementation of guidelines).

Feedback can be delivered in different ways, which can be categorized in terms of the source (for example, administrators, senior colleagues or peers), the recipients (for example, individuals or groups), formats (for example, verbal or written), frequency (for example, monthly or yearly), and content (for example, including level of aggregation of data, type of comparison, clarity of message and action plan). The feedback of performance information can be performed in ways that involve varying amounts of interaction or engagement with recipients, depending on the level of interest and availability of resources.

Audits can be a prerequisite for accreditation and certification (*see* Chapter 8), and feedback can be linked to economic incentives (*see* Chapter 14). Furthermore, performance data can be made publically available to contribute to informed patient choice (*see* Chapter 13). However, in most cases feedback is confidential rather than public. In contrast to other quality improvement strategies, such as accreditation, certification and supervision (*see* Chapter 8), which are focused on healthcare organizations or institutions, audit and feedback is most often focused on improving performance of health professionals.

10.2 Why should audit and feedback contribute to healthcare quality?

Health professionals are usually assumed to be highly motivated individuals dedicated to providing high-quality care. However, it is well documented that many patients do not receive recommended care and that there are great variations in medical practice (Ash et al., 2006; Wennberg, 2014), which cannot be explained by illness, patient preferences or medical science. Part of the explanation for this phenomenon is likely that professionals have a limited ability to accurately assess their own performance (Davis et al., 2006). Therefore, information about how they perform compared to descriptive or normative standards can be an important motivator for change amongst health professionals (Godin et al., 2008).

Like many other quality improvement strategies, audit and feedback has been conceptualized as a cyclical process that involves five steps (*see* Fig. 10.1): (1) preparing for audit; (2) selecting criteria; (3) measuring performance; (4) making improvements; and (5) sustaining improvements (Benjamin, 2008). Roughly the first half of the cycle is concerned with auditing of professional performance, while the second half of the cycle starts with feeding this information back to professionals. However, audit and feedback will result in quality improvements only if the feedback leads to changes that improve clinical practice.

Whether or not practice changes take place depends on various factors, which have been explored qualitatively in numerous studies (*see* Brown et al., 2016). Many theories exist to explain how audit and feedback may lead to changes in

Fig. 10.1 *The audit and feedback cycle*

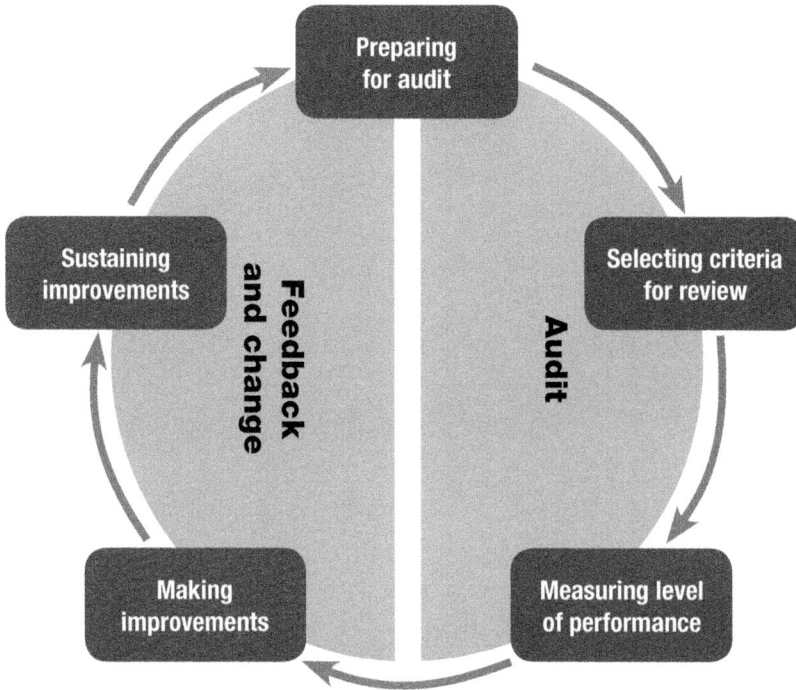

Source: based on Benjamin, 2008, with modifications

professional practice. Some theories focus on change within the professionals, others on change within the social setting or within the organizational and economic context (Grol et al., 2007). According to these theories, audit and feedback may change the awareness of the recipients and their beliefs about current practice, which will subsequently result in changes of clinical practice. In addition, audit and feedback may change perceived social norms and direct attention to a specific set of tasks or subgoals (Ivers et al., 2012).

The extent to which audit and feedback successfully accomplishes this desired reaction depends upon the features of the intervention itself, the targeted behaviour change, and how these interact with features of the recipient and their environment (*see* below). Well designed feedback considers all these factors and seeks to minimize emotional responses of defensiveness while shifting the recipient's attention towards the specific, achievable tasks needed to achieve best possible patient outcomes (Payne & Hysong, 2016).

10.3 What is being done in Europe?

The UK and the Netherlands are the countries in Europe that have the longest history of audit and feedback. In both countries audit and feedback initiatives

Table 10.1 A selection of some audit and feedback programmes in Europe

Country	Programme/ responsible institution	Focus of programme			Audited information (data sources)	Indicators	Type of feedback	Comments
		Care area	Quality dimension(s)	Types of providers				
Finland	Conmedic (31 health centres which provide services for one fifth of the population)	Prevention, acute, chronic care	Effectiveness	Primary health centres	Electronic patient records	Process	Feedback report and web page for potential exchange between health centres	
Germany	External Quality Assurance for Inpatient Care (esQS)/Federal Joint Committee	30 acute care areas (2014)	Effectiveness, patient safety	Inpatient care	Specifically documented quality assurance data, administrative data	416 process and outcome indicators (33% risk-adjusted) (2014), for example, inpatient mortality of cholecystectomy patients or antibiotics initiated within 8 hours for community-acquired pneumonia	Benchmark report to hospital (with comparison to national average performance)	Mandatory programme, combined with peer review process in case of suspected quality problems, public reporting of about 70% of indicators
	Initiative Qualitätsmedizin (IQM) (non-profit association)	Acute care	Effectiveness, safety	Inpatient care	Administrative data sources	Outcome indicators (for example, inpatient mortality per condition)	Benchmark report to hospitals	Voluntary programme, combined with systematic peer review
Ireland	National office of clinical audit	Six different audits for secondary and tertiary care	Effectiveness, safety	Hospitals	Hospital records	Structure, process, outcome	Benchmark report, comparing with similar providers	
Italy	Emilia-Romagna region	Primary care	Effectiveness, patient-centredness	GPs	Administrative data sources	Structure, process, outcome	GPs are mandated to join a primary care team to collaborate and share information	A primary care team includes on average 15 members; goal is to promote teamwork and create a culture of quality, not to be punitive

Country	Programme/responsible institution	Focus of programme			Audited information (data sources)	Indicators	Type of feedback	Comments
		Care area	Quality dimension(s)	Types of providers				
Netherlands	Dutch Institute for Clinical Auditing	23 different treatments	Effectiveness, patient safety, patient-centredness	Hospitals, medical teams	Hospital records	Structure, process, outcome	Regular (at least monthly) feedback to providers, usually combined with PDCA (plan-do-check-act) cycles	Indicators are selected yearly together with scientific associations, hospital organizations and patients
United Kingdom	National Clinical Audit Programme/ Healthcare Quality Improvement Partnership (HQIP)	30 clinical conditions, including acute (for example, emergency laparotomy) and chronic conditions (for example, diabetes)	Effectiveness, safety and patient experience	Specialist inpatient and outpatient service providers	Questionnaires on hospital structures, patient surveys, patient clinical data review, analyses of administrative databases	Structures (for example, staff availability), processes (for example, percentage of patients with foot examinations), outcomes (for example, incidence of hypoglycemic episodes and patient experience)	Benchmark reports for local trusts	
	Quality and Outcomes Framework	Primary care (prevention, acute and chronic care)	Effectiveness, safety, patient experience	GP practices	Clinical records	81 (2014/15) different indicators: structures (disease registers), processes, outcomes (limits on blood pressure)	Results and payment information only	Primarily a financial rewards programme, not to be used as sole input for clinical audit (because of exception reporting, which might hide clinically relevant cases)

Source: authors' compilation, based on an email survey in 2012 and desk research using available online sources in 2016/2017

developed on a voluntary basis in the 1970s and 1980s. Later, from 1991, the UK was the first country that required hospital doctors to participate in audit. Within a few years other health professionals were required to join multiprofessional clinical audits. In Germany and France audit and feedback initiatives emerged mostly in the 1990s. Table 10.1 provides an overview about some prominent audit and feedback programmes in Europe.

In the UK various actors are active in the field of audit and feedback. The National Clinical Audit Programme is run by the Healthcare Quality Improvement Partnership (HQIP). National audits are performed for about 30 clinical conditions, including acute (for example, emergency laparotomy) and chronic conditions (for example, diabetes). These audits focus mostly on specialist inpatient and outpatient service providers, who are assessed with regard to all three dimensions of quality: effectiveness, patient safety and patient experience. Audits rely on various data sources, and assess performance in relation to numerous indicators of structures, processes and outcomes. Benchmark reports are provided to local trusts and annual reports are published for each of the clinical conditions. In the area of primary care the most important national audit programme is the Quality and Outcomes Framework (QOF). However, the main purpose of QOF is to distribute financial incentives (representing around 15% of GP income), and indicators were developed externally. GPs are also required to undertake audit and feedback as part of their revalidation scheme, which was launched in 2012. Furthermore, medical students are taught audit, and there is some teaching for GP trainees. Finally, there is a National Quality Improvement and Clinical Audit Network (NQICAN), which brings together 15 regional clinical audit/effectiveness networks from across England. NQICAN supports staff working in quality improvement and clinical audit in different health and social care organizations, providing practical guidance and support.

In the Netherlands audit and feedback activities historically started in primary care and were initiated by GPs. More recently, audit and feedback has expanded also to secondary inpatient and outpatient care and is more embedded in broader quality assurance initiatives. A Dutch Institute for Clinical Audit (DICA) was set up in 2009 and medical specialist societies use DICA to measure quality and communicate about it. DICA runs registers for cancer patients (colorectal, breast, upper gastrointestinal and lung), collects patient-reported outcome measures, and provides feedback reports to professionals. Almost all hospitals have established quality improvement strategies based on feedback reports from DICA, which also allow them to measure improvements over time. In addition, a comprehensive clinical and organizational audit is part of primary care practice accreditation. Furthermore, almost all GPs are part of one of 600 educational pharmacotherapy groups existing in the country, each consisting of GPs and pharmacists. These groups use audits of prescribing data as a starting point for discussions.

In Germany audit and feedback efforts also exist at several levels of the healthcare system. The most important audit and feedback initiative is the mandatory external quality assurance programme introduced for all hospitals in 2001. It is the responsibility of the Federal Joint Committee, which includes representatives of providers (for example, hospitals) and sickness funds. By 2014 the programme covered 30 specific areas of inpatient care (for example, cholecystectomy, or community-acquired pneumonia), which were assessed on the basis of more than 400 process and outcome indicators, including also patient-safety indicators (AQUA, 2014). Providers have to comply with specific quality documentation requirements in order to provide data for the audits. Collected data are analysed and forwarded to professional expert sections who may initiate a peer review process if the data suggest potential quality problems. Public disclosure of data was introduced in 2007. Smaller programmes cover amongst other things disease management programmes (DMPs) and ambulatory dialysis. In addition, professional associations may have their own audit systems, for example, for reproductive medicine, producing annual reports and providing feedback to providers.

In Italy the Emilia-Romagna region requires GPs to join a Primary Care Team. GPs are mandated to collaborate and share information and to engage in improving the quality of healthcare services provided to patients. Primary Care Teams receive quality reports featuring structure, process and outcome indicators computed on the basis of data from the regional healthcare administrative database, an anonymous comprehensive and longitudinal database linkable at the patient and provider level. The GPs in each team are asked to identify at least one critical area of the report and initiate quality improvement activities in their practice accordingly. The reports are not meant to be "punitive"; rather, the reports are intended to promote teamwork and coordination, and encourage clinical discussion. GPs seem to have a positive view of the reports (Maio et al., 2012; Donatini et al., 2012).

In Finland audit and feedback is used mostly in health centres. One fifth of all health centres participate in yearly quality measurements, based on two-week samples of treatment of patients, organized by Conmedic, a primary care quality consortium. Quality measurement always includes indicators for diabetes and cardiovascular care but also several other areas of care, which may vary from year to year based on decisions of health centres. Measured care areas have included fracture prevention, smoking cessation, interventions for risky alcohol consumption, dementia and self-care. The purpose of the audit and feedback is to inform local quality improvement activities. In addition, all intensive care units collect information on all patients, and the information is reported back to the professionals. Both audit and feedback systems started in 1994. The audit and feedback is voluntary, driven by health professionals. Audit data are fed back at group level. Another interesting initiative in Finland is the evidence-based decision support system (EBMeDS) developed by Duodecim, the Finnish Medical Society. EBMeDS is linked to many patient record systems and provides direct feedback and decision support to practitioners.

In Ireland a National Office of Clinical Audit (NOCA) was established in 2012. Its objective is to maintain clinical audit programmes at national level. They offer different audit programmes (major trauma, national intensive care unit, national orthopaedic register, hip fracture and hospital mortality) and publish national reports on some audit areas. National clinical audits are ongoing reviews of clinical practice that use structural, process and outcome measures to find room for improvement. NOCA emphasizes the importance of action based on audit output and supports hospitals in learning from their audit cycles. The comprehensiveness of data has improved over the years; for example, the most recent report on hip fractures contains data from all 16 eligible hospitals.

At the European level, guidelines on clinical audit for medical radiological practices, including diagnostic radiology, nuclear medicine and radiotherapy, were published by the EU Commission in 2010. These provide recommendations on how to approach clinical audit in radiological practice and suggest the inclusion of structure, process and outcome indicators for comprehensive audits. However, it remains unclear how far these guidelines have been implemented at national level.

To our knowledge, no systematic research has been conducted to assess or compare the use of audit and feedback across European healthcare systems. However, the informal overview provided in this section illustrates the large variation not only in terms of what is audited, but also how the feedback is delivered and ownership of the programmes.

10.4 The effectiveness and cost-effectiveness of audit and feedback

A systematic review from Cochrane on the effects of audit and feedback was first published in 2000 and has since been updated twice (2006 and 2012). Table 10.2 summarizes characteristics of 140 studies included in the 2012 update of the review (Ivers et al., 2012). Almost half of all studies were conducted in the USA. In most studies audit and feedback was combined with other quality improvement strategies such as clinician education, educational outreach (also called academic detailing) or reminder systems, and the targeted professionals were most often physicians.

Audited information included mostly process indicators; it was mostly focused on aggregate patient data (for example, proportions of patients not receiving guideline consistent care), and on individual providers instead of groups of

Table 10.2 *Characteristics of 140 audit and feedback intervention trials included in Ivers et al., 2012*

Country		USA (49%), UK or Ireland (15%), Canada (8%), Australia or New Zealand (7%), other (21%)
Setting		Outpatient (67%), inpatient (26%), other/unclear (7%)
Intervention		Audit and feedback alone (35%), with clinician education (34%), with educational outreach/academic detailing (20%), with clinician reminders or decision support (12%)
Clinical topic		Diabetes/cardiovascular disease management (21%), laboratory testing/radiology (15%), prescribing (22%), other (41%)
Targeted professionals		Physicians (86%), nurses (11%), pharmacists (4%), other (2%)
Audited information	Assessed indicators	Processes (79%), outcomes (14%), other (for example, costs, 32%)
	Focus of analysis	Individual patient cases (for example, patients who did not receive a particular test, 25%), aggregate of patient cases (for example, proportion not receiving guideline consistent care, 81%)
	Level of analysis	Performance of individual provider (81%), performance of provider group (64%)
Feedback characteristics	Format	Written (60%), verbal and written (23%), verbal (9%), unclear (8%)
	Source	Investigators/unclear (80%), supervisor/colleague (9%), employer (11%)
	Frequency	Once only (49%), less than monthly (26%), monthly (14%), weekly (8%)
	Lag time	Days (4%), weeks (16%), months (33%), years (2%), mix (1%), unclear (44%)
	Target	Individuals (51%), groups (18%), both (16%), unclear (14%)
	Comparison	Others' performance (49%), guideline (11%), own previous performance (4%), other or combination (10%), unclear (26)
Required change		Increase current behaviour (41%), decrease current behaviour (21%), mix or unclear (39%)
Instructions for change		Goal setting (8%), action planning (29%), both (3%), neither (60%)

Source: based on Ivers et al., 2012, Brehaut et al., 2016, and Colquhoun et al., 2017

providers. Feedback was usually provided in writing, and in almost half of the studies it was provided only once. In more than half of the studies feedback was provided to individuals and it mostly showed comparisons with the performance of peers. In response to the feedback, professionals were required to either increase (41%) or decrease (21%) their behaviour, but they usually did not receive detailed instructions about how to change their behaviour.

Table 10.3 provides an overview of the main results of the meta-analyses performed as part of the 2012 Cochrane review of audit and feedback trials. The largest number of studies reported results comparing the compliance of professionals with desired practice using dichotomous outcomes (for example, the proportion of professionals compliant with guidelines). These studies found a small to moderate effect of audit and feedback. The median increase of compliance with desired practice was 4.3% (interquartile range (IQR) 0.5% to 16%).

Table 10.3 *Main results of audit and feedback studies included in Ivers et al., 2012*

Outcome	Outcome measure	Comparisons included in meta-analysis	Results (weighted median-adjusted RD or change)*	Conclusions (certainty of evidence)
Any audit and feedback intervention compared with usual care				
Compliance with desired practice	Dichotomous outcomes, for example, proportion compliant with guidelines	82 comparisons from 49 studies	4.3% (IQR 0.5% to 16%) absolute increase in desired practice	Audit and feedback leads to small but potentially important improvements in professional practice (moderate) (low)
	Continuous outcomes, for example, number of lab tests	26 comparisons from 21 studies	1.3% (IQR 1.3% to 29%) increase in desired practice	
Patient outcomes	Dichotomous outcomes, for example, smoking status	12 comparisons from 6 studies	0.4% (IQR –1.3% to 1.6%)	
	Continuous outcomes, for example, blood pressure	8 comparisons from 5 studies	17% (IQR 1.5% to 17%)	
Audit and feedback alone compared with usual care				
Compliance with desired practice	Dichotomous outcomes, for example, proportion compliant with guidelines	32 comparison from 26 studies	3.0% (IQR 1.8% to 7.7%)	The difference between audit and feedback alone versus audit and feedback combined with other interventions is statistically significant only for studies with continuous outcomes but not with dichotomous outcomes
Compliance with desired practice	Continuous outcomes, for example, number of lab tests	14 comparisons from 13 studies	1.3% (IQR 1.3% to 11.0%)	
Audit and feedback combined with other interventions compared with usual care				
Compliance with desired practice	Dichotomous outcomes, for example, proportion compliant with guidelines	50 comparisons from 32 studies	5.5% (IQR 0.4% to 16%)	
Compliance with desired practice	Continuous outcomes, for example, number of lab tests	12 comparisons from 11 studies	26.1% (IQR 12.7% to 26.1%)	
Additional results based on meta-regression				
• Effect appears to be (significantly) larger when: • baseline performance is low • feedback source is supervisor or senior colleague • feedback delivered both verbally and written	• feedback provided more than once • required change is to decrease current behaviour • intervention targets prescribing • includes both explicit targets and an action plan			

Source: based on Ivers et al., 2012

Notes: * For dichotomous outcomes the adjusted risk difference (RD) was calculated as the difference in adherence after the intervention minus the difference before the intervention. For continuous outcomes the adjusted change relative to the control group was calculated as the post-intervention difference in means minus the baseline difference in means divided by the baseline control group mean. Effect size was weighted by the number of health professionals involved in the trial reported to ensure that very small trials did not contribute the same to the overall estimate as larger trials.

Although the median effect may be perceived as relatively small, a quarter of the studies included in the primary analysis showed larger than 16% absolute improvement in health professionals' compliance with desired behaviour.

Relatively few studies reported effects of audit and feedback on patient outcomes, including dichotomous outcomes (for example, smoking status) or continuous outcomes (for example, blood pressure). Studies reporting dichotomous outcomes found a minimal discernible effect, while studies reporting continuous outcomes found a comparatively large positive outcome (17%). In summary, the review confirmed the conclusions of earlier reviews that audit and feedback can be a useful and effective intervention for improving professional practice and potentially patient outcomes.

The large variation in reported results, with a quarter of studies reporting relatively large effects (i.e. absolute improvements in desired practice >16%), suggests that audit and feedback, when optimally designed, delivered and implemented, can play an important role in improving professional practice. However, it also implies that poorly designed audit and feedback schemes will have a minimal or no effect. This underlines the need to focus attention on the design and implementation of audit and feedback schemes.

A meta-regression included in the Cochrane review showed that baseline performance, characteristics of the feedback and the type of change in practice required by the intervention can explain part of the variation in effect size (*see* Table 10.3). For example, when feedback is presented both verbally and in written format, the median effect is 8% higher than when feedback is presented only verbally. Similar differences in effect sizes exist if the feedback is delivered by a supervisor or senior colleague compared to the investigators, when the frequency is increased from once only to weekly and when the feedback contains both an explicit, measurable target and a specific action plan. However, all the findings of the meta-regression should be taken as tentative, as they are based on indirect analyses and ecological bias.

Not surprisingly, the meta-regression also found that the effect of audit and feedback is larger among health professionals with low baseline performance. In addition, it seems that feedback is more effective for less complex changes in professional behaviour (such as prescriptions) than for more complex ones (such as the overall management of patients with chronic disease), although it is plausible that feedback may be useful if it targets very specific behaviour changes related to chronic disease management.

Furthermore, the meta-regression showed that sources of feedback associated with the lowest effect size are "professionals' standards review organization" and "representative of the employer or purchaser". This is an important finding in line with previous qualitative work, which suggested that feedback with a punitive tone is less effective than constructive feedback (Hysong, Best & Pugh, 2006). Also, Feedback Intervention Theory (Kluger & DeNisi, 1996) suggests that feedback directing attention towards acceptable and familiar tasks (as opposed to feedback that generates emotional responses or causes deep self-reflection) is more likely to lead to improvements.

Finally, Table 10.3 presents separately results from studies where audit and feedback was carried out alone and results for interventions where audit and feedback was combined with other interventions. Although combined interventions appeared to have a larger median effect size than studies where audit and feedback was implemented alone, the difference was not statistically significant. These findings are consistent with other reviews (O'Brien et al., 2007; Forsetlund et al., 2009; Squires et al., 2014), which found that there is no compelling evidence that multifaceted interventions are more effective than single-component ones. Therefore, it remains unclear whether it is worth the additional resources and costs to add other interventions to audit and feedback.

The cost-effectiveness of audit and feedback in comparison with usual care has not been evaluated in any review to date. In general, cost-effectiveness analyses are rare in the quality improvement literature (Irwin, Stokes & Marshall, 2015). However, it is clear that the costs of setting up an audit and feedback programme will vary depending on how the intervention is designed and delivered. Local conditions, such as the availability of reliable routinely collected data, have an important impact on the costs of an intervention. If accurate data are readily available, audit and feedback may prove to be cost-effective, even when the effect size is small.

Only very few reviews investigating the effectiveness of audit and feedback compared with other quality improvement strategies are available. The Cochrane review included 20 direct comparisons between audit and feedback and other interventions but it remained unclear whether audit and feedback works better than reminders, educational outreach, opinion leaders, other educational activities or patient-mediated interventions. One review compared the influence of 11 different quality improvement strategies, including audit and feedback, on outcomes of diabetes care (Tricco et al., 2012). Findings consistently indicated across different outcome measures (HbA1c, LDL levels, systolic and diastolic blood pressure) that complex interventions, such as team changes, case management and promotion of self-management, are more effective than audit and feedback in improving outcomes. However, cost-effectiveness was not considered in this review. The greater effectiveness of complex, system-level interventions compared to audit and feedback suggests that audit and feedback does not work well if the desired patient-level outcomes are not exclusively under the control of the provider receiving the feedback.

In summary, substantial evidence shows that audit and feedback improves care across a variety of clinical settings and conditions; further trials comparing audit and feedback with no intervention are not needed. However, given that the effect size differs widely across different studies, it is important to focus future research on understanding how audit and feedback systems can be designed and implemented to maximize the desired effect.

10.5 How can audit and feedback be implemented? What are the organizational and institutional requirements?

Different recommendations exist to provide guidance for the design of best practice audit and feedback schemes (Copeland, 2005; Ivers et al., 2014a; Brehaut et al., 2016; McNamara et al., 2016). Copeland (2005) is a practical handbook for clinical audit published by NHS England. Ivers (2014a, 2014b) made recommendations based on findings from the Cochrane review and the collective experience of a wide range of experts working in audit and feedback who gathered at a meeting in 2012. Brehaut et al. (2016) summarize recommendations that build upon findings from Ivers (2014a, 2014b) and add evidence from an additional series of interviews with experts from a range of disciplines. Finally, McNamara (2016) is a report prepared for the Agency for Healthcare Research and Quality in the United States that summarizes all the above, and incorporates real-world experience of those who have implemented audit and feedback strategies. Table 10.4 summarizes the main recommendations of the four sources, although the evidence supporting these statements is sometimes relatively weak.

The first step of an audit and feedback process is to identify the problem and the local resources to solve it in order to define the focus of the intervention. The topic should be a priority for the organization and the patients it serves – and be perceived as a priority by the recipients of the feedback – and typically involves high-volume, high-risk and/or high-cost issues where there is known variation in performance. In addition, the audit should focus on care areas where there is clear evidence about what care is effective and appropriate, and for whom, implying that audits should focus on clinical practices for which strong recommendations according to the GRADE approach (Grading of Recommendations Assessment, Development and Evaluation) exist (Guyatt et al., 2008).

Concerning the audit component, it is important that the audited data are perceived to be valid and that the indicators assess structure, processes and/or outcomes that the recipients of feedback would have expected and/or intended to

Table 10.4 *Tentative "best practices" when designing and implementing audit and feedback*

Focus of intervention	Care areas that are a priority for the organization and for patients and are perceived as important by the recipients of the feedback
	Care areas with high volumes, high risks (for patients or providers), or high costs
	Care areas where there is variation across healthcare providers/organizations in performance and where there is substantial room for improvement
	Care areas where performance on specific measures can be improved by providers because they are capable and responsible for improvements (for example, changing specific prescribing practices rather than changing the overall management of complex conditions)
	Care areas where clear high-quality evidence about best practice is available
Audit component	Indicators include relevant measures for the recipient (this may include structure, processes and/or outcomes of care, including patient-reported outcomes) that are specific for the individual recipient
	Indicators are based on clear high-quality evidence (for example, guidelines) about what constitutes good performance
	Data are valid and perceived as credible by the report recipients
	Data are based on recent performance
	Data are about the individual/team's own behaviour(s)
	Audit cycles are repeated at a frequency informed by the number of new patient cases with the condition of interest such that new audits can capture attempted changes
Feedback component	Presentation is multimodal including either text and talking or text and graphical materials
	Delivery comes from a trusted, credible source (for example, supervisor or respected colleague), with open acknowledgement of potential limitations in the data
	Feedback includes a relevant comparator to allow the recipient to immediately identify if they are meeting the desired performance level
	A short, actionable declarative statement should describe the discrepancy between actual and desired performance, followed by detailed information for those interested
Targets, goals and action plan	The target performance is provided; the target may be based on peer data or on a consensus-approved benchmark
	Goals for target behaviour are specific, measurable, achievable, relevant and time-bound
	A clear action plan is provided when discrepancies are evident
Organizational context	Audit and feedback is part of a structured programme with a local lead
	Audit and feedback is part of an organizational commitment to a constructive, non-punitive approach to continuous quality improvement
	Recipients have or are provided with the time, skills and/or resources required to analyse and interpret the data available
	Teams are provided with the opportunity to discuss the data and share best practices

Sources: Copeland, 2005; Ivers, 2014a, 2014b; Brehaut, 2016; McNamara, 2016

achieve and that they would feel capable of improving within the measurement interval. If goal-commitment and/or self-efficacy to achieve high performance in the indicator are not present, co-interventions may be needed for the feedback to achieve its desired results (Locke & Latham, 2002). It has been suggested that the key source of information for audits should be the medical record and routinely collected data from electronic systems (Akl et al., 2007). However, medical records are not always available or suitable for extracting the data needed, and it is necessary to pay attention to the reliability and validity of the data as well as to the appropriateness of the sample. In particular, the validity of records can vary depending on the type of information being extracted (Peabody et al., 2004), especially in outpatient settings. In some cases clinical vignettes or case reports have been shown to be a more valid source of information about practice behaviours than records (Peabody et al., 2004; Stange et al., 1998). In other cases, the use of patient-reported experience or outcome measures might be a promising approach, so long as the measures are validated and perceived as actionable (Boyce, Browne & Greenhalgh, 2014).

Concerning the feedback component, feedback is likely to be more effective when it is presented both verbally and in writing than when using only one modality and when the source (*i.e.*, the person delivering the feedback) is a respected colleague rather than unknown investigators or employers of purchasers of care. Source credibility matters a great deal (Ferguson, Wakeling & Bowie, 2014).

Audit and feedback schemes should always include clear targets and an action plan specifying the steps necessary to achieve the targets (Gardner et al., 2010). Ideal targets are commonly considered to be specific, measurable, achievable, relevant and time-bound (Doran, 1981). In addition, feedback should include a comparison with achievable but challenging benchmarks (for example, comparing performance to the top 10% of peers) (Kiefe et al., 2001).

Furthermore, audit and feedback requires a supportive organizational context. This includes commitment to a constructive (i.e. non-punitive) approach to continuous quality improvement and to iterative cycles of measurement at regular, predictable intervals (Hysong, Best & Pugh, 2006). In addition, many mediating structural factors may impact on care and on the likelihood of clinical audit to improve care, such as staffing levels, staffing morale, availability of facilities and levels of knowledge. Finally, the recipients may require skills and/ or resources to properly analyse and interpret the audited data and they need to have the capacity to act upon it. This is especially true if the feedback does not provide patient-level information with clear suggestions for clinical action (meaning resources may be needed to conduct further analyses) or if the feedback highlights indicators that require organizational changes to address (such that change-management resources may be needed).

It is rarely possible to design each component of an audit and feedback scheme in an optimal way. Therefore, it is useful to perceive the individual components outlined in Table 10.4 as "levers" to be manipulated when working within setting-specific constraints. For example, if circumstances dictate that the delivery of feedback cannot be repeated in a reasonable timeframe, extra attention should be paid to other aspects of the intervention, such as the source of the feedback. In addition, co-interventions, tailored to overcome identified barriers and boost facilitators, may help if feedback alone seems unlikely to activate the desired response (Baker et al., 2010).

10.6 Conclusions for policy-makers

Audit and feedback is a quality strategy that is widely used in European countries in various ways. The various programmes presented in Table 10.1 may provide inspiration for policy-makers aiming to introduce similar programmes in their countries. The available evidence suggests that audit and feedback can contribute to improving quality measured in terms of processes (for example, adherence to guidelines) or outcomes (for example, reduction in blood pressure) (*see* Table 10.3). Recently, a number of large-scale initiatives using audit and feedback have shown success with a focus on safety in the prescription of medicines (Guthrie et al., 2016; Dreischulte et al., 2016).

Several aspects have to be taken into account when implementing audit and feedback (*see* Table 10.4). Feedback is more effective when baseline performance is low since the room for improvement of practice is greater and because the mechanism of action requires a noteworthy discrepancy between desired and expected performance. The effect of feedback is greater when the source of feedback is a respected colleague, when it is provided regularly both verbally and in written reports, and when it includes both measurable targets and an action plan for changing practice (Ivers et al., 2012, 2014b).

There is inconclusive evidence about the effectiveness of audit and feedback compared with other quality improvement strategies, such as reminders, educational outreach, opinion leaders, other educational activities or patient-mediated interventions. In addition, it remains somewhat unclear whether audit and feedback is more effective when combined with other interventions, and whether the cost of these additional interventions can be justified. In general, cost-effectiveness of audit and feedback in comparison with other strategies remains largely unexplored.

Ultimately, most decisions about audit and feedback must largely be guided by local circumstances, barriers and facilitators, and pragmatic considerations. Organizational support, including time and resources for professionals as well as provision of data, is crucial. When audit and feedback is utilized, careful attention to the way it is designed and delivered may increase its effectiveness.

In summary, it would be fair to say that, in comparison to most other quality improvement or implementation strategies, a strong answer *does* exist to the question of "Should audit and feedback be implemented to improve processes of care?" In most circumstances the correct answer is Yes! Small to moderate absolute improvements in desired practice are achievable, depending on the measures in the audit and the design of the feedback. However, a strong answer to the question "How could policy-makers best implement audit and feedback and how should it be combined with other interventions?" cannot be given in light of the available evidence. Most likely, the correct answer is: It depends!

This chapter offers a series of tentative recommendations and best practices based on the current evidence base and relevant theory. To guide policy-makers, a shift is needed in the implementation research towards a comparative effectiveness paradigm, prioritizing studies that assess not whether audit and feedback works, but how best to conduct feedback and how best to combine it with other interventions (Ivers et al., 2014b). Whenever policy-makers are planning to implement audit and feedback initiatives, they could partner with researchers to prospectively test different approaches and iteratively improve the impact of their programmes while contributing in important ways to the implementation science literature (Ivers & Grimshaw, 2016).

References

Akl EA et al. (2007). NorthStar, a support tool for the design and evaluation of quality improvement interventions in healthcare. *Implementation Science*, 2:19.

AQUA (2014). Qualitätsreport 2014. Göttingen: Institut für Qualitätsförderung und Forschung im Gesundheitswesen (AQUA).

Ash S et al. (2006). Who is at greatest risk for receiving poor-quality health care? *New England Journal of Medicine*, 354(24):2617–19.

Baker R et al. (2010). Tailored interventions to overcome identified barriers to change: effect on professional practice and health care outcomes. *Cochrane Database of Systematic Reviews*, (3):CD005470.

Benjamin A (2008). Audit: how to do it in practice. *BMJ*, 336(7655):1241–5.

Brehaut J et al. (2016). Practice Feedback Interventions: 15 Suggestions for Optimizing Effectiveness. *Annals of Internal Medicine*, 164(6):435–41.

Boyce MB, Browne JP, Greenhalgh J (2014). The experiences of professionals with using information from patient-reported outcome measures to improve the quality of healthcare: a systematic review of qualitative research. *BMJ Quality and Safety*, 23(6):508–18.

Brown B et al. (2016). A meta-synthesis of findings from qualitative studies to audit and feedback interventions. UK: National Institute of Health Research.

Colquhoun H et al. (2017). Reporting and design elements of audit and feedback interventions: a secondary review. *BMJ Quality and Safety*, (1):54–60.

Copeland G (2005). A Practical Handbook for Clinical Audit. London: Clinical Governance Support Team, Department of Health Publications.

Davis D et al. (2006). Accuracy of physician self-assessment compared with observed measures of competence: a systematic review. *Journal of the American Medical Association*, 296(9):1094–102.

Donatini A et al. (2012). Physician Profiling in Primary Care in Emilia-Romagna Region, Italy: a Tool for Quality Improvement. *Population Health Matters* (formerly *Health Policy Newsletter*), 25(1):10.

Doran G (1981). There's a S.M.A.R.T. way to write management's goals and objectives. *AMA Management Review*, 70:35–6.

Dreischulte T et al. (2016). Safer Prescribing – A Trial of Education, Informatics, and Financial Incentives. *New England Journal of Medicine*, 374:1053–64.

Ferguson J, Wakeling J, Bowie P (2014). Factors influencing the effectiveness of multisource feedback in improving the professional practice of medical doctors: a systematic review. *BMC Medical Education*, 14:76.

Forsetlund L et al. (2009). Continuing education meetings and workshops: effects on professional practice and health care outcomes. *Cochrane Database of Systematic Reviews*, (2):CD003030.

Foy R. et al. (2002). Attributes of clinical recommendations that influence change in practice following audit and feedback. *Journal of Clinical Epidemiology*, 55(7):717–22.

Gardner B et al. (2010). Using theory to synthesise evidence from behaviour change interventions: the example of audit and feedback. *Social Science and Medicine*, 70(10):1618–25.

Godin G et.al (2008). Healthcare professionals' intentions and behaviours: a systematic review of studies based on social cognitive theories. *Implementation Science*, 3:36.

Grol R et al. (2007). Planning and studying improvement in patient care: the use of theoretical perspectives. *Millbank Quarterly*, 85(1):93–138.

Guthrie B et al. (2016). Data feedback and behavioural change intervention to improve primary care prescribing safety (EFIPPS): multicentre, three arm, cluster randomised controlled trial. BMJ (Clinical Research Edition), 354:i4079.

Guyatt G et al. (2008). GRADE: an emerging consensus on rating quality of evidence and strength of recommendations. *BMJ (Clinical Research Edition)*, 336(7650):924–6.

Hysong S, Best R, Pugh J (2006). Audit and feedback and clinical practice guideline adherence: making feedback actionable. *Implementation Science*, 1:9.

Irwin R, Stokes T, Marshall T (2015). Practice-level quality improvement interventions in primary care: a review of systematic reviews. *Primary Health Care Research and Development*, 16(6):556–77.

Ivers N, Grimshaw J (2016). Reducing research waste with implementation laboratories. *Lancet*, 388(10044):547–8.

Ivers N et al. (2012). Audit and feedback: effects on professional practice and healthcare outcomes. *Cochrane Database of Systematic Reviews*, (6):CD000259.

Ivers N et al. (2014a). Growing literature, stagnant science? Systematic review, meta-regression and cumulative analysis of audit and feedback interventions in health care. *Journal of General Internal Medicine*, 29(11):1534–41.

Ivers N et al. (2014b). No more "business as usual" with audit and feedback interventions: towards an agenda for a reinvigorated intervention. *Implementation Science*, 9:14.

Kiefe C et al. (2001). Improving quality improvement using achievable benchmarks for physician feedback: a randomized controlled trial. *Journal of the American Medical Association*, 285(22):2871–9.

Kluger A, DeNisi A (1996). The Effects of Feedback Interventions on Performance: a Historical Review, a Meta-Analysis, and a Preliminary Feedback Intervention Theory. *Psychological Bulletin*, 119(2):254–84.

Locke E, Latham G (2002). Building a Practically Useful Theory of Goal Setting and Task Motivation; a 35-Year Odyssey. *American Psychologist*, (9):705–17.

McNamara et al. (2016). Confidential physician feedback reports: designing for optimal impact on performance. Rockville, Maryland: AHRQ.

Maio V et al. (2012). Physician Profiling in Primary Care in Emilia-Romagna Region, Italy: A Tool for Quality Improvement. *Population Health Matters* (formerly *Health Policy Newsletter*), 25(1):Article 10.

O'Brien M et al. (2007). Educational outreach visits: effects on professional practice and health care outcomes. *Cochrane Database of Systematic Reviews*, (4): CD000409.

Payne V, Hysong S (2016). Model depicting aspects of audit and feedback that impact physicians' acceptance of clinical performance feedback. *BMC Health Services Research*, 16:260.

Peabody J et al. (2004). Measuring the quality of physician practice by using clinical vignettes: a prospective validation study. *Annals of Internal Medicine*, 141(10):771–80.

Squires J et al. (2014). Are multifaceted interventions more effective than single-component interventions in changing health-care professionals' behaviours? An overview of systematic reviews. *Implementation Science*, (9):152.

Stange K et al. (1998). How valid are medical records and patient questionnaires for physician profiling and health services research? A comparison with direct observation of patient visits. *Medical Care*, 36(6):851–67.

Tricco A et al. (2012). Effectiveness of quality improvement strategies on the management of diabetes: a systematic reviews and meta-analysis. *Lancet*, 379(9833):2252–61.

Wennberg J (2014). Forty years of unwanted variation – and still counting. *Health Policy*, 114(1):1–2.

Chapter 11

Patient safety culture as a quality strategy

Cordula Wagner, Solvejg Kristensen, Paulo Sousa, Dimitra Panteli

Summary

What are the characteristics of the strategy?

In every health system not all care is as safe as it could be. Patient harm as a result of healthcare interventions is of great concern. As discussed in the first two chapters of this book, the dimension of safety is one of the cornerstones of quality of care; there is, however, a persistent challenge in defining the interplay between patient safety as a discipline and quality as a goal for healthcare services and systems. For the purpose of this book, we understand patient safety as one of the indispensable ingredients and a prerequisite of quality. Therefore, a safety problem is by definition also a quality problem. Safety is not a single strategy that can be employed to improve the quality of health services, but rather a discipline encompassing a number of different levels and possible initiatives that can support improvement. These initiatives can be viewed as cogs that can be used in an overall system to enable safer care. This chapter presents an overview of safety initiatives and then focuses on patient safety culture as a catalyst for safer, better quality care. "Culture" in this context is understood as the shared values, attitudes, norms, beliefs, practices, policies and behaviours about safety issues in daily practice.

What is being done in European countries?

The 2009 EU Council Recommendation on patient safety included four cornerstone areas of action: national safety plans; adverse events reporting systems; patient empowerment; and safety-sensitive training for the health workforce. The implementation of the Recommendation was evaluated in 2014; findings showed progress along all four areas of action but also ample room for improvement in many countries, particularly regarding patient empowerment and workforce education. While the Council recommendations had raised awareness on safety at political and provider levels, concrete action had not been triggered to the same extent. At the same time, just over half of surveyed EU citizens thought it likely that patients could be harmed by healthcare in their country. Regarding patient safety culture specifically, an investigation of the use of patient safety culture surveys in 2008–2009 collected information on the use of patient safety culture instruments in 32 European countries and recommended fitting tools for future use. There is no newer overview of country practices in the EU, although an increasing volume of work, mainly from the Netherlands, focuses on the effects of patient safety culture.

What do we know about the effectiveness and cost-effectiveness of the strategy?

Regarding patient safety in general, it was determined that approximately 15% of hospital expenditure and activity in OECD countries was attributable to addressing safety failures, while most of the financial burden is linked to a definite number of common adverse events, including healthcare-associated infections, venous thromboembolism, pressure ulcers, medication errors and wrong or delayed diagnoses. Accordingly, the most cost-effective safety interventions would target those occurrences first. Empirical evidence on the link between safety culture and patient outcomes is scarce. The relationship between culture, behaviours and clinical outcomes is thought to be circular, with changes in behaviours and outcomes also improving safety culture. Research from the Netherlands has shown that improvements in patient safety culture can increase incident reporting in general practice, but a systematic review demonstrated variable results and weak evidence quality regarding the effectiveness of changes in patient safety culture on patient outcomes.

How can the strategy be implemented?

Bearing in mind the complex and dynamic causes of patient harm, it is not surprising that system- and organizational-level safety interventions are important, including professional education and training, clinical governance systems, safety standards, and person and patient engagement strategies. Regarding patient safety culture, organizations should start out by discussing, defining and communicating their safety values, set strategies to match their values, and a mission statement in enhancement of patient safety and patient safety culture, then assess and link the strengths and weaknesses of the patient safety culture and the chosen patient safety outcome measures. Strengthening leadership can act as a significant catalyst for patient safety culture improvement. As the perception of safety climate differs between professional groups, tailored approaches seem reasonable overall.

Conclusions for policy-makers

A range of interventions at different levels are available to improve patient safety. At the national level, countries should adopt patient safety strategies based on a systems perspective, encouraging and coordinating different programmes – in other words, safety culture should already start at this level. Professional education, clear evidence-based safety standards and the possibility for blame-free reporting of adverse events are indispensable in this respect. From the efficiency perspective, investments in identifying and addressing the most burdensome adverse events in different settings (acute care, primary care, long-term care) are crucial. Recent work clearly demonstrates that the costs of prevention are lower than those of failure. To effectively, sustainably and adaptively address patient safety issues, leadership across all levels of healthcare systems will be of the utmost importance. National safety strategies should entail making the necessary arsenal available to stakeholders across the healthcare system.

11.1 Introduction: the characteristics of patient safety

In every health system not all care is as safe as it could be. Patient harm as a result of healthcare interventions is of great concern. A growing body of evidence indicates that around 10% of patients may be harmed during hospital care, and that half of these incidents are preventable (Schwendimann et al., 2018). Patient safety was firmly anchored on the policy agenda, first in the United States and then internationally, following the publication of the landmark Institute of Medicine (IOM) Report, *To Err is Human: Building a Safer Health System* (Kohn, Corrigan & Donaldson, 2000; *see* Box 11.1). The report demonstrated that mortality from medical errors in hospitals was higher than from vehicular accidents, breast cancer and AIDS combined – three causes of death that were considered major public health issues at the time. The realization that the risk of patient harm was high in hospitals had begun to gain traction a decade earlier, with the Harvard Medical Practice Study, which recognized the persistent problem of (partially preventable) adverse events; it also systematized the methods for measuring and evaluating them (Brennan et al., 1991; Leape et al., 1991). The IOM built on the approach developed in the Harvard study to carry out the work behind *To Err is Human*.

Beyond further substantiating the serious problem with adverse events, the IOM's report also galvanized the concept that systemic errors were a significant contributing factor to patient harm, removing the full weight of responsibility from individual practitioners: "the problem is not bad people in health care; it is that good people are working in bad systems that need to be made safer".

Box 11.1 *Definitions of patient safety, adverse events and errors*

Patient safety

- **Kohn, Corrigan & Donaldson, 2000:** Patient safety relates to the reduction of risk and is defined as "freedom from accidental injury due to medical care, or medical errors".
- **Emanuel et al., 2008:** Patient safety is a discipline in the healthcare sector that applies safety science methods towards the goal of achieving a trustworthy system of healthcare delivery. Patient safety is also an attribute of healthcare systems; it minimizes the incidence and impact of, and maximizes recovery from, adverse events.
- **Slawomirski, Auraaen & Klazinga, 2017:** Patient safety is the reduction of risk of unnecessary harm associated with healthcare to an acceptable minimum; [this minimum is defined based on] the collective notions of current knowledge, resources available and the context in which care was delivered and weighed against the risk of non-treatment or alternative treatment.

Errors and adverse events (from Kohn, Corrigan & Donaldson, 2000; *see also* Walshe, 2000)

- An error is defined as the failure of a planned action to be completed as intended (i.e., error of execution) or the use of a wrong plan to achieve an aim (i.e., error of planning) (Reason, 1990).
- An adverse event is an injury caused by medical management rather than the underlying condition of the patient. An adverse event attributable to error is a "preventable adverse event" (Brennan et al., 1991). Negligent adverse events represent a subset of preventable adverse events that satisfy legal criteria used in determining negligence (i.e., whether the care provided failed to meet the standard of care reasonably expected of an average physician qualified to take care of the patient in question) (Leape et al., 1991).

Examples of adverse events related to level of care and generic possible causes

Level of care	Adverse event related to level of care	General drivers of adverse events (unrelated)
Primary care	• Adverse drug events/ • medication errors • Diagnostic error/ • delayed diagnosis	• Communication and information deficits
Long-term care	• Adverse drug events • Pressure injury • Falls	• Insufficient skills/knowledge • Inadequate organizational culture and misaligned incentives
Hospital care	• Healthcare-associated • infections • Venous thromboembolism • Adverse drug events • Pressure injury • Wrong site surgery	

Source: Slawomirski, Auraaen & Klazinga, 2017

The prevailing notion until that point was that adverse events were attributable to human failure on the part of clinicians. Seminal work by James Reason in 1990 had already described upstream factors affecting safety outcomes in other contexts. Reason's "Swiss cheese" model of accidents occurring in an organizational setting (like a hospital) demonstrates how upstream errors can lead to incidents downstream, i.e. at the point of care. The latter is considered "active error", as it occurs at the point of human interface with a complex system and the former "latent error", which represents failures of system design. Reason's safety management model (Fig. 11.1) shows the relationship between distant latent factors like management decisions (for example, on the number of nurses on a patient ward), to contextual factors on the ward (for example, having no structured handover at shift changes), to human active factors (for example, forgetting a patient's new medication). Adverse events can be linked to overuse, underuse and misuse of healthcare services (Chassin & Galvin, 1998) as well as a lack of care coordination (Ovretveit, 2011).

As Emanuel et al. (2008) point out, the propagation of this understanding in the IOM report led to the realization that blame culture was pointless as long as the underlying causes of errors remained unaddressed. Thus, *To Err is Human* essentially catalysed the establishment of patient safety as a discipline and shifted the focus from professional education alone to targeting organizational and contextual factors as well. It spurred a considerable international response, demonstrated by the creation of the WHO's and the OECD's World Alliance for Patient Safety in 2004 and a number of European initiatives. These included the Safety Improvement for Patients in Europe (SImPatIE) project, which systematized nomenclatures and identified appropriate indicators and other safety improvement tools, and the European Network for Patient Safety (EUNetPaS), which introduced a collaborative network for a range of stakeholders in EU Member States. In 2009 the Council of the European Union issued its first Recommendation on Patient Safety, urging Member States to take action along several axes. Following a sobering evaluation on the extent of its implementation in 2014 (*see* below), the European Parliament adopted its "Resolution on safer healthcare in Europe: improving patient safety and fighting antimicrobial resistance (2014/2207(INI))", which reiterated the importance of advancing patient safety and urged Member States to redouble efforts even in light of financial constraints. It stressed the importance of training and multidisciplinarity, but also of adequate reporting systems and a unified, validated set of patient safety indicators. It also highlighted the necessity of cross-country collaboration. Later on, the European Union Network for Patient Safety and Quality of Care (PaSQ) Joint Action aimed to advance these goals through knowledge exchange. It united representatives of the European medical community and the institutional partners involved in Patient Safety and Quality of Care in the Member States of the European Union.

Fig. 11.1 *Reason's accident causation model*

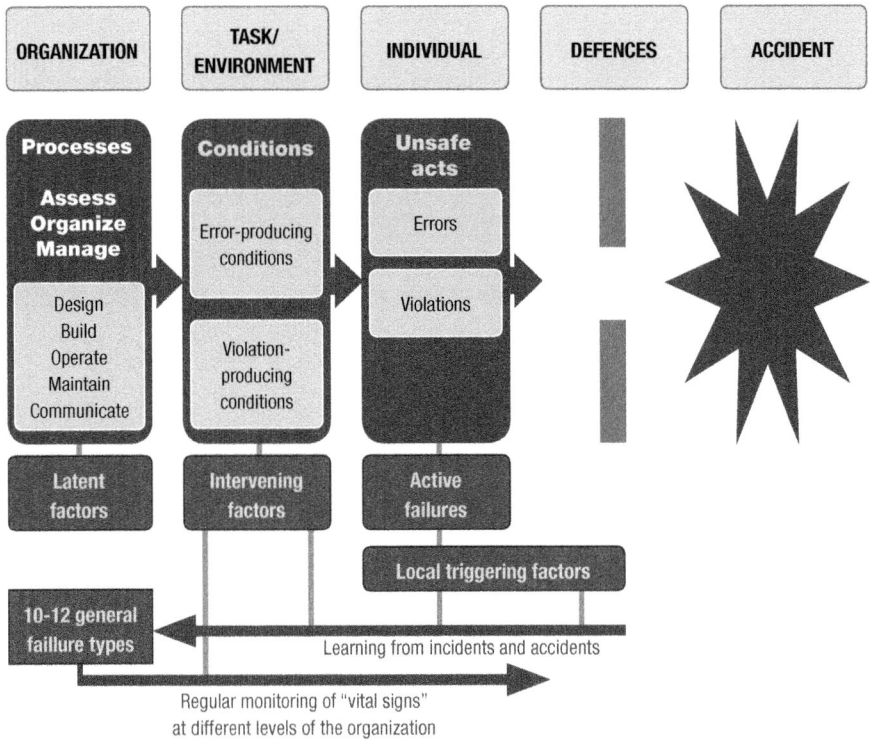

Source: Reason, Hollnagel & Paries, 2006

11.2 Why should patient safety contribute to healthcare quality?

As discussed in the first two chapters of this book, the dimension of safety is one of the cornerstones of quality of care. The IOM also viewed safety as a critical component of good quality care in *To Err is Human*. However, there is a persistent challenge in defining the interplay between patient safety as a discipline and quality as a goal for healthcare services and systems. While some patient safety scholars consider it important to retain a delineation between quality and safety, perhaps in recognition of the latter's importance and multifacetedness, others "dismiss [this distinction] as an exercise in semantics" (Emanuel et al., 2008). The former stance is reflected in the names of a number of initiatives, such as the PaSQ Joint Action mentioned above and the British Medical Journal's Quality and Safety Forum. For the purpose of this book, we understand patient safety as one of the indispensable ingredients and a prerequisite of quality. Therefore,

Fig. 11.2 *Three levels of patient safety initiatives*

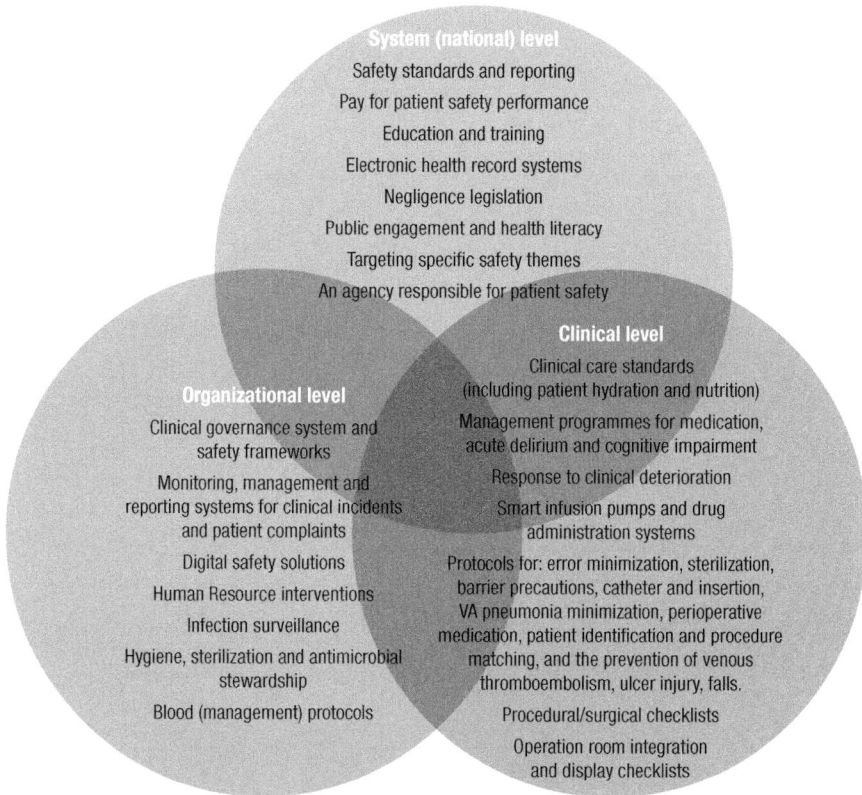

System (national) level
Safety standards and reporting
Pay for patient safety performance
Education and training
Electronic health record systems
Negligence legislation
Public engagement and health literacy
Targeting specific safety themes
An agency responsible for patient safety

Clinical level
Clinical care standards
(including patient hydration and nutrition)

Organizational level

Management programmes for medication,
acute delirium and cognitive impairment

Clinical governance system and
safety frameworks

Response to clinical deterioration

Monitoring, management and
reporting systems for clinical incidents
and patient complaints

Smart infusion pumps and drug
administration systems

Digital safety solutions

Protocols for: error minimization, sterilization,
barrier precautions, catheter and insertion,
VA pneumonia minimization, perioperative
medication, patient identification and procedure
matching, and the prevention of venous
thromboembolism, ulcer injury, falls.

Human Resource interventions

Infection surveillance

Hygiene, sterilization and antimicrobial
stewardship

Blood (management) protocols

Procedural/surgical checklists

Operation room integration
and display checklists

Source: based on Slawomirski, Auraaen & Klazinga, 2017

a safety problem is by definition also a quality problem. However, we also note that safety is not a single strategy that can be employed to improve the quality of health services, but rather a discipline encompassing a number of different levels and possible initiatives that can support improvement. Indeed, in its 2013 report on patient participation in reducing healthcare-related safety risks, WHO points out that "patient safety is about managing [the risk from accidental injury due to medical care or medical errors] using a variety of methods and instruments" (WHO, 2013).

In 2017 the OECD published a report on the economics of patient safety which identified a broad range of initiatives and interventions that foster safety of care and classified them based on their level of application (system, organizational and clinical levels; *see* Fig. 11.2 and Slawomirski, Auraaen & Klazinga, 2017). Looking at these approaches through the lens of the five-lens framework for quality of care presented in Chapter 2, it becomes clear that while they invariably and unsurprisingly focus on patient safety and most pertain to acute and potentially chronic care settings, they have different targets (for example, provider organizations or clinicians) and focus on different activities (for example, setting standards or monitoring progress). The authors of the OECD report projected their taxonomy of initiatives on Donabedian's structure-process-outcome triad, further highlighting the complementarity of different approaches towards achieving the overall goal of patient safety (Fig. 11.3).

Indeed, these initiatives should not be viewed in isolation but rather as cogs that can be used in an overall system to enable safer care. WHO described such an integrated approach for patient safety as a cycle (Fig. 11.4), which combines measuring incidents and adverse events, getting insight into the causes of incidents and adverse events, finding solutions, setting up improvement projects, and evaluating the impact of these projects (WHO, 2008). Important prerequisites for such an approach include the necessary systems for reporting and analysing incidents that have occurred, with and without patient harm, carrying out prospective analyses to identify potential for risk within an organization, proactively encouraging a patient safety culture which incorporates open communication and reflection, and ensuring multidisciplinary workforce training (for example, to improve teamwork, communication and, as a result, handovers; *see also* Box 11.2).

Fig. 11.3   *Patient safety and Donabedian's structure-process-outcome framework*

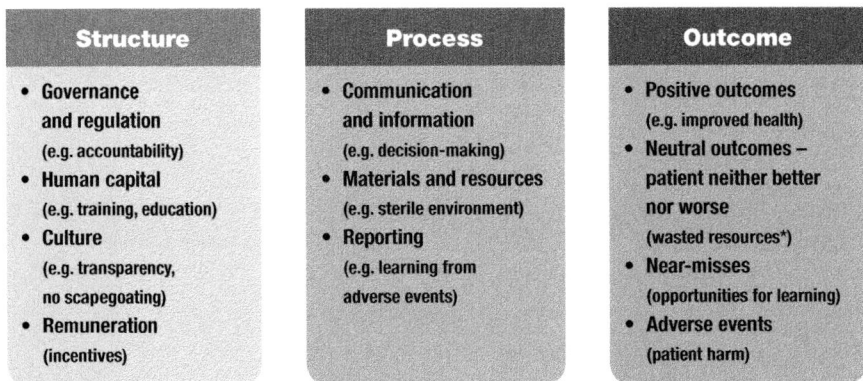

Structure	Process	Outcome
• Governance and regulation (e.g. accountability) • Human capital (e.g. training, education) • Culture (e.g. transparency, no scapegoating) • Remuneration (incentives)	• Communication and information (e.g. decision-making) • Materials and resources (e.g. sterile environment) • Reporting (e.g. learning from adverse events)	• Positive outcomes (e.g. improved health) • Neutral outcomes – patient neither better nor worse (wasted resources*) • Near-misses (opportunities for learning) • Adverse events (patient harm)

Source: from Slawomirski, Auraaen & Klazinga, 2017

*Authors' note: when the aim is to sustain outcomes, neutral outcomes do not constitute a waste of resources.

More recently, the ambition to learn and improve has shifted from learning from incidents and adverse events (Safety I) to learning from the comparison of "work-as-imagined" as described in guidelines and procedures, and "work-as-done" in daily practices and ever-changing contexts (Safety II). Safety II is based on complexity theory and the idea that interactions between various parts in the system determine the outcome, instead of a cause-effect chain in a linear way. In the same situation the outcome might be good or bad, and resilience to daily changes should be recognized and trained to make healthcare safer (Hollnagel,

2014; Dekker, 2011). This line of thought is new in healthcare and instruments for implementation have still to be developed, alongside the change in culture needed to think from inside-out during incident analyses.

Fig. 11.4 *WHO Safety improvement cycle*

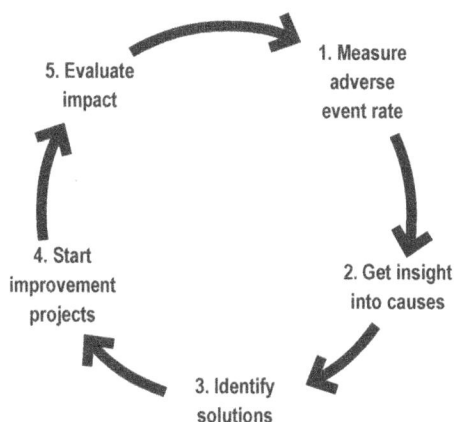

Source: adapted from WHO, 2008

11.3 What is being done in Europe and what do we know about cost-effectiveness?

The 2009 EU Council Recommendation on patient safety included four cornerstone areas of action (national safety plans; adverse events reporting systems; patient empowerment; and safety-sensitive training for the health workforce) which are very much in line with the integrated approach described above. The European Commission evaluated the implementation of the Recommendation in 2014 and compared it to the snapshot assessment that had been carried out two years previously. It found progress along all four areas of action but also that many countries still had a long way to go, particularly in regard to patient empowerment and workforce education (*see* Table 11.1). The Commission's report found that among 28 reporting countries, 26 had developed patient safety strategies or programmes, and patient safety standards were mandatory in 20 (compared to 11 in 2012). Almost twice as many countries had adverse event reporting and learning systems in 2014 (a total of 27), mostly at national and provider levels. While important progress was also recorded in the extent to which countries empower patients by informing them about patient safety standards, safety measures to reduce or prevent errors, the rights to informed consent to treatment, complaint procedures and available redress (20 countries reported related action in 2014 compared to only five in 2012), there was still ample room for improvement. Overall, respondents indicated that while the Council recommendations had raised awareness on safety at political and

Table 11.1 *Member State action in the four domains of the 2009 Council Recommendation, 2014*

Country	Education and training of healthcare workers	Reporting incidents and learning systems	Patient empowerment	Policies and programmes on patient safety
Austria	No	Partial	No	Yes
Belgium	No	Yes	No	Partial
Bulgaria	No	Partial	Partial	No
Croatia	No	Partial	Partial	Yes
Cyprus	No	Partial	Partial	No
Czechia	No	Partial	No	Yes
Denmark	No	Yes	No	Yes
Estonia	No	Yes	Partial	Partial
Finland	No	Partial	No	Yes
France	Partial	No	Yes	Partial
Germany	No	Partial	Yes	Yes
Greece	No	Partial	No	No
Hungary	No	Partial	Partial	Yes
Ireland	Yes	Yes	Partial	Yes
Italy	No	Yes	No	Partial
Latvia	Partial	No	Yes	No
Lithuania	No	No	Partial	Yes
Luxembourg	No	Partial	No	No
Malta	No	Partial	No	No
Netherlands	No	Yes	Partial	Partial
Poland	No	Partial	No	Partial
Portugal	No	Partial	No	Yes
Romania	No	No	No	No
Slovakia	No	Partial	No	Partial
Slovenia	No	Partial	No	No
Spain	No	Partial	No	Yes
Sweden	No	Partial	No	Partial
United Kingdom	Partial	Partial	Partial	Yes

Source: European Commission, 2014b

provider levels, concrete action had not been triggered to the same extent. This led to the reiteration of the importance of continued attention in the European Parliament's Resolution of 2015 (*see* above).

A concurrent Eurobarometer survey found that just over half of surveyed EU citizens thought it likely that patients could be harmed by healthcare in their country – a slight increase since 2009. The share was slightly higher for hospital care than for ambulatory care and the variation between countries was substantial. The survey also recorded a significant increase in the proportion of adverse events that were reported by those who experienced them or by their families – from 28% in 2009 to 46% in 2013. This can be interpreted to mean that pathways to report adverse events are more accessible to care recipients and may also indicate a change in culture. At the same time, the most likely outcome of reporting an adverse event was lack of action (37%), with only one in five respondents receiving an apology from the doctor or nurse and even fewer (17%) an explanation for the error from the healthcare facility. These results further underlined the need for continued action and attention to safety culture and patient empowerment (European Commission, 2014a).

The 2017 OECD report on the economics of patient safety reviewed available evidence and surveyed relevant policy and academic experts to identify cost-effective interventions (Slawomirski, Auraaen & Klazinga, 2017). It found that approximately 15% of hospital expenditure and activity in OECD countries was attributable to addressing safety failures, while the overall cost of adverse events would also need to consider indirect elements, such as productivity loss for patients and carers. Furthermore, the report illustrates that most of the financial burden is linked to a definite number of common adverse events, including healthcare-associated infections (HAI), venous thromboembolism (VTE), pressure ulcers, medication errors, and wrong or delayed diagnoses. Accordingly, the most cost-effective safety interventions would target those occurrences first, and the OECD report summarizes sound evidence to support this notion. However, bearing in mind the complex and dynamic causes of patient harm (as described earlier in this chapter), it is not surprising that the importance of system- and organizational-level interventions was highlighted in the report and that such approaches were short-listed as "best buys" to cost-effectively address safety overall, including professional education and training, clinical governance systems, safety standards, and person and patient engagement strategies. Policy and academic experts surveyed for the purposes of the report also highlighted the critical contribution of developing a culture conducive to safety to anchor individual interventions. In accordance with these results, Box 11.2 summarizes information on incident reporting systems and root cause analysis, which are indispensable for framing necessary action at the organizational level. The second part of the chapter focuses on safety culture as a quality improvement strategy.

Box 11.2 *Incident reporting systems and analysis*

An incident is an unexpected and unwanted event during the healthcare process which could have harmed or did harm the patient. In various countries national, regional or local incident reporting systems have been introduced (Smits et al., 2009; Wagner et al. 2016). The first reporting systems in healthcare were introduced in the 2000s, following the examples of other high-risk industries such as aviation and nuclear power. Analysing incidents as well as near misses can provide valuable information for detecting patient safety problems and might help professionals to prevent harming patients in the future and improve quality of care. Incident reporting systems are considered a fairly inexpensive although incomplete means for monitoring patient safety and, when combined with systematic interventions, potentially effective in reducing preventable adverse events (Simon et al., 2005). Other methods of incident tracking include morbidity and mortality conferences and autopsy, malpractice claims analysis, administrative data analysis, chart review, applications embedded in electronic medical records, observation of patient care and clinical surveillance including staff interviews (Thomas & Petersen, 2003). Some are more geared towards the detection of active and some latent errors.

A well known national reporting system is the National Reporting and Learning System in the UK (Howell et al., 2015). Established in 2003, it received over a million reports in a period of five years, mainly from acute care hospitals. In 2010 it became mandatory for National Health Service (NHS) trusts in England to report all serious patient safety incidents to the central Care Quality Commission. As a result of considerations about the extent to which the results of national reporting systems are applicable to hospital units, the very places where changes and improvements have to be implemented, the government and healthcare providers in the Netherlands have opted for a local and decentralized unit-based approach. The advantage of a centralized system is the possibility to discover rare but important problems (Dückers et al., 2009), whereas decentralized reporting systems might increase the sense of urgency because all reported incidents have actually happened in a recognizable context. Indeed, national figures on incident types and root causes do not necessarily reflect the risks of a specific hospital unit or unit type. Team engagement in improvement projects may suffer if the reporting does not match their practice needs (Wagner et al., 2016). The European Commission's Reporting and Learning Subgroup published an overview of reporting systems in European countries in 2014 (European Commission, 2014b).

Despite the considerable effort that has been put into establishing incident reporting and learning systems in healthcare in many countries and settings, under-reporting of incidents is estimated to be considerable (*see*, for example, Archer et al., 2017). Barach & Small (2000) put it at 50% to 96% annually in the US (Barach & Small, 2000), a figure that is still used as an orientation point today. Nevertheless, there is evidence that the willingness to report has increased over the years in hospitals (Verbeek-van Noord et al., 2018). Common barriers to reporting incidents among doctors are due to a negative attitude, a non-stimulating culture or a perceived lack of ability to fulfill related tasks and include lack of clarity about what constitutes an incident, fear of reprisal, unfavourable working conditions involving colleagues and supervisors, code of silence (reporting as a sign of lack of loyalty), loss of reputation, additional work based on user-unfriendly platforms, and lack of feedback or action when incidents are reported (Martowirono et al., 2012). On the other hand, features of an organization that encourage incident reporting are: flat hierarchy, staff participation in decision-making, risk management procedures, teamwork, and leadership ability and integrity (Firth-Cozens, 2004). Research shows that mandatory reporting may result in lower error rates than voluntary reporting, while the reporting profession (for example, nurses vs. physicians) and the mode of reporting (paper-based vs. web-based) may also play a role in how effective reporting systems are. An increase in incident reporting is positively correlated with a more positive safety culture (Hutchinson et al., 2009). Reporting should be non-punitive, confidential or anonymous, independent, timely, systems oriented and responsive (*see* also Leape, 2002).

Root cause analysis (RCA) can give insight into the origination of incidents which have already happened and have been reported; it is a method to analyse adverse events and to generate interventions, in order to prevent recurrence. RCA is generally employed to uncover latent errors underlying an adverse event (*see* Fig. 11.1) and consists of four major steps: first, a team of managers, physicians and/or experts from the particular field as well as representatives from involved staff collect relevant data concerning the event; the RCA team then organizes and analyses possible causal factors using a root-cause tree or a sequence diagram with logic tests that describe the events leading up to an occurrence, plus the conditions surrounding these events (there is rarely just one causal factor – events are usually the result of a combination of contributors); the third step entails the identification of the underlying reason for each causal factor, so all problems surrounding the occurrence can be addressed; finally, the RCA team generates recommendations for changes in the care process. Clearly, the effectiveness of RCA depends on the actions taken based on its outputs. If the analysis reveals an underlying problem, solutions need to be discussed and implemented, a process which can be as difficult as any requiring that professionals change their behaviour. Thus, the impact of RCA on patient safety outcomes is indirect and difficult to measure. Nevertheless, insights from RCA can help to prioritize improvement areas and solutions. Overall, an easily accessible, comprehensive reporting system combined with awareness of and training in RCA are prerequisites for learning and safety improvements.

For the proactive, prospective identification of potential process failures, Failure Mode Effects Analysis (FMEA) was developed for the aviation industry and has also been used in a healthcare context. Its aim is to look at all possible ways in which a process can fail, analyse risks and make recommendations for changes in the process of preventing adverse events. A few variations exist, like Failure Mode Effects and Criticality Analysis (FMECA) and Healthcare Failure Mode Effects Analysis (HFMEA). Despite the importance of a proactive approach, FMEA in its entirety was considered cumbersome to implement at clinical or organizational level, and showing results of not unequivocal validity (Shebl, Franklin & Barber, 2012; Shebl et al., 2012). However, it was recognized that it may have potential as a tool for aiding multidisciplinary groups in mapping and understanding a process of care (Shebl et al., 2012). A newly developed risk identification framework (Simsekler, Ward & Clarkson, 2018), which incorporates FMEA elements, still needs to be tested for usability and applicability.

11.4 Patient safety culture as a quality strategy

11.4.1 What are the characteristics of the strategy?

Beginning in the 1980s, industries and researchers have paid substantial attention to the contribution of organizational and cultural factors to safety of operations. Accumulating evidence indicated that organizational and cultural aspects were underlying causal factors of accidents, and the 1986 Chernobyl disaster triggered the fusion of the concepts of safety and culture. Today it is an acknowledged fact that within any organization where operations may involve human risk, a culture of safety should be accounted for when planning quality improvement. "Culture" in this context is understood as the shared values, attitudes, norms, beliefs, practices, policies and behaviours about safety issues in daily practice (Verbakel et al., 2014; Scott et al., 2003). When adapted to healthcare, (patient) safety culture has been described as the product of individual and group values, attitudes, perceptions, competencies and patterns of behaviour that determine the commitment to, and the style and proficiency of, an organization's health and safety management (Verbakel et al., 2016; Sammer et al., 2010). It is characterized by shared behavioural patterns regarding a number of subthemes such as communication, teamwork, job satisfaction, stress recognition, perceptions of management, working conditions, organizational learning and outcome measures (for example, the perceived patient safety level and the frequency of adverse event reporting). However, despite a growing body of work on patient safety culture for both the hospital and the primary care setting, no universally accepted definition of what it entails or its constituent subcultures exists in the literature. Across all the definitions and concepts used to describe patient safety culture, there is agreement that it represents, broadly put, "the way we do things around here in relation to a patient's exposure to risks". The Health Foundation summarized these notions as follows: "Safety culture refers to the way patient safety is thought about, structured and implemented in an organisation. Safety climate is a subset of this, focused on staff attitudes about patient safety." (Health Foundation, 2011). Thus a safe culture in healthcare is one where staff within an organization have a constant and active awareness of the potential for things to go wrong and affect the quality of care delivered. Recognizing such cultural attributes and the potential impact that cultural weaknesses have on safety outcomes, creating a sound culture of safety is regarded as an imperative to any type of safety improvement programme in healthcare. This was substantiated by the latest survey presented in the 2017 OECD report (Slawomirski, Auraaen & Klazinga, 2017). In essence, patient safety culture can contribute to quality of care by providing the environment for safety-conscious design and behaviours, thus influencing structures, processes and, ultimately, outcomes of care.

11.4.2 What is being done in Europe?

Early quantitative patient safety culture assessment instruments for the healthcare sector adapted versions of questionnaires developed in other industries. In recent years a large number of quantitative instruments with varying characteristics have been developed and used. In Europe the use of patient safety culture surveys has been investigated through the European Network for Patient Safety (EUNetPaS) project, which collected information on the use of patient safety culture instruments in 32 European countries in 2008–2009. More than 90 European experts in the field of patient safety contributed to the survey. Based upon the survey responses, a literature review and an extensive consensus-building process, three instruments were recommended for use in European Member States. These were:

a. The Hospital Survey on Patient Safety Culture (HSPSC): this questionnaire was created by the Agency for Healthcare Research and Quality in the USA (AHRQ, 2018). Healthcare organizations can use this survey instrument to: (1) assess patient safety culture, (2) track changes in patient safety over time, and (3) evaluate the impact of patient safety interventions. With the HSPSC, seven unit-level and three hospital-level aspects of safety culture, together with four outcome variables, can be surveyed. The survey is also available in versions for nursing homes and medical offices. They all have extensive material for guiding users in all processes of the assessment.

b. The Safety Attitudes Questionnaire (SAQ): this tool originated at the University of Texas and the Johns Hopkins University in the USA (Sexton et al., 2006). SAQ can be applied at the level of team, unit, department and/or hospital and investigates seven subcultures, and can be used for the same three purposes as the HSPSC. SAQ surveys also have extensive material for guiding users in all processes of the assessment. For most purposes the generic version of SAQ is recommended.

c. The Manchester Patient Safety Framework (MaPSaF): this tool from the University of Manchester in the UK (University of Manchester, 2006) is a process instrument designed to help organizations to assess and reflect on, as well as develop, the safety culture. The MaPSaF is a qualitative assessment instrument carried out in workshops. The MaPSaF uses nine dimensions of patient safety culture. This method also has extensive material for guiding users in all processes of assessing the patient safety culture in different settings, from acute hospital care to mental care.

Comparative work showed similarities between the first two instruments and concluded that survey length, content, sensitivity to change and the ability to benchmark should determine instrument choice (Etchegaray & Thomas, 2012). There is no newer overview of country practices in the EU. Most research on the implementation and effectiveness of patient safety culture in Europe comes from the Netherlands (*see* below).

11.4.3 Is patient safety culture (cost-) effective?

Empirical research on the link between safety culture and patient outcomes is scarce. According to a systematic overview compiled by the Health Foundation in 2011, existing evidence included mixed findings and was of variable quality, focusing primarily on hospitals and examining single time periods and often single institutions. Few of the studies included in the review found a relationship between safety culture or climate and hospital morbidity, adverse events and readmission rates, while others showed no impact. Improving safety culture seemed to affect staff safety behaviours and injury rates (Health Foundation, 2011). The study concluded that the relationship between culture, behaviours and clinical outcomes could be circular, with changes in behaviours and outcomes also improving safety culture.

Since then, research from the Netherlands has shown that improvements in patient safety culture (for example, using professional education and workshops) can increase incident reporting in general practice (Verbakel et al., 2015), but that its role in influencing the number of incidents in hospitals could not be proven (Smits et al., 2012). In general, patient safety culture in the Netherlands has developed to a more open and safety supporting culture. This might be related to an extensive five-year national programme on patient safety in all Dutch hospitals (Verbeek-van Noord et al., 2018). Recent work from the US found that it may be possible to improve catheter-associated infection rates without making significant changes in safety culture (Meddings et al., 2017), contradicting previous work on the issue. A systematic review published by Weaver at al. in 2013 also demonstrated variable results and weak evidence quality regarding the effectiveness of changes in patient safety culture on patient outcomes (Weaver et al., 2013).

11.4.4 How can the strategy be implemented?

Since the 1990s many cross-sectional studies assessing patient safety culture in different settings in healthcare have been carried out. However, relatively little research has focused on how new practices can be delivered with an acceptable trade-off between high quality of care, organizational efficiency and cost-effectiveness and a lot remains to be found about how to overcome barriers to the

Fig. 11.5 *The Safety Culture Pyramid*

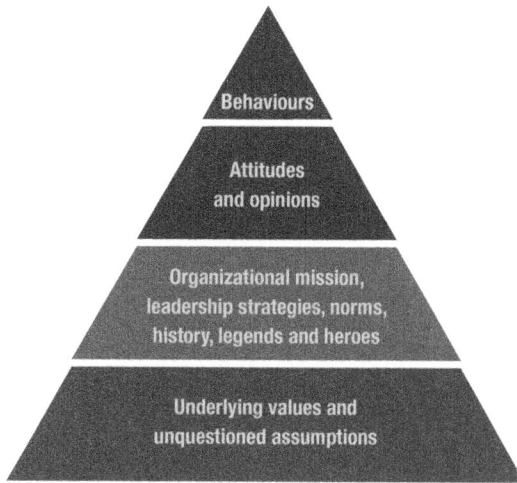

Source: Patankar & Sabin, 2010

successful implementation of new evidence, harness staff motivation and best practice, sustain good results, and spread such results to other organizational units or healthcare settings. Safety culture must be viewed as a highly dynamic and multidimensional concept. It is influenced by a wide variety of individual and group-related personal and professional, organizational, ethical and social factors. Patankar & Sabin (2010) suggested a Safety Culture Pyramid as a way of describing and developing the dynamic balance and linkage between four stacked layers with different safety attributes (Fig. 11.5). In this sense, organizations should start out by discussing, defining and communicating their safety values, set strategies to match their values, and a mission statement in enhancement of patient safety and patient safety culture, then assess and link the strengths and weaknesses of the patient safety culture and the chosen patient safety outcome measures. This process should be followed by appropriate interventions to bridge the gap between weaknesses in patient safety culture and safety performance.

A large cross-European study involving frontline staff and clinical leaders found positive associations between implementation of quality management systems and teamwork and safety climate. Further, a difference in perception between clinical leaders and frontline staff was identified for both teamwork and safety climate, as more clinical leaders than frontline clinicians have a positive perception of teamwork and safety climate (Kristensen et al., 2015b). Senior leadership accountability has been found to be imperative for an organization-wide culture of safety, and patient safety WalkRounds™ (i.e. a systematic approach entailing an informal method for hospital leaders to talk with frontline staff about safety issues; *see* Frankel et al., 2003) have been reported as an effective tool for engaging leadership, identifying safety issues and supporting a culture of safety (*see*, for example, Sølvtofte, Larsen & Laustsen, 2017). A systematic review showed that classroom-based team training can improve patient safety culture (Verbeek-van Noord et al., 2014).

Weaver et al. (2013) identified and evaluated interventions to foster patient safety culture in acute care settings. Most studies included team training or communication initiatives, executive or inter-disciplinary walk-rounds, and multicomponent, unit-based interventions were also investigated. In all, 29 studies reported some improvement in safety culture (or patient outcomes, *see* above), but considerable heterogeneity was observed and the strength of evidence was low. Thus, the review only tentatively concluded that interventions can improve perceptions of safety culture and potentially reduce patient harm. Evidence on interventions to enhance safety culture in primary care was largely also inconclusive due to limited evidence quality (Verbakel et al., 2016). A Danish study found that strengthening leadership can act as a significant catalyst for patient safety culture improvement. To broaden knowledge and strengthen leadership skills, a multicomponent programme consisting of academic input, exercises, reflections and discussions, networking and action learning was implemented among clinical leaders. The proportion of frontline staff with positive attitudes improved by approximately five percent for five of seven patient safety culture dimensions over time. Moreover, frontline staff became more positive on almost all cultural dimensions investigated (Kristensen et al., 2015a).

A survey of healthcare professionals, on the other hand, found them to be positive about feedback on patient safety culture and its effect on stimulating improvement, especially when it is understandable and tailored to specific hospital departments (Zwijnenberg et al., 2016). A different survey demonstrated that the perception of safety climate differs between professional groups (higher for clinical leaders compared to frontline clinicians) and suggested that the implementation of quality management systems can be supportive in fostering shared values and behaviours. As perceptions have also been shown to differ among professionals in primary care (Verbakel et al., 2014), tailored approaches seem reasonable overall. Organizational-level initiatives aimed at building a positive culture may include training and development, team-building and communication strategies, inclusive management structures, staff culture surveys and safety awards (Slawomirski, Auraaen & Klazinga, 2017). An example of such a multifaceted approach is the TeamSTEPPS system developed by the Agency for Healthcare Research and Quality in the USA (AHRQ, 2018).

For the training component towards more safety-sensitive care, curricula based on the Crew Resource Management (CRM) concept created for aviation have been adopted in healthcare as well (see, for example, McConaughey, 2008; Verbeek-van Noord et al., 2014; Eddy, Jordan & Stephenson, 2016). CRM promotes and reinforces situational awareness and team learning by emphasizing six key areas: managing fatigue; creating and managing teams; recognizing adverse situations (red flags); cross-checking and communication; decision-making; and performance feedback. Classroom and simulation-based team trainings of this kind are expected to improve cooperation, communication and handovers between professionals. However, evidence on their implementation shows that results might be time-consuming to achieve (Sax et al., 2009). Overall, the importance of teamwork is gaining recognition along with the impact of team training on attitudes of healthcare providers and team communication (*see*, for example, Frankel et al., 2017).

11.5 Conclusions for policy-makers

For as long as medicine has been practised, unnecessary and unintended harm to patients has been a reality. The increasing complexity of health increases the risk of harm and necessitates greater vigilance and an increased commitment to ensuring patient safety. A range of interventions at different levels is available to improve patient safety. At the national level, countries should adopt patient safety strategies based on a systems perspective, encouraging and coordinating different programmes – in other words, safety culture should already start at this level. Professional education, clear evidence-based safety standards and the possibility for blame-free reporting of adverse events are indispensable in this respect. From the efficiency perspective, investments in identifying and addressing the most burdensome adverse events in different settings (acute care, primary care, long-term care) are crucial. Recent work clearly demonstrates that the costs of prevention are lower than those of failure. To effectively, sustainably and adaptively address patient safety issues, leadership across all levels of the healthcare systems will be of the utmost importance.

In their assessment of the two decades since *To Err is Human*, Bates & Singh (2018) point out that a lot still remains to be done, including stimulating a multidisciplinary understanding of safety and the development of corresponding mechanisms for improvement, optimizing reporting and measurement to be comprehensive and sustainable, enabling a "learning health system" approach to safety (i.e. one where continuously and routinely measuring incidents consistently leads to improvement), and rising to emerging priority areas such as harm in outpatient care and in the context of digitalized healthcare. They, too, highlight the importance of safety culture for the success of safety interventions. Assessing safety culture is a process which can contribute to positive culture changes by enabling organizations to see the features of their practice and providing insights for transformation. However, depending on the setting, the instrument and approach for evaluating its existing attributes and catalysing cultural change should be carefully monitored. National safety strategies should entail making the necessary arsenal available to stakeholders across the healthcare system.

References

AHRQ (2018). Hospital Survey on Patient Safety Culture. Rockville, Maryland: Agency for Healthcare Research and Quality.

Archer S et al. (2017). Development of a theoretical framework of factors affecting patient safety incident reporting: a theoretical review of the literature. *BMJ Open*, 7(12):e017155.

Barach P, Small SD (2000). Reporting and preventing medical mishaps: lessons from non-medical near miss reporting systems. *BMJ*, 320(7237):759–63.

Bates D, Singh H (2018). Two Decades Since *To Err is Human*: an Assessment of Progress and Emerging Priorities in Patient Safety. *Health Affairs*, 37(11):1736–43.

Brennan TA et al. (1991). Incidence of adverse events and negligence in hospitalized patients: results of the Harvard Medical Practice Study I. *New England Journal of Medicine*, 324:370–7.

Chassin MR, Galvin RW (1998). The urgent need to improve health care quality. Institute of Medicine National Roundtable on Health Care Quality. *Journal of the American Medical Association*, 280(11):1000–5.

Dekker S (2011). Drift info failure. From hunting broken components to understanding complex systems. Farnham: Ashgate.

Dückers M et al. (2009). Safety and risk management interventions in hospitals: a systematic review of the literature. *Medical Care Research and Review*, 66(6 Suppl):90S–119S.

Eddy K, Jordan Z, Stephenson M (2016). Health professionals' experience of teamwork education in acute hospital settings: a systematic review of qualitative literature. *JBI Database of Systematic Reviews and Implementation Reports*, 14(4):96–137.

Emanuel L et al. (2008). What Exactly Is Patient Safety? In: Henriksen K et al. (eds.). Advances in Patient Safety: New Directions and Alternative Approaches (Vol. 1: Assessment). Rockville, Maryland: Agency for Healthcare Research and Quality.

Etchegaray JM, Thomas EJ (2012). Comparing two safety culture surveys: safety attitudes questionnaire and hospital survey on patient safety. *BMJ Quality and Safety*, 21(6):490–8.

European Commission (2014a). Special Eurobarometer 411: "Patient Safety and Quality of Care". Wave EB80.2. Brussels: European Commission/TNS Opinion & Social.

European Commission (2014b). Key findings and recommendations on Reporting and learning systems for patient safety incidents across Europe. Report of the Reporting and learning subgroup of the European Commission PSQCWG. Brussels: European Commission.

Firth-Cozens (2004). Organisational trust: the keystone to patient safety. *Quality and Safety in Health Care*, 13(1):56–61.

Frankel A et al. (2003). Patient safety leadership WalkRounds. *Joint Commission Journal on Quality and Safety*, 29(1):16–26.

Frankel A et al. (2017). A Framework for Safe, Reliable, and Effective Care. White Paper. Cambridge, Mass.: Institute for Healthcare Improvement and Safe & Reliable Healthcare.

Health Foundation (2011). Does improving safety culture affect outcomes? London: Health Foundation.

Hollnagel, E (2014). Safety-I and Safety-II. The past and future of safety management. Farnham: Ashgate.

Howell AM et al. (2015). Can Patient Safety Incident Reports Be Used to Compare Hospital Safety? Results from a Quantitative Analysis of the English National Reporting and Learning System Data. *PloS One*, 10(12):e0144107.

Hutchinson A et al. (2009). Trends in healthcare incident reporting and relationship to safety and quality data in acute hospitals: results from the National Reporting and Learning System. *BMJ Quality & Safety*, 18:5–10.

Kohn LT, Corrigan JM, Donaldson MS (eds.) (2000). To Err is Human: Building a Safer Health System. Washington, DC: National Academies Press.

Kristensen S et al. (2015a). Strengthening leadership as a catalyst for enhanced patient safety culture: a repeated cross-sectional experimental study. *BMJ Open*, 6:e010180.

Kristensen S et al. (2015b). Quality management and perceptions of teamwork and safety climate in European hospitals. *International Journal for Quality in Health Care*, 27(6):499–506.

Leape LL (2002). Reporting of adverse events. New England Journal of Medicine, 347(20):1633–8.

Leape LL et al. (1991). The nature of adverse events in hospitalized patients. Results of the Harvard Medical Practice Study II. *New England Journal of Medicine*, 324:377–84.

McConaughey E (2008). Crew resource management in healthcare: the evolution of teamwork training and MedTeams. *Journal of Perinatal and Neonatal Nursing*, 22(2):96–104.

Martowirono K et al. (2012). Possible solutions for barriers in incident reporting by residents. *Journal of Evaluation in Clinical Practice*, 18(1):76–81.

Meddings J et al. (2017). Evaluation of the association between Hospital Survey on Patient Safety Culture (HSOPS) measures and catheter-associated infections: results of two national collaboratives. *BMJ Quality and Safety*, 26(3):226–35.

Ovretveit J (2011). Widespread focused improvement: lessons from international health for spreading specific improvements to health services in high-income countries. *International Journal for Quality in Health Care*, 23(3):239–46.

Patankar MS, Sabin EJ (2010). The Safety Culture Perspective. In Salas E and Maurino D (eds.). Human Factors in Aviation (Second Edition). San Diego: Academic Press.

Reason J (1990). Human error. New York: Cambridge University Press.

Reason J, Hollnagel E, Paries J (2006). Rethinking the "Swiss Cheese" Model of Accidents. EEC Note No. 13/06. Brussels: European Organization for the Safety of Air Navigation.

Sammer CE et al. (2010). What is patient safety culture? A review of the literature. *Journal of Nursing Scholarship*, 42(2):156–65.

Sax HC et al. (2009). Can aviation-based team training elicit sustainable behavioral change? *Archives of Surgery*, 144(12):1133–7.

Schwendimann R et al. (2018). The occurrence, types, consequences and preventability of in-hospital adverse events – a scoping review. *BMC Health Services Research*, 18(1):521.

Scott T et al. (2003). The quantitative measurement of organizational culture in health care: a review of the available instruments. *BMC Health Services Research*, 38(3):923–45.

Sexton JB et al. (2006). The Safety Attitudes Questionnaire: psychometric properties, benchmarking data, and emerging research. *BMC Health Services Research*, 6:44.

Shebl N, Franklin B, Barber N (2012). Failure mode and effects analysis outputs: are they valid? *BMC Health Services Research*, 12:150.

Shebl N et al. (2012). Failure Mode and Effects Analysis: views of hospital staff in the UK. *Journal of Health Services Research & Policy*, 17(1):37–43.

Simon A et al. (2005). Institutional medical incident reporting systems: a review. Edmonton, Alberta: Heritage Foundation for Medical Research.

Simsekler M, Ward JR, Clarkson PJ (2018). Design for patient safety: a systems-based risk identification framework. *Ergonomics*, 61(8):1046–64.

Slawomirski L, Auraaen A, Klazinga N (2017). The economics of patient safety. Paris: OECD Publishing.

Smits M et al. (2009). The nature and causes of unintended events reported at ten emergency departments. *BMC Emergency Medicine*, 9:16.

Smits M et al. (2012). The role of patient safety culture in the causation of unintended events in hospitals. *Journal of Clinical Nursing*, 21(23–24):3392–401.

Sølvtofte AS, Larsen P, Laustsen S (2017). Effectiveness of Patient Safety Leadership WalkRounds™ on patient safety culture: a systematic review protocol. *JBI Database of Systematic Reviews and Implementation Reports*, 15(5):1306–15.

Thomas EJ, Petersen LA (2003). Measuring errors and adverse events in health care. *Journal of General Internal Medicine*, 18(1):61–7.

University of Manchester (2006). Manchester Patient Safety Framework (MaPSaF). Manchester: University of Manchester.

Verbakel NJ et al. (2014). Exploring patient safety culture in primary care. *International Journal for Quality in Health Care*, 26(6):585–91.

Verbakel NJ et al. (2015). Effects of patient safety culture interventions on incident reporting in general practice: a cluster randomised trial. *British Journal of General Practice: the Journal of the Royal College of General Practitioners*, 65(634):e319–29.

Verbakel NJ et al. (2016). Improving Patient Safety Culture in Primary Care: A Systematic Review. *Journal of Patient Safety*, 12(3):152–8.

Verbeek-van Noord I et al. (2014). Does classroom-based Crew Resource Management training improve patient safety culture? A systematic review. *Sage Open Medicine*, 2:2050312114529561.

Verbeek-van Noord I et al. (2018). A nation-wide transition in patient safety culture: a multilevel analysis on two cross-sectional surveys. *International Journal for Quality in Health Care*. doi: 10.1093/intqhc/mzy228 [Epub ahead of print].

Wagner C et al. (2016). Unit-based incident reporting and root cause analysis: variation at three hospital unit types. *BMJ Open*, 6(6):e011277.

Walshe K (2000). Adverse events in health care: issues in measurement. *Quality in Health Care*, 9(1):47–52.

Weaver SJ et al. (2013). Promoting a culture of safety as a patient safety strategy: a systematic review. *Annals of Internal Medicine*, 158(5 Pt 2):369–74.

WHO (2008). World Alliance for Patient Safety: Research for Patient Safety – Better Knowledge for Safer Care. Geneva: World Health Organization.

WHO (2013). Exploring patient participation in reducing healthcare-related safety risks. Copenhagen: WHO Regional Office for Europe.

Zwijnenberg NC et al. (2016). Healthcare professionals' views on feedback of a patient safety culture assessment. *BMC Health Services Research*, 16:199.

Chapter 12

Clinical pathways as a quality strategy

Thomas Rotter, Robert Baatenburg de Jong,
Sara Evans Lacko, Ulrich Ronellenfitsch, Leigh Kinsman

Summary

What are the characteristics of the strategy?

Clinical pathways (CPWs) are tools used to guide evidence-based healthcare. Their aim is to translate clinical practice guideline recommendations into clinical processes of care within the unique culture and environment of a healthcare institution. A CPW is a structured multidisciplinary care plan with the following characteristics: (1) it is used to translate guidelines or evidence into local structures; (2) it details the steps in a course of treatment or care in a plan, pathway, algorithm, guideline, protocol or other "inventory of actions"; and (3) it aims to standardize care for a specific clinical problem, procedure or episode of healthcare in a specific population.

What is being done in European countries?

The use of clinical pathways has been growing in Europe since the 1990s, beginning in the UK, and pathways are currently used in most European countries. In some European countries (for example, Belgium, Bulgaria, Germany, the Netherlands) there are increasing activities in the development and implementation of clinical pathways. The European Pathways Association (EPA), the world's largest CPW professional organization, was founded in 2004 with the aim of supporting the development, implementation and evaluation of clinical/care pathways in Europe. In 2018 the EPA reported members in more than 50 countries, covering both national health systems and SHI systems.

What do we know about the effectiveness and cost-effectiveness of the strategy?

A review of the Cochrane Collaboration including 27 studies involving 11 398 participants showed reductions in length of stay and hospital costs for the CPW group(s) compared with usual care. Meta-analysis showed that CPWs are associated with reduced in-hospital complications and two studies reported improved professional documentation. No effects on hospital readmission or in-hospital mortality were shown. The majority of studies reported a reduction in in-hospital costs.

How can the strategy be implemented?

Evidence on successful clinical pathway implementation is sparse. Successful CPW uptake and implementation is a complex process and requires careful consideration about facilitators and barriers to change provider behaviour in the specific setting. An active process that maximizes the input is essential, and support of both managers and clinicians is required to overcome the inherent resistance often apparent in the implementation of CPWs. Top-down strategies that do not actively involve the relevant professionals have little or no impact. It is also pivotal to carefully select the group of patients targeted by the CPW. Compliance with evidence-based recommendations should always be measured prior to CPW development and implementation in order to demonstrate the presence of, and extent of, impact on clinical practice.

Conclusions for policy-makers

CPWs are associated with improved patient outcomes and could play an important role in patient safety. They may also act as a managerial intervention to tackle the challenges associated with case-mix systems (i.e. DRGs) in healthcare reimbursement. For local healthcare providers and policy-makers, the choice of implementing CPW strategies should be based upon considerations of their likely costs and benefits. It should be noted that the development and implementation of CPWs consumes a considerable amount of resources when done as recommended in an active process – but it will likely have positive effects on patient outcomes, while also reducing hospital costs.

12.1 Introduction: the characteristics of clinical pathways

Clinical pathways (CPWs) are tools used to guide evidence-based healthcare; their use has been widespread since the 1980s. CPWs aim to translate clinical practice guideline recommendations (*see* Chapter 9) into clinical processes of care within the unique culture and environment of the healthcare institution, thereby maximizing patient safety and clinical efficiency.

CPWs should be developed based on the best available evidence, such as clinical practice guidelines or a systematic review. Thus, they have the potential to streamline clinical practice for a specific group of patients with a particular diagnosis or undergoing a particular procedure. In other words, CPWs can be described as structured multidisciplinary care plans which detail essential steps in the care of patients with a specific clinical problem.

In daily practice and research, widespread confusion exists as to what constitutes a CPW and there is a lack of agreement regarding an internationally agreed CPW definition. In fact, a recent study revealed 84 different terms that may refer to a CPW, including (among others) care map, critical pathway, protocol and integrated care pathway (De Bleser et al., 2006).

However, several definitions vary in the content criteria described. *See* Box 12.1 for the European Pathways Association (EPA) definition of a CPW.

Box 12.1 *EPA Definition of a clinical pathway*

"A care pathway is a complex intervention for the mutual decision making and organisation of care processes for a well-defined group of patients during a well-defined period. Defining characteristics of care pathways include: An explicit statement of the goals and key elements of care based on evidence, best practice, and patients' expectations and their characteristics; the facilitation of communication among team members and with patients and families; the coordination of the care process by coordinating the roles and sequencing the activities of the multidisciplinary care team, patients and their relatives; the documentation, monitoring, and evaluation of variances and outcomes, and the identification of the appropriate resources" (EPA, 2018a).

The EPA definition lacks specificity, i.e. it does not allow CPWs to be distinguished from similar concepts or strategies. Such a distinction is necessary when addressing the issue of effectiveness of the strategy.

Independent of the terminology used, the concept of CPWs is defined by the characteristics and content of the strategy. Based on a synthesis of published definitions and descriptions, an operational definition of CPWs has been proposed (Kinsman et al., 2010; Rotter et al., 2010; Rotter et al., 2013).

Therefore, a CPW is a structured multidisciplinary care plan with the following characteristics:

1. It is used to translate guidelines or evidence into local structures.

2. It details the steps in a course of treatment or care in a plan, pathway, algorithm, guideline, protocol or other "inventory of actions" (i.e. the intervention has time-frames or criteria-based progression).

3. It aims to standardize care for a specific clinical problem, procedure or episode of healthcare in a specific population.

In theory, CPWs could be implemented in any area of healthcare, i.e. preventive, acute, chronic and palliative care. They mainly focus on processes in relation to effectiveness, patient-safety and/or patient-centredness. CPWs are strongly linked to recommendations from clinical guidelines (*see* Chapter 9), if available for the specific condition.

This chapter follows the common structure of all chapters in Part 2 of this book. The underlying rationale of why CPWs should contribute to healthcare quality is described, along with an overview of what is being done in European countries in respect to the specific quality strategy, while the following section provides an overview of the available evidence with regard to the effectiveness and cost-effectiveness of the specific strategy. The next section addresses questions of implementation, and the final section provides conclusions for policy-makers, bringing together the available evidence and highlighting lessons for implementation of the strategy.

12.2 Why should clinical pathways contribute to healthcare quality?

The main aim of clinical pathway implementation is to align clinical practice with guideline recommendations (*see* Chapter 9) in order to provide high-quality care within an institution. CPWs may serve as useful tools to reduce variations in clinical practice, thereby maximizing patient outcomes and clinical efficiency. They have the capacity to promote safe, evidence-based care by providing locally oriented recommendations for the management of a specific condition, disease or reason to demand healthcare (Kiyama et al., 2003; Aizawa et al., 2002; Choong et al., 2000; Delaney et al., 2003; Marelich et al., 2000). CPWs also contribute to the reduction of complications and treatment errors (Rotter et al., 2010).

CPWs structure the flow of services for a group of patients with a particular diagnosis or undergoing a particular procedure and they guide the patient through the treatment process. They also support the translation of clinical guideline recommendations or evidence available in other forms into local protocols and clinical practice (Campbell et al., 1998). Whilst clinical guidelines provide generic recommendations, CPWs institutionalize best practices to bring evidence to the bedside for all the health professionals involved (Campbell et al., 1998; Kinsman et al., 2010). (For more information on professionals' education, *see* Chapter 5.)

As an example, a clinical guideline recommendation for an outpatient rehabilitation programme will be implemented locally in a clinical pathway in much more detail, such as when to submit the referral and to whom it should be submitted. Thus CPWs aim to standardize clinical processes of care within the unique culture and environment of the healthcare institution. As a result of standardizing clinical practice according to evidence-based clinical practice guidelines, CPWs have the potential to reduce treatment errors and improve patient outcomes.

An example of a CPW for the management of elderly inpatients with malnutrition is provided in Fig. 12.1.

Another rationale (for policy-makers and healthcare institutions) for implementing and using CPWs is that they have also been proposed as a strategy to optimize resource allocation and cost-effectiveness. Within the trend towards the economization of healthcare, as evidenced by the prevalence of case mix (CM) systems worldwide, there is also evidence of the increased promotion of clinical pathway interventions to tackle these dramatic changes in healthcare reimbursement methods (Delaney et al., 2003).

12.3 What is being done in Europe?

The use of CPWs has been growing in Europe since the 1990s, beginning in the UK (Zander, 2002), and spreading to most European countries (Vanhaecht et al., 2006; Knai et al., 2013).

The European Pathways Association (EPA), the world's largest CPW professional organization, was founded in 2004 with the aim of supporting the development, implementation and evaluation of clinical/care pathways within Europe (*see* Box 12.2). In 2018 the EPA reported members in more than 50 countries, covering both national health systems and SHI systems (EPA, 2018a). CPWs are being used in countries with public not-for-profit and with private for-profit healthcare providers.

In 2006 the EPA network published its first international survey and overview on the reported use and dissemination of CPWs in 23 countries (Vanhaecht et al., 2006). CPW prevalence was defined as the number of individual patients reported to be on a pathway. The study found that reported estimates of CPW use were low and that when CPWs were used it was mainly in acute care settings. Pathway utilization was low (1–5%) in Belgium, the Netherlands, Germany and Spain, whereas in Wales and Scotland it was found to be higher (6–10%), and in the rest of the UK the estimate was 11–15% (Vanhaecht et al., 2006). The

Fig. 12.1 *A clinical pathway for the management of elderly inpatients with malnutrition*

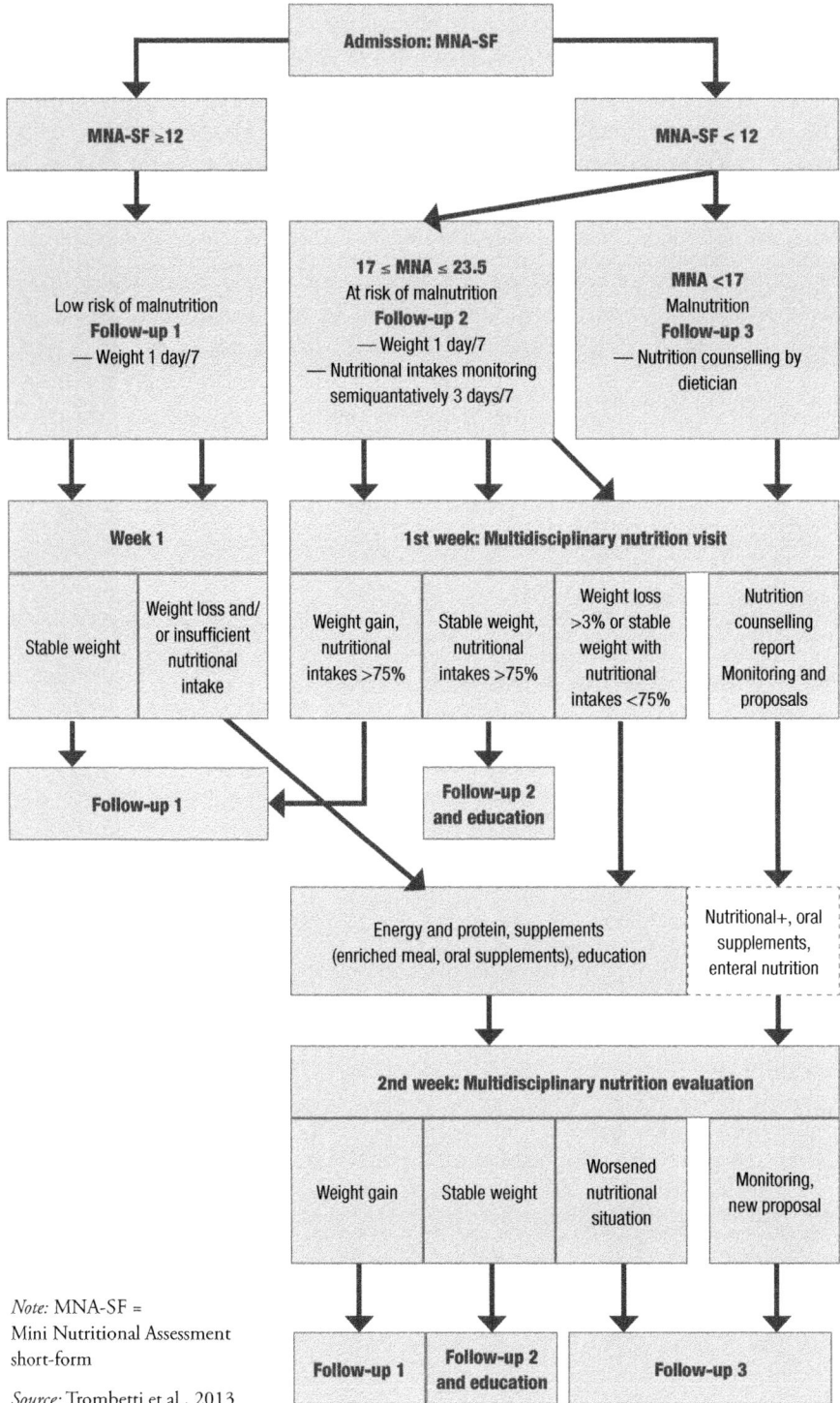

Admission: MNA-SF

MNA-SF ≥12

MNA-SF < 12

Low risk of malnutrition
Follow-up 1
— Weight 1 day/7

17 ≤ MNA ≤ 23.5
At risk of malnutrition
Follow-up 2
— Weight 1 day/7
— Nutritional intakes monitoring
semiquantatively 3 days/7

MNA <17
Malnutrition
Follow-up 3
— Nutrition counselling by
dietician

Week 1

1st week: Multidisciplinary nutrition visit

Stable weight

Weight loss and/
or insufficient
nutritional
intake

Weight gain,
nutritional
intakes >75%

Stable weight,
nutritional
intakes >75%

Weight loss
>3% or stable
weight with
nutritional
intakes <75%

Nutrition
counselling
report
Monitoring and
proposals

Follow-up 1

**Follow-up 2
and education**

Energy and protein, supplements
(enriched meal, oral supplements), education

Nutritional+, oral
supplements,
enteral nutrition

2nd week: Multidisciplinary nutrition evaluation

Weight gain

Stable weight

Worsened
nutritional
situation

Monitoring,
new proposal

Follow-up 1

**Follow-up 2
and education**

Follow-up 3

Note: MNA-SF =
Mini Nutritional Assessment
short-form

Source: Trombetti et al., 2013

> **Box 12.2** *The European Pathways Association (EPA)*
>
> "The purpose of the association is
>
> (1) To conduct international research into the quality and efficiency of organizing healthcare and methods for the coordination of primary healthcare and care pathways.
>
> (2) To set up an international network for pooling know-how and the international training initiatives that go with it.
>
> (3) To foster international cooperation between healthcare researchers, managers and healthcare providers from European countries and the wider international community.
>
> (4) To advise policy-makers within the area of healthcare management."
>
> EPA network activities are organized by country in the form of EPA national sections, but not all European countries are represented. EPA runs a summer school and a clinical pathway conference, held on a yearly basis. EPA also edits the *International Journal of Care Pathways* and is developing a standardized set of indicators to evaluate CPWs in clinical practice (EPA, 2018a).

investigation concluded that CPWs were primarily used as an inter-professional tool to improve the quality of care.

The cross-sectional survey (n = 76 respondents) reflects limited representation and is at high risk of self-selection bias (Vanhaecht et al., 2006), so this information should be considered with caution.

In 2013 the EPA network published a follow-up cross-sectional survey. The investigators collected 163 responses from 39 countries with a 25% response rate (Knai et al., 2013). In this update the authors clearly stated that it was not a representative survey and no prevalence estimates were reported (Knai et al., 2013). Neither survey addressed the issue of which pathway conditions were reported and included in the responses.

In some European countries (*see* below) there are increasing activities in the development and implementation of CPWs. The examples show that there is an increasing number of activities in this field, but little can be said about the actual usage and content of the CPWs.

12.3.1 Belgium and the Netherlands

The Belgian Dutch Clinical Pathway (BDCP) Network (*Netwerk klinische Paden*) was launched in March 2000 by a multidisciplinary team under the leadership of the Centre for Health Services and Nursing Research, School of Public Health, at the Catholic University of Leuven, Belgium (BDCP Network, 2018).

The network aims to support Belgian and Dutch hospital organizations in the development, implementation and evaluation of CPWs.

The main activities are: (1) to provide education sessions on CPWs, patient safety, quality management and evidence-based medicine; (2) to support multidisciplinary teamwork; and (3) to foster international research and collaboration. Since 2003 the network has closely collaborated with the Dutch Institute for Healthcare Improvement (CBO). By 2018 more than 57 healthcare organizations were members of the BDCP Network (including acute hospital trusts, rehabilitation centres and home-care organizations) (BDCP Network, 2018). Within the Network more than 1000 projects are under development or have been implemented.

In 2003 the Dutch Ministry of Health initiated a complementary national quality improvement collaborative called Faster Better. The purpose of the programme was to realize a significant improvement in patient safety and patient flow in 20% of Dutch hospitals within four years. One of the specific aims of the programme was to shorten the total duration of the diagnostic process and treatment by between 40% and 90%. CPWs were used to achieve this. During the first year of the programme the participating hospitals achieved a reduction of 32% (Consortium-Sneller-Beter-Pijler 3, 2006).

The Dutch government has been pushing responsibility for improving healthcare to healthcare facilities, insurance companies and patients. In 2011 one of the largest Dutch insurance companies and various healthcare providers jointly created the Lean Network in Healthcare (LIDZ) knowledge network. The goal of this network is to make process improvement an integral and daily part of healthcare by creating and sharing knowledge (LidZ, 2012). The approach of the network is complementary to CPW and directly refers to the Lean methodology. The network comprises more than 60 healthcare organizations.

12.3.2 England

CPWs have been promoted in several government health policy reports and it is likely that the use of CPWs in the NHS is increasing (Darzi, 2008, 2009; Department of Health, 2007). The growing focus in the NHS, especially during the current budget constraints, is on evidence-based practice and improving quality of care. As a result, CPWs have been identified as tools which could play an important role in reducing costly variations in care in addition to improving patient safety (Darzi, 2009). Several tools and resources have been developed to facilitate the use and implementation of CPWs within the NHS. An online pathway tool aims to provide easy access for NHS staff to clinical evidence and best practice. The pathway database is hosted at the National Institute for Health and Care Excellence (NICE). The NICE database offers generic information about CPWs for all NHS staff, jurisdictions and stakeholders including quality standards, technology appraisals, clinical and public health guidance and NICE implementation tools (NICE, 2012). In addition, the Releasing Time To Care® programme in the NHS is a complementary approach but it has a much broader scope and directly refers to the Lean Methodology.[1] Releasing Time to Care (also known as the productive ward) provides a systematic approach to delivering safe, high-quality care to patients within the NHS. It has been widely implemented in NHS trusts and entities to respond to the needs of the community and to ensure that standards of healthcare are high (Wilson, 2009).

CPWs have the potential to stimulate social movements such as the demand for shared decision-making, the continuing development of the "information society", advances in treatment, and the changing expectations of patients and the workforce in the UK. There have been several success stories of CPW implementation in England thus far, for example the stroke care pathway originally highlighted by Lord Darzi's report (Intercollegiate Stroke Working Party, 2011). Nevertheless, despite the noted benefits of several CPW initiatives and support among key stakeholders, a recent report by the King's Fund and Nuffield Trust highlights several barriers to implementation of CPWs within the NHS, and makes recommendations for calls to action in order to support and facilitate CPWs "at scale and pace" (Goodwin et al., 2012). Although this is an important issue and should guide future efforts, it is not unique to the UK (Greenhalgh et al., 2004; Evans-Lacko et al., 2010).

More recently, there has been growing emphasis on better integration of patient and public involvement in the development and implementation of CPWs in the NHS. Resources such as the Smart Guides to Engagement (Maher, 2013), which support Clinical Commissioning Groups in employing strategies for pathway development involving and clearly reflecting the values of patients, caregivers and family members in order to promote appropriateness and efficiency (NHS England, 2016) of CPWs, play an important role.

12.3.3 Germany

Before 2008 the implementation of CPWs had been proposed and endorsed by many stakeholders in the German healthcare system. Several professional societies had recommended that CPWs should be used in everyday practice, but their development was left to single institutions and cross-linking and exchange of ideas between them was rare and often cumbersome. Many healthcare professionals

---

1   Lean Management (LM) in healthcare is based upon the principles of reducing waste and wait-times and improving the quality of care. The Lean Methodology is a complex multicomponent intervention and refers to standard work in the form of clinical protocols and clinical pathways.

therefore perceived an increasing need for an umbrella organization which allows single professionals to bundle forces and share knowledge with peers, and to enhance their negotiating power with hospital administrations, policy-makers, colleagues and other professional organizations.

In 2008 the German Society for Clinical Process Management (DGKPM) was founded. Its principal goal is to scientifically assess and improve processes in clinical medicine, with the ultimate aim of improving the quality of patient care (DGKPM, 2008). To that end, the society intensively promotes the use of CPWs and engages in their development, implementation and scientific evaluation. The DGKPM does not want to compete with the single medical professional societies but, rather, wants to cooperate with them and offer mutual support.

DGKPM members have published theoretical papers on CPWs but also assessed quality effects of pathway projects. For example, a classification for development levels of CPWs has been proposed (Uerlich et al., 2009). Moreover, a systematic review on the utilization of CPWs in surgery (Ronellenfitsch et al. 2008) and a qualitative study on success factors for development and implementation of CPWs (De Allegri et al., 2011) have been conducted. The DGKPM is a co-host of the annual workshop "Clinical Pathways in Surgery", which serves as an exchange platform for clinicians, nurses and administrators interested in working with CPWs. In recent years the society has also cooperated with commercial companies to provide advice and support in the development of software solutions for clinical decision support, which incorporate several elements of CPWs. In the near future the DGKPM will establish a curriculum to train healthcare professionals as clinical process managers. This curriculum comprises a dedicated part on implementation and everyday usage of CPWs.

12.3.4 Bulgaria

In Bulgaria so-called "clinical pathways" are being used in case-based payments. Since 2001 hospitals have been reimbursed with a single flat rate per pathway. A set number of diagnoses are grouped and reimbursed according to a "clinical pathway" (more than 250 in 2017) where the costs of up to two outpatient medical examinations after hospital discharge are included. As an attempt to optimize hospital activity, CPWs for outpatient procedures were also introduced in 2016. There are 42 outpatient procedures (for example, cataract surgery, chemotherapy) and four different procedures which require a length of stay up to 24 hours (for example, intensive treatment of new-borns with assisted breathing) (Dimova et al., 2018).

The Bulgarian approach illustrates the widespread confusion as to what constitutes a clinical pathway but it also shows a potential benefit of CPWs in the move to standardizing and optimizing hospital care.

12.4 The effectiveness and cost-effectiveness of clinical pathways

Effectiveness

As with any other intervention in healthcare, the question is whether CPWs achieve what they aim for, whether they ultimately contribute to improve the outcomes of healthcare, and at what cost this is achieved. Rotter et al. (2012) addressed the effects of CPWs on professional practice, patient outcomes, length of stay and hospital costs for the hospital setting in a Cochrane systematic review (Rotter et al., 2012). The methodology of the review is summarized in Box 12.3. The review represents the most comprehensive database in terms of the available quantitative literature; an update has been submitted to the Cochrane Library for publication.

Box 12.3 *Methodology of systematic review*

Sources and Search

The authors searched the EPOC Register, the Cochrane CENTRAL Register of Controlled Trials, and bibliographic databases including Medline, EMBASE, CIHNAL, NHS EED and Global Health. Other sources were hand-searched journals, reference lists and the ISI Web of Science; in addition, they contacted authors and experts in the field of clinical pathway research.

Selection Criteria

Randomized controlled trials (RCTs) and non-randomized trials (for example, controlled clinical trials, controlled before and after studies and interrupted time series studies) were included.

Outcomes measures

Objectively measured patient outcomes included mortality, hospital readmission, complications, adverse events, length of stay (LOS) and hospital costs. Professional practice outcomes included documentation in medical records, patient satisfaction and time to mobilization post-surgery.

Data Synthesis

The authors presented the results of their studies in tabular form and made an assessment of the effects of the studies. Primary studies were statistically pooled and the results depicted if there were enough comparable primary studies.

Rotter et al. (2012) observed considerable clinical and methodological heterogeneity, with a broad range of disparate outcomes measured, many different settings in which care is delivered, and a wide range of diagnoses and types of patient included in the different study designs. Study outcomes reported were in-hospital complications, in-hospital mortality, hospital readmission, length of stay and hospital costs (Kinsman et al., 2010).

Out of the 3214 studies identified, 27 involving 11 398 participants met the Effective Practice and Organization of Care (EPOC) eligibility and study quality criteria for inclusion. Twenty studies compared CPWs with usual care and seven studies compared CPWs as part of a multifaceted intervention with usual care. Nineteen randomized controlled trials (RCTs) and eight non- randomized controlled trials met the selection criteria and many different hospital settings were included in the systematic review. The majority of studies (13) were conducted in the United States (Bauer et al., 2006; Bookbinder et al., 2005; Brook et al., 1999; Delaney et al., 2003; Falconer et al., 1993; Gomez et al., 1996; Johnson et al., 2000; Kim et al., 2002; Kollef et al., 1997; Marelich et al., 2000; Philbin et al., 2000; Roberts et al., 1997; Tilden & Shepherd, 1987), four in Australia (Choong et al., 2000; Doherty & Jones, 2006; Dowsey et al., 1999; Smith et al., 2004), three in Japan (Aizawa et al., 2002; Kiyama et al., 2003; Usui et al., 2004), two each in the United Kingdom (Sulch et al., 2000, 2002; Chadha et al., 2000) and Canada (Cole et al., 2002; Marrie et al., 2000), and one each in Thailand (Kampan, 2006), Taiwan (Chen et al., 2004) and Norway (Brattebo et al., 2002).

Due to the high level of clinical and statistical heterogeneity (I square), length of stay (LOS) and hospital cost data were not suitable for pooling among those studies.

Table 12.1 depicts the main results of the meta-analysis of primary studies, which compared care with and without CPWs.

Despite the different settings and investigations included in the systematic review, it was striking that the majority of studies reported reductions in both length of stay and hospital costs for the CPW group(s) compared with usual care. Meta-analysis showed that CPWs are associated with a reduction in in-hospital complications and two studies reported on improved professional documentation (*see* Table 12.1).

In-hospital complications were measured in five studies of pathways for invasive interventions (both elective and non-elective), concerning a total of 664 participants. All studies reported improved outcomes for the CPW group (Aizawa et al., 2002; Choong et al., 2000; Delaney et al., 2003; Kiyama et al., 2003; Marelich et al., 2000). Fig. 12.2 provides details about the meta-analytic comparison.

Table 12.1   *Effectiveness of CPWs compared to usual care*

Outcome	Number of studies (patients) included	Event rate %		OR (95% CI)
		CPW	UC	
In-hospital complications	5 (664)	9.3%	15%	0.58 (0.36 to 0.94)
In-hospital mortality at 26 weeks	3 (1187)	22%	25%	0.84 (0.64 to 1.11) *
Hospital readmission	6 (672)	5.5%	8.5%	0.6 (0.32 to 1.13) *
Professional documentation	2 (240)	84%	52%	11.95 (4.72 to 30.3)

Source: Rotter et al., 2012

Notes: *NS = not significant; NNT = number needed to treat; NNT and CI calculated from review data; UC = Usual care; OR = Odds Ratio; CI = Confidence Interval

Aizawa et al. (2002) tested a clinical pathway for transurethral resection of the prostate (TURP), Choong et al. (2000) assessed a CPW for femoral neck fracture, Delaney et al. (2003) tested a CPW for laparotomy and intestinal resection, Kiyama et al. (2003) a CPW for gastrectomy, and Marelich et al. (2000) a clinical pathway for mechanical ventilation. In-hospital complications assessed were wound infections, bleeding and pneumonia (Aizawa et al., 2002; Choong et al., 2000; Delaney et al., 2003; Kiyama et al., 2003; Marelich et al., 2000). The results indicate that in order to avoid one hospital complication it would be necessary to include 18 patients in a CPW (i.e. number needed to treat = 18).

However, both groups did not differ for in-hospital mortality and hospital readmission within six months after discharge (the longest follow-up period reported.)

Fig. 12.2   *Clinical pathway vs. usual care, outcome: in-hospital complications*

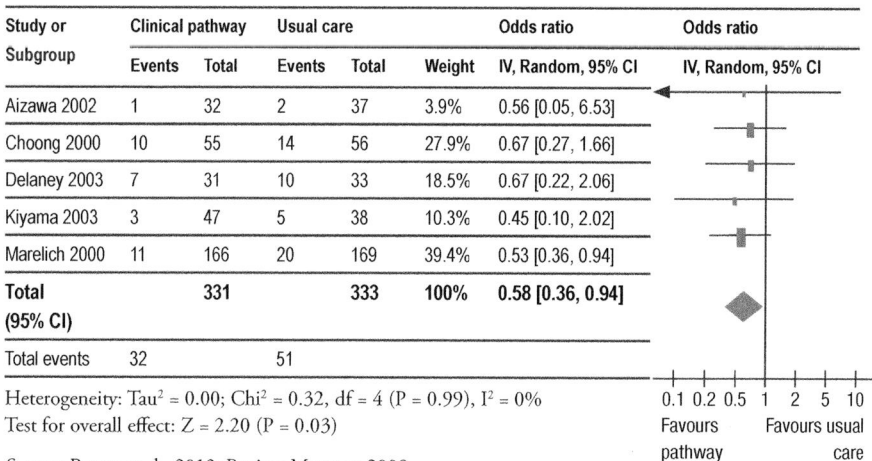

Study or Subgroup	Clinical pathway		Usual care			Odds ratio	Odds ratio
	Events	Total	Events	Total	Weight	IV, Random, 95% CI	IV, Random, 95% CI
Aizawa 2002	1	32	2	37	3.9%	0.56 [0.05, 6.53]	
Choong 2000	10	55	14	56	27.9%	0.67 [0.27, 1.66]	
Delaney 2003	7	31	10	33	18.5%	0.67 [0.22, 2.06]	
Kiyama 2003	3	47	5	38	10.3%	0.45 [0.10, 2.02]	
Marelich 2000	11	166	20	169	39.4%	0.53 [0.36, 0.94]	
Total (95% CI)		**331**		**333**	**100%**	**0.58 [0.36, 0.94]**	
Total events	32		51				

Heterogeneity: Tau^2 = 0.00; Chi^2 = 0.32, df = 4 (P = 0.99), I^2 = 0%

Test for overall effect: Z = 2.20 (P = 0.03)

0.1 0.2 0.5 1 2 5 10

Favours pathway   Favours usual care

Sources: Rotter et al., 2012; Review-Manager 2008

Significant variations across studies prevented further meta-analysis and limited conclusions. In terms of the transferability and generalizability of the review results, four RCTs were conducted in medical units (Brook et al., 1999; Cole et al., 2002; Kampan, 2006; Philbin et al., 2000), three RCTs in surgical units (Aizawa et al., 2002; Delaney et al., 2003; Kiyama et al., 2003), three RCTs in medical or surgical intensive care, two RCTs in emergency departments (Kim et al., 2002b; Roberts et al., 1997), two RCTs in stroke rehabilitation wards (Falconer et al., 1993; Sulch et al., 2000) and five RCTS in other hospital settings (Bauer et al., 2006; Chen et al., 2004; Dowsey et al., 1999; Johnson et al., 2000; Marrie et al., 2000).

12.4.1 Cost-effectiveness

Hospital cost data were reported as direct hospital costs and as total costs (direct costs and indirect costs) including administration or other overhead costs. Due to the low number of high-quality studies evaluating hospital costs, the study investigated all objective cost data available, such as hospital charges (i.e. DRGs) or country-specific insurance points (Rotter et al., 2010). This highly variable set of reported cost measures precluded further economic evaluation and we concentrated therefore on the direct cost-effects of CPWs rather than their cost-effectiveness. Table 12.2 presents an overview of the costing method used and which costs/charges were included and excluded in the calculations (as far as reported).

Most studies reported a reduction in in-hospital costs. The adjusted cost effects (weighted mean difference in US dollars standardized to the year 2000) ranged from additional costs of US$261 per case for a protocol-directed weaning from mechanical ventilation (Kollef et al., 1997) to savings of US$4 919 per case for an emergency department-based protocol for rapidly ruling out myocardial ischemia (Gomez et al., 1996). Significant clinical and methodological heterogeneity prevented a meta-analysis of the reported cost results. In summary, CPWs are associated with improved patient outcomes and could play an important role in patient safety, but considerable clinical and methodological heterogeneity prohibited further economic investigation of the reported effect measures and benefits.

It should be noted that the development and implementation of CPWs consumes a considerable amount of resources. This corresponds to the fact that truly achievable cost savings depend on the number of cases (volume) of the condition targeted by the pathway. According to a cost analysis from Comried (1996), inflation-adjusted costs for the development and implementation of the pathway for the indication "Caesarian section" amounted to more than US$26 000 while the costs for the development and implementation of a CPW for the indication "uncomplicated vaginal delivery" were estimated at approximately US$10 000

Table 12.2   *Evidence on cost-effectiveness of CPWs*

Study ID	Cost measure	Country	Costs/charges included	Costs/ charges excluded	Cost effects of CPWs compared to usual care
Comparison 1: CPW intervention vs. usual care Mean/median difference					
Aizawa et al., 2002	Insurance points (including direct and indirect costs)	Japan	Dosage, injection, treatment, operation and anaesthesia, examination, diagnostic, room, medical care	Not reported	– 6 941.30 Hospital insurance points
Falconer et al., 1993	Median hospital charges to proxy direct costs of rehabilitation	USA	Charges for hospital bed days, medical and rehabilitation services (including professional fees), equipment, drugs and procedures (radiographs, laboratory tests, injections)	Not reported	+ 25 US$ Favours usual care
Gomez et al., 1996	Mean hospital charges	USA	Room, nursing care, laboratory tests, therapy	Physician fees	– 4 919.18 US$
Johnson et al., 2000	Mean hospital charges	USA	Room, medication, laboratory tests and respiratory therapy	Physician fees	– 743.08 US$
Kim et al., 2002	Mean hospital costs (direct costs)	USA	Remains unclear, only "total direct costs" reported	Professional fees	– 836.00 US$
Kiyama et al., 2003	Mean hospital costs (direct costs)	Japan	Total medical costs including medication and examination (physician fees)	Fixed costs	– 2 771.94 US$
Kollef et al., 1997	Mean hospital costs	USA	Not reported	Physician fees	+ 261 US$ Favours usual care
Roberts et al., 1997	Mean hospital costs (direct and indirect costs)	USA	Professional fees	Not reported	– 641.54 US$
Usui et al., 2004	Insurance points (including direct costs)	Japan	Treatment (antibiotic infusion), laboratory and radiography tests	Fixed costs	– 9 710.00 Hospital insurance points
Comparison 2: Multifaceted intervention including a CPW vs. usual care					
Bauer et al., 2006	Mean hospital costs (direct costs)	USA	Not reported	Not reported	– 3 316.19 US$
Kampan, 2006	Mean hospital costs (remains unclear if direct and indirect costs have been used, only "mean costs" reported)	Thailand	Not reported	Not reported	– 52.63 US$
Philbin et al., 2000	Mean hospital charges	USA	Not reported	Not reported	– 887.03 US$

Legend: Mean costs/charges data in US dollars standardized to the year 2000
Source: Rotter et al., 2010

(Comried, 1996). However, since normally 20% of diagnoses cover 80% of cases (Schlüchtermann et al., 2005), a considerable percentage of medical services can be dealt with using a relatively small number of CPWs.

12.5 How can the strategy be implemented? What are the organizational and institutional requirements?

The implementation of CPWs needs to be an active process that considers barriers to clinician usage of the CPW. While any change to processes and systems has its challenges, there is particular resistance to the implementation of CPWs as they are often described as "cook-book medicine" by clinicians who may fear a loss of autonomy. However, check-lists and CPWs are being increasingly demonstrated as improving professional practice and patient outcomes (Rotter et al., 2010; de Vries et al., 2010) so strategies to enhance clinician compliance with CPWs need to be considered and built into implementation strategies.

Passive, top-down approaches to CPW implementation have little or no impact (Kinsman & James, 2001) as opposed to a growing evidence-base for participative implementation processes. These processes include use of an implementation team and "local champions". Identifying barriers to change, clinician involvement in design and implementation, identification of local evidence-practice gaps, optimizing the evidence-base of the CPW content, adaptation of evidence to the local circumstances, staff education sessions, incorporation of reminder systems, and audit and feedback (*see* Chapter 10) regarding CPW compliance and outcomes are key success factors (Cluzeau et al., 1999; Doherty & Jones, 2006; Grimshaw, 1998; Grimshaw et al., 2001; Kinsman, James & Ham, 2004).

12.5.1 CPW implementation strategies

Implementation strategies have been too poorly reported in the literature to allow for identifying specific characteristics that contribute to the uptake of CPWs by clinicians. Most CPW evaluations focused on effectiveness measures rather than on CPW uptake or adherence to the evidence-based recommendations and evidence underpinning which implementation strategies are the most successful remains scarce.

By definition, CPWs support the involvement of patients in clinical practice but this aspect was rarely reported in over 3 000 primary studies that have been critically appraised in the systematic review presented above (Rotter et al. 2012). However, more patient involvement in the clinical decision-making process in terms of CPW-guided hospital care is pivotal because the patient should play a central role in this process (van der Weijden et al., 2012). Implementation research has shown that patient involvement is a crucial factor for the success or failure of clinical pathway interventions in terms of the quality of care provided as well as clinical efficiency, for example in pediatric hospital settings (Cene et al., 2016). A plain language version of a CPW for guidance of the patient and shared decision-making is therefore a crucial element in increasing compliance and patient safety.

However, among the 27 studies included in our systematic review that showed generally positive outcomes from CPWs, the most commonly reported implementation strategies were use of an implementation team, identification of evidence-practice gaps, audit and feedback, and education sessions. This supports evidence reported for the successful implementation of research into practice via other strategies such as clinical guidelines (Grimshaw & Thomson, 1998; Bero et al., 1998).

This evidence indicates that planning and resources need to be directed at implementation strategies in conjunction with the development of the CPW itself. The quality of the CPW is irrelevant if it is not accepted and adopted by clinicians. An active process that maximizes the input and support of both managers and clinicians is required to overcome the inherent resistance often apparent in the implementation of CPWs.

12.6 Conclusions for policy-makers

This chapter has shown that although the clinical pathway concept is not a "silver bullet" for improving healthcare practice in Europe, it has the potential to promote quality of care and to maximize clinical efficiency. From a patient perspective, CPWs provide better guidance and understanding of what patients should expect throughout the care episode.

CPWs may also act as a managerial intervention to tackle the challenges associated with the globalization of case-mix systems (i.e. DRGs) in healthcare reimbursement. Therefore, CPWs may be promoted for reasons relating to management or cost-containment even though clinicians may have negative attitudes in terms of standardization of healthcare practice (Evans-Lacko et al., 2010). In fact, the clinical pathway concept is a tool to translate guideline recommendations and to organize clinical care differently but it does not necessarily interfere with clinical decision-making.

Many countries and professional bodies embrace the clinical pathway concept. Examples are the United Kingdom, Canada and Australia (EPA, 2018b; Huckson & Davies, 2007; Grimshaw et al., 2007). CPWs may serve as useful and evidence-based management tools to reduce variations in clinical practice and to decrease costs and length of stay. The reported effects on in-hospital complications are promising and the pathway concept seems to be effective for large groups of patients, especially those receiving invasive procedures. Thus CPW implementation is likely to become increasingly emphasized in Europe (Evans-Lacko et al., 2010) although much more experience with CPW implementation is needed to fully understand this quality improvement concept.

Evidence on successful clinical pathway implementation is sparse and varies significantly in how healthcare organizations implement CPWs. Successful CPW uptake and implementation is a complex process and requires careful consideration about facilitators and barriers in order to change provider behaviour (Grimshaw et al., 2001). The clinical pathway concept is by definition a multidisciplinary approach and should include all involved professions. Passive, top-down strategies to promote and implement CPWs have little or no impact. Engagement of both clinical and management staff in the development and adoption of CPWs is required and multifaceted strategies should be used to implement this concept. It is pivotal to carefully select the targeted group of patients and a setting-specific and tailored implementation strategy is most likely to be effective (Evans-Lacko et al., 2010). The planned implementation strategy could be also adopted from complementary studies investigating clinical practice guidelines or surgical checklists (Bosch et al., 2007). Compliance with clinical guideline recommendations should always be measured prior to CPW development and implementation in order to improve clinical practice.

CPWs are not new and are complementary to clinical practice guidelines, disease-management programmes (DMPs) and clinical checklists or protocols. They are based on clinical guidelines and available evidence and are tailored to suit the organizational requirements. It is also striking that similar interventions such as DMPs often include CPWs, and that their successful implementation strategies also refer to an implementation team, audit and feedback, patient involvement and education sessions.

For local healthcare providers and policy-makers, the choice of implementing clinical pathway strategies should be also based upon considerations of the expected costs and benefits of pathway interventions. It should be noted that the development and implementation of CPWs consumes a considerable amount of resources. This corresponds to the fact that truly achievable cost savings depend on the number of cases (volume) of the condition targeted by the pathway.

References

Aizawa T et al. (2002). Impact of a clinical pathway in cases of transurethral resection of the prostate. *Japanese Journal of Urology*, 93(3):463–8.

Bauer MS et al. (2006). Collaborative care for bipolar disorder: part I (& II) Intervention and implementation in a randomized effectiveness trial. *Psychiatric Services*, 57(7):927–6.

BDCP Network (2018). Belgian Dutch Clinical Pathway Network. Available at: https://www.kuleuven.be/samenwerking/ligb/reseachlines/belgian-dutch-clinical-pathway-network, accessed 27 June 2018.

Bero LA et al. (1998). Closing the gap between research and practice: an overview of systematic reviews of interventions to promote the implementation of research findings. The Cochrane Effective Practice and Organization of Care Review Group. *BMJ*, 317(7156):465–8.

Bookbinder M et al. (2005). Improving end-of-life care: development and pilot-test of a clinical pathway. *Journal of Pain and Symptom Management*, 29(6):529–43.

Bosch M et al. (2007). Tailoring quality improvement interventions to identified barriers: a multiple case analysis. *Journal of Evaluation in Clinical Practice*, 13(2):161–8.

Brattebo G et al. (2002). Effect of a scoring system and protocol for sedation on duration of patients' need for ventilator support in a surgical intensive care unit. *BMJ*, 324(7350):1386–9.

Brook AD et al. (1999). Effect of a nursing-implemented sedation protocol on the duration of mechanical ventilation. *Critical Care Medicine*, 27(12):2609–15.

Campbell H et al. (1998). Integrated care pathways. *BMJ*, 316(7125):133–7.

Cene CW et al. (2016). A Narrative Review of Patient and Family Engagement: The "Foundation" of the Medical "Home". *Medical Care*, 54(7): 697-705.

Chadha Y et al. (2000). Guidelines in gynaecology: evaluation in menorrhagia and in urinary incontinence. *BJOG: An International Journal of Obstetrics and Gynaecology*, 107(4):535–43.

Chen SH et al. (2004). The development and establishment of a care map in children with asthma in Taiwan. *Journal of Asthma*, 41(8):855–61.

Choong PF et al. (2000). Clinical pathway for fractured neck of femur: a prospective, controlled study. *Medical Journal of Australia*, 172(9):423–6.

Cluzeau FA et al. (1999). Development and application of a generic methodology to assess the quality of clinical guidelines. *International Journal of Quality in Health Care*, 11(1):21–8.

Cole MG et al. (2002). Systematic detection and multidisciplinary care of delirium in older medical inpatients: a randomized trial. *Canadian Medical Association Journal*, 167(7):753–9.

Comried LA (1996). Cost analysis: initiation of HBMC and first CareMap. *Nursing Economics*, 14(1):34–9.

Consortium Sneller Beter Pijler 3 (2006). Sneller Beter werkt! Resultaten van het eerste jaar. Den Haag.

Darzi A (2008). High quality care for all: NHS Next Stage Review final report. London: Department of Health.

Darzi A (2009). The first year of high quality care for all. *Health Service Journal*, 119(6162):17.

De Allegri M et al. (2011). Which factors are important for the successful development and implementation of clinical pathways? A qualitative study. *BMJ Quality and Safety*, 20(3):203–8.

De Bleser L et al. (2006). Defining pathways. *Journal of Nursing Management*, 14:553–63.

de Vries EN et al. (2010). Effect of a comprehensive surgical safety system on patient outcomes. *New England Journal of Medicine*, 363:1928–37.

Delaney CP et al. (2003). Prospective, randomized, controlled trial between a pathway of controlled rehabilitation with early ambulation and diet and traditional postoperative care after laparotomy and intestinal resection. *Diseases of the Colon and Rectum*, 46(7):851–9.

Department of Health (2007). Our NHS Our future: NHS next stage review – interim report. London: Department of Health.

DGKPM (2008). German Society for Clinical Process Management. Available at: www.dgkpm.de, accessed 04 May 2012.

Dimova A et al. (2018). Bulgaria: Health system review. *Health Systems in Transition*: 20(4).

Doherty SR, Jones PD (2006). Use of an 'evidence-based implementation' strategy to implement evidence-based care of asthma into rural district hospital emergency departments. *Rural and Remote Health*, 6(1):1.

Dowsey MM et al. (1999). Clinical pathways in hip and knee arthroplasty: a prospective randomised controlled study. *Medical Journal of Australia*, 170(2):59–62.

EPA (2018a). EPA Care Pathways. Available at: http://e-p-a.org/care-pathways/, accessed 27 June 2018.

EPA (2018b). Health Quality Ontario. Evidence and Health Quality Ontario. Available at: http://www.hqontario.ca/Evidence-to-Improve-Care/Evidence-and-Health-Quality-Ontario, accessed 29 June 2018.

Evans-Lacko S et al. (2010). Facilitators and barriers to implementing clinical care pathways. *BMC Health Services Research*, 10:182.

Falconer JA et al. (1993). The critical path method in stroke rehabilitation: lessons from an experiment in cost containment and outcome improvement. *QRB Quality Review Bulletin*, 5(1):8–16.

Gomez MA et al. (1996). An emergency department-based protocol for rapidly ruling out myocardial ischemia reduces hospital time and expense: results of a randomized study (ROMIO). *Journal of the American College of Cardiology*, 28(1):25–33.

Goodwin N et al. (2012). A report to the Department of Health and the NHS Future Forum. Available at: http://www.kingsfund.org.uk/sites/files/kf/integrated-care-patients-populations-paper-nuffield-trust-kings-fund-january-2012.pdf, accessed 05 December 2018.

Greenhalgh T et al. (2004). Diffusion of innovations in service organizations: systematic review and recommendations. *Milbank Quarterly*, 82(4):581–629.

Grimshaw J (1998). Evaluation of four quality assurance initiatives to improve out-patient referrals from general practice to hospital. Aberdeen: University of Aberdeen.

Grimshaw JM, Thomson MA (1998). What have new efforts to change professional practice achieved? Cochrane Effective Practice and Organization of Care Group. *Journal of the Royal Society of Medicine*, 91(Suppl 35):20–5.

Grimshaw JM et al. (2001). Changing provider behaviour: an overview of systematic reviews of interventions. *Medical Care*, 39(8 – suppl 2).

Grimshaw JM et al. (2007). Looking inside the black box: a theory-based process evaluation alongside a randomised controlled trial of printed educational materials (the Ontario printed educational message, OPEM) to improve referral and prescribing practices in primary care in Ontario, Canada. *Implementation Science*, 2:38.

Huckson S, Davies J (2007). Closing evidence to practice gaps in emergency care: the Australian experience. *Academic Emergency Medicine*, 14(11):1058–63.

Intercollegiate Stroke Working Party (2011). National Sentinel Stroke Clinical Audit 2010 Round 7: Public Report for England, Wales and Northern Ireland. London: Royal College of Physicians.

Johnson KB et al. (2000). Effectiveness of a clinical pathway for inpatient asthma management. *Pediatrics*, 106(5):1006–12.

Kampan P (2006). Effects of counseling and implementation of clinical pathway on diabetic patients hospitalized with hypoglycemia. *Journal of the Medical Association of Thailand*, 89(5):619–25.

Kim MH et al. (2002). A prospective, randomized, controlled trial of an emergency department-based atrial fibrillation treatment strategy with low-molecular-weight heparin (Structured abstract). *Annals of Emergency Medicine*, 40:187–92.

Kinsman L, James EL (2001). Evidence based practice needs evidence based implementation. *Lippincott's Case Management*, 6(5):208–19.

Kinsman L, James E, Ham J (2004). An interdisciplinary, evidence-based process of clinical pathway implementation increases pathway usage. *Lippincott's Case Management*, 9(4):184–96.

Kinsman L et al. (2010). What is a clinical pathway? Development of a definition to inform the debate. *BMC Medicine*, 8(31).

Kiyama T et al. (2003). Clinical significance of a standardized clinical pathway in gastrectomy patients (Structured abstract). *Journal of Nippon Medical School*, 70:263–9.

Knai C et al. (2013). International experiences in the use of care pathways. *Journal of Care Services Management*, 7(4):128–35.

Kollef MH et al. (1997). A randomized, controlled trial of protocol-directed versus physician-directed weaning from mechanical ventilation. *Critical Care Medicine*, 25(4):567–641.

LidZ (2012). Stichting Lean in de zorg. Website: http://www.lidz.nl, accessed 20 May 2019.

Maher L (2013). Developing pathways: using patient and carer experiences. London: NHS Networks.

Marelich GP et al. (2000). Protocol weaning of mechanical ventilation in medical and surgical patients by respiratory care practitioners and nurses: effect on weaning time and incidence of ventilator-associated pneumonia. *Chest*, 118(2):459–67.

Marrie TJ et al. (2000). A controlled trial of a critical pathway for treatment of community-acquired pneumonia. CAPITAL Study Investigators. Community-Acquired Pneumonia Intervention Trial Assessing Levofloxacin. *Journal of the American Medical Association*, 283:749–55.

NHS England (2016). Involving our patients and public in improving London's healthcare: NHS England (London) participation and engagement review 2015/16. Available at: https://www.england.nhs.uk/london/wp-content/uploads/sites/8/2016/12/improv-londons-healthcare.pdf, accessed 29 June 2018.

NICE (2012). NICE database clinical pathways. Available at: http://pathways.nice.org.uk/, accessed 14 April 2019.

Philbin EF et al. (2000). The results of a randomized trial of a quality improvement intervention in the care of patients with heart failure. The MISCHF Study Investigators. *American Journal of Medicine*, 109(6):443–9.

Review Manager (RevMan) [Computer program] (2008). Version 5.0. Copenhagen, The Nordic Cochrane Centre.

Roberts RR et al. (1997). Costs of an emergency department-based accelerated diagnostic protocol vs hospitalization in patients with chest pain: a randomized controlled trial. *Journal of the American Medical Association*, 278(20):1670–6.

Ronellenfitsch U et al. (2008). Clinical Pathways in surgery: should we introduce them into clinical routine? A review article. *Langenbeck's Archives of Surgery*, 393(4):449–57.

Rotter T et al. (2010). Clinical pathways: effects on professional practice, patient outcomes, length of stay and hospital costs. *Cochrane Database of Systematic Reviews*, 17(3):CD006632.

Rotter T et al. (2012). The effects of clinical pathways on professional practice, patient outcomes, length of stay, and hospital costs. Cochrane systematic review and meta-analysis. *Evaluation and the Health Professions*, 35(1): 3–27.

Rotter T et al. (2013). Clinical pathways for primary care: effects on professional practice, patient outcomes, and costs. *Cochrane Database of Systematic Reviews*, 8:CD010706.

Schlüchtermann J et al. (2005). Clinical Pathways als Prozesssteuerungsinstrument im Krankenhaus. *In:* Oberender P (ed.). Clinical pathways: Facetten eines neuen Versorgungsmodells. Stuttgart: Kohlhammer Verlag.

Smith et al. (2004). Impact on readmission rates and mortality of a chronic obstructive pulmonary disease inpatient management guideline. *Chronic Respiratory Disease,* 1(1):17–28.

Sulch D et al. (2000). Randomized controlled trial of integrated (managed) care pathway for stroke rehabilitation. *Stroke*, 31(8):1929–34.

Sulch D et al. (2002). Integrated care pathways and quality of life on a stroke rehabilitation unit. *Stroke*, 33(6):1600–4.

Tilden VP, Shepherd P (1987). Increasing the rate of identification of battered women in an emergency department: use of a nursing protocol. *Research in Nursing and Health*, 10(4):209–24.

Trombetti A et al. (2013). A critical pathway for the management of elderly inpatients with malnutrition: effects on serum insulin-like growth factor-I. *European Journal of Clinical Nutrition*, 67(11):1175–81.

Uerlich M et al. (2009). Clinical Pathways – Nomenclature and levels of development. *Perioperative Medicine*, 1(3):155–63.

Usui K et al. (2004). Electronic clinical pathway for community acquired pneumonia (e-CP CAP). *Nihon Kokyuki Gakkai zasshi (The Journal of the Japanese Respiratory Society)*, 42(7):620–4.

van der Weijden T et al. (2012). Clinical practice guidelines and patient decision aids. An inevitable relationship. *Journal of Clinical Epidemiology*, 65(6):584–9.

Vanhaecht K et al. (2006). Prevalence and use of clinical pathways in 23 countries – an international survey by the European Pathway Association. *Journal of Integrated Care Pathways*, 10:28–34.

Wilson G (2009). Implementation of Releasing Time to Care – the productive ward. *Journal of Nursing Management*, 17(5):647–54.

Zander K (2002). Integrated Care Pathways: eleven international trends. *Journal of Integrated Care Pathways*, 6:101–7.

Chapter 13

Public reporting as a quality strategy

Mirella Cacace, Max Geraedts, Elke Berger

Summary

What are the characteristics of the strategy?

Public reporting as a quality strategy is characterized by (1) the reporting of quality-related information to the general public about (2) non-anonymous, identifiable professionals and providers (for example, individuals, institutions), (3) using systematically gathered comparative data. Public reporting is expected to contribute to improvements in effectiveness, safety and/or responsiveness, depending on the measured and reported indicators through two pathways. First, it may enable patients to select high-quality providers and professionals (selection pathway), and second, it may provide incentives to providers and professionals to improve their quality of care (change pathway).

What is being done in European countries?

An increasing number of countries in Europe uses public reporting of quality of care provided by hospitals, GPs or specialists. Relatively elaborated public reporting initiatives have been implemented in the United Kingdom (nhs.uk), the Netherlands (kiesbeter, "Make better Choices"), Germany (weisse-liste.de "White List"), and Denmark (sundhed.dk, "Health"). However, many other countries also report quality information but usually initiatives cover a smaller proportion of providers or report on a more restricted set of quality indicators. Public reporting is less frequent in countries that joined the EU in 2004 or later.

What do we know about the effectiveness and cost-effectiveness of the strategy?

Several reviews found that public reporting is associated with a small reduction in mortality, although the quality of available evidence is moderate or low. Larger effects were observed in studies that did not have a control group and in those that focused on cardiovascular mortality. There is evidence of some unintended effects, such as changed coding and readmission practices. Public reporting has been found to be more effective if baseline performance is low. Studies have generally found low utilization rates of public reporting by patients. Populations with lower socioeconomic status – just like older adults – are less likely to make use of publicly reported information. Evidence on costs and cost-effectiveness is missing.

How can the strategy be implemented?

Implementation strategies have to be adjusted to the respective aims and target groups of public reporting. It is important to involve all relevant stakeholders, such as patients/patient organizations and providers/staff at all levels of organization. In addition, both clinical and non-clinical indicators should be reported, and information should be available at different levels of aggregation. Combining the use of composite indicators, which summarize quality information available from different indicators, with the option to obtain information about these individual indicators, allows users to receive information tailored to their needs.

Conclusions for policy-makers

While use of publicly reported information by patients is (still) relatively low, public reporting may lead to improvements in the quality of care by incentivizing providers and professionals to improve their practice. To be effective, information has to be easily accessible and indicators should be valid and reliable. Strong regulations may support achieving high coverage of providers and high quality of data.

13.1 Introduction: the characteristics of public reporting

Public reporting about the quality of care has been increasing in many European countries over the past 20 years (OECD, 2019). The strategy aims to promote transparency and informed choice of providers, to stimulate quality improvement, and to hold providers accountable for the care they deliver. We define public reporting as the reporting of performance-related information to the general public about non-anonymous, identifiable professionals and providers (for example, individuals, institutions), using systematically gathered comparative data.

This definition does not consider all publicly available information on providers to be public reporting. First and foremost, reporting must allow for the identification of individual providers. This excludes initiatives that report performance as summary indicators at the level of geographic areas, as happens in France. In addition, our definition excludes open comments by healthcare users in the mass media because this information is not systematically collected. However, the definition includes public reporting of patient satisfaction based on systematic surveys or rating websites. Finally, non-public feedback from insurers to providers is not considered if this information is not disclosed to the public (Marshall, Romano & Davies, 2004).

Public reporting as a quality strategy focuses on the reporting of quality-related information about effectiveness, safety and responsiveness of care, measured in terms of structure, process or outcome indicators. Public reporting may be used to address quality in different areas of care, i.e. primary prevention, acute care, chronic care or palliative care. In this chapter we focus only on hospital care and on physician practices, which – depending on the healthcare system under consideration – are predominantly single or group practices. Although several European countries also provide public reports for nursing homes (Rodrigues et al., 2014), considering these activities here would go beyond the scope of the chapter.

Public reporting requires the systematic and reliable measurement of a range of relevant and meaningful quality indicators (*see* also Chapter 3). It may be combined with audit and feedback strategies (*see* Chapter 10) and external assessment strategies (*see* Chapter 8) with the aim of strengthening incentives for improvement of quality.

The chapter follows the common structure of most chapters in Part 2 of this book. The next section describes the underlying rationale of why public reporting should contribute to healthcare quality, followed by a review of approaches to public reporting in European countries in order to identify context, relevant actors, scope and the range of indicators used. While the interest in public reporting is continuously growing in Europe, evaluations of public reporting instruments are scant. We therefore derive information on effectiveness and (cost-)effectiveness and on the implementation requirements by including experiences from other continents, in particular from the United States. In synthesizing these experiences, we conclude by summarizing the lessons learned and by deriving potential conclusions and recommendations for policy-makers.

13.2 Why should public reporting contribute to healthcare quality?

Berwick, James & Coye (2003) identify two principal pathways through which quality measurement and public reporting can lead to the improvement of healthcare services. Fig. 13.1 shows the two pathways of change and their interaction based on motivational and reputational factors. In the first pathway, "improvement through selection", comparative information enables users to exercise informed choice and to select providers according to quality criteria. By "voting with their feet" consumers are supposed to select good performers and discard bad ones, thus triggering competitive processes (Hirschman, 1970). For this mechanism to work effectively the option of "exit" is necessary, which means that the respective healthcare system needs to offer at least some choice of provider (Dixon, Robertson & Bal, 2010). Furthermore, effective choice is also a question of regional supply. In particular in rural areas, low density of medical care providers can be a restricting factor, and choice will depend on the willingness and ability of patients to invest time and financial resources to exert their choices.

However, instead of simply dropping out of the market, providers with low performance can improve on it by changing their behaviour, which brings us to the second pathway, "improvement through change". In this pathway, quality information allows providers to identify areas of underperformance relative to their peers. Making individuals or provider organizations aware of their own performance and allowing them to compare to some form of "expected" level then acts as a stimulus, motivating providers to improve (Shekelle, 2009).

At first sight, the change pathway may work also without disclosing this quality information to the general public. Indeed, revealing the divergence between own and peer group performance might suffice for intrinsically motivated providers to stimulate behaviour change, which is the basic idea of audit and feedback strategies (*see* Chapter 10). The role for public reporting, however, results from the fact that the threat of reputational damage provides additional incentives to institutions and individuals to improve the quality of care by changing clinical practices and the organization of care (Hamblin, 2008). Therefore, public reporting is often combined with audit and feedback strategies and also with external assessment strategies, such as accreditation, certification and supervision (*see* Chapter 8).

Fig. 13.1 *Two pathways of change through public reporting*

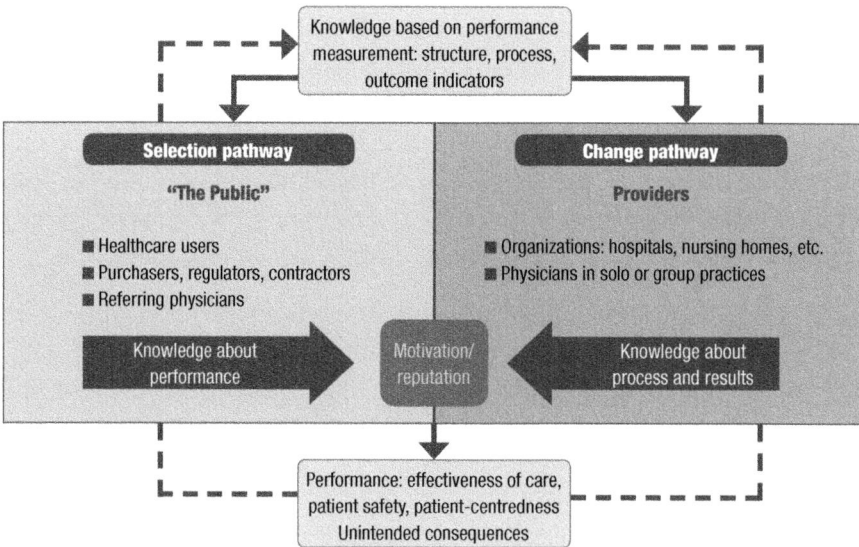

Source: adapted from Berwick, James & Coye, 2003

Both pathways are interlinked through the provider's self-awareness and the intention to maintain or increase reputation and, in a competitive context, market share (Berwick, James & Coye, 2003; Werner & Asch, 2005). It is worth noting that through the second pathway quality improvement may occur even if patients make limited use of provider choice, slightly releasing the link between choice and exit as a prerequisite for change (Cacace et al., 2011). Schlesinger (2010) argues that "voice", i.e. the critical dialogue exerted by the informed and empowered patient, is complementary, and in some cases also alternative, to "exit". This is particularly important for healthcare settings in which voice seems the more promising strategy in achieving quality gains compared to exit, for example in primary care, where the continuity of the physician-patient relationship is an objective in its own right. Admittedly, however, voice is much more powerful if there is an exit option and a credible threat that consumers will exert their choice.

13.3 What is being done in Europe?

The interest in public reporting is continuously growing across European countries. In the OECD Health Systems Characteristics Survey, more than half of the 21 countries surveyed in 2016 reported the public release of the results of monitored quality metrics at provider level (OECD, 2019). Table 13.1 presents an overview of public reporting initiatives in 10 European countries and indicates whether they are focused on GPs, specialists and/or hospitals. This overview does not claim to be exhaustive, but considers the most important public reporting strategies identified at the time of writing. The table shows that most public reporting initiatives focus on quality in the hospital sector, while there are fewer public reporting initiatives that cover GPs and/or specialists.

In some countries, such as Germany, the Netherlands and the UK, several different initiatives exist for the hospital sector and there are at least two that cover GPs and specialists. Relatively few initiatives cover both ambulatory care (GPs and specialists) and hospital care. Interestingly, all reviewed public reporting initiatives end at the borders of the respective country. To our knowledge, there is no public reporting system supporting cross-border care in Europe.

Relatively elaborated public reporting initiatives have been implemented in the United Kingdom (nhs.uk, former *NHS Choices*), the Netherlands (kiesbeter.nl, "Make better Choices"), Germany (weisse-liste.de "White List"), and Denmark (sundhed.dk, "Health"). These initiatives cover either all or at least a majority of providers in the respective country and report on large sets of quality indicators in multiple sectors of the healthcare system, including general and specialist care in hospitals and physician practices, and optionally also nursing homes as well as dental care providers.

In some countries public reporting is combined with financial incentives in a Pay-for-Quality (P4Q) approach (*see also* Chapter 14), such as the Quality and Outcomes Framework (QOF) in the UK or the Quality Bonus Scheme (QBS) in Estonia. In the UK the QOF was introduced in 2004 for rewarding GP practices for providing quality care. It systematically rewards and reports an array of clinical and non-clinical performance indicators at the level of GP practices and therefore goes far beyond the usually reported data on GP practices in other countries.

Many other countries also have public reporting initiatives but these are usually less systematic and cover a smaller proportion of providers for a variety of reasons. For example, in some more decentralized healthcare systems, such as Sweden, the implementation of public reporting initiatives and the detail of publicly released information vary greatly between regional units. The same applies to Italy, where measures of the National Evaluation Programme (*Programma Nazionale Esiti*, PNE) are publicly reported at hospital level in some regions, for example, in the Regional Programme for the Evaluation of Healthcare Outcomes (P.Re.Val.E) in Lazio (PNE, 2019). As with many other policy innovations, regions can serve as "laboratories for experimentation" for quality reporting with the potential for national scale-up (Cacace et al., 2011).

So far, few public reporting activities have been identified in the countries that joined the EU in 2004 or later (for example, Bulgaria, the Czech Republic, Romania, Slovakia, Slovenia). Only the Baltic countries have recently introduced some initiatives: in Estonia, the Quality Bonus Scheme (QBS) publishes information about the achieved quality points per practice. In Latvia a pilot project

Table 13.1   *Overview of public reporting initiatives in Europe (2019)*

Country	Website	Focus			Sponsorship
		GPs	Specialists	Hospitals	
Austria	kliniksuche.at			✓	public
	docfinder.at	✓	✓		private
Denmark	esundhed.dk	✓	✓		public
	sundhed.dk			✓	public
	sundhetskvalitet.dk			✓	public
Estonia	Quality Bonus Scheme (QBS)[d]	✓			public
France	scopesante.fr			✓	public
Germany	AOK Gesundheitsnavigator[e]	✓	✓	✓	public
	deutsches-krankenhaus-verzeichnis.de			✓	private
	g-ba-qualitaetsberichte.de			✓	public
	jameda.de[b]	✓	✓		private
	qualitätskliniken.de[c]			✓	private
	weisse-liste.de	✓	✓	✓	private
Italy	P.Re.Val.E[e]			✓	public
Netherlands	independer.nl	✓	✓	✓	private
	kiesbeter.nl			✓	public
	ziekenhuischeck.nl			✓	private
	zorgkaartnederland.nl	✓	✓		private
Norway	helsenorge.no	✓	✓	✓	public
Sweden	öppna jämforelser [f]			✓	public
	vantetider.se			✓	public
United Kingdom	cqc.org.uk	✓	✓	✓	public
	Hospital Scorecard Scotland[g]			✓	public
	nhs.uk[h]	✓	✓	✓	public
	Quality & Outcomes Framework (QOF)[i]	✓			public

Note: a: "AOK Health Navigator", one example of a sickness fund-led initiative based on results of weisse-liste.de;

b: one example of an array of physician rating sites in Germany, see for example, Emmert & Meszmer (2018) for more information;

c: in the beginning also covering hospitals, now only rehabilitation clinics are covered;

d: website: haigekassa.ee;

e: for registered users only and only for the region of Lazio: Programma Regionale Valutazione degli Esiti degli Interventi Sanitari ("Regional Programme Evaluation of Healthcare Outcomes"), website: https://bit.ly/2BtrebL;

f: "Open comparisons", website: socialstyrelsen.se/oppnajamforelser;

g: only in Scotland and only for NHS registered users, website: Isdscotland.org;

h: former NHS Choices;

i: relaxed in Wales, dropped in Scotland, running in England and Northern Ireland, website: qof.digital.nhs.uk

Source: Authors' compilation

of public reporting on both hospitals' and GPs' performance has been initiated recently which – depending on its success – might be scaled up in the future. In Lithuania quality indicators are publicly reported for both hospitals and GPs by the six sickness funds (OECD, 2018). However, as detailed information is unavailable, the initiative is not included in Table 13.1.

Finally, it needs to be acknowledged that for some countries information is not available in international publications and that, in contrast to other quality strategies (*see* Chapters 12 and 8), no organization or association exists that unites different national organizations responsible for public reporting. Furthermore, public reporting in European countries is constantly changing, with new initiatives being implemented, and others being dropped, renamed and/or incorporated into new ones. Therefore, the overview of public reporting initiatives does not claim to be exhaustive, but considers the most important public reporting strategies identified at the time of writing.

13.3.1 Regulation and sponsorship

In all European countries the state plays at least a minimal role in quality management, which is also reflected in the funding, provision and regulation of public reporting. Regulatory frameworks differ with respect to more centralized or decentralized approaches. In England and the Nordic countries the government plays a decisive role in regulating, funding and reporting quality information. In countries where public reporting is combined with financial incentives, the regulatory framework is particularly important and also more elaborated as it overlaps with the regulation of the financial incentive.

In several countries regulation on public reporting differs across healthcare sectors. Often public reporting is mandatory for hospital care but not for ambulatory care. For example, in the Netherlands reporting on selected quality indicators is mandatory for hospital inpatient and outpatient care (Zorginstituut, 2019), while no such regulation exists for primary care. Likewise in Germany federal legislation requires only hospitals to engage in external quality management and to publish annual quality reports, which are the basis of many German public reporting initiatives.

Even though most initiatives in Europe – sponsored either publicly or privately – are governmentally regulated, legislation does not limit the number of public reporting initiatives in a country and does not restrict sponsorship of public reporting. As a consequence, in several countries multiple and diverse public, private non-profit and for-profit sponsors are involved in public reporting. For example, in Germany 18 differently regulated public reporting initiatives on hospital care (Emmert et al., 2016) and 29 physician rating websites have been identified (Emmert & Meszmer, 2018).

A range of different public – and sometimes private – actors play a role in the governance of reporting initiatives in hospital care. In Denmark (sundhedskvalitet. dk), for example, the municipalities and regions, the National Board of Health and the Ministry of the Interior and Health are involved. The Dutch kiesbeter. nl is operated by the National Quality Institute, which was founded in 2013, to bundle different existing activities related to quality in healthcare (van den Hurk, Buil & Bex, 2015). In the German social insurance system, sickness funds play a major role in the regulation of public reporting through their representation in the Federal Joint Committee (Gemeinsamer Bundesausschuss, G-BA), which is the highest decision-making body in healthcare. Furthermore, sickness funds are obliged to make data from hospital quality reports accessible for users on the internet (*see*, for example, AOK *Gesundheitsnavigator*, "AOK Health Navigator"). In addition, some hospitals report performance data on the basis of membership in a (private) quality initiative, such as the German qualitaet-skliniken.de, which is, however, restricted to rehabilitation care. Reporting in this case is more self-regulated and also (self-)selective, as non-members do not contribute to quality reporting.

At the level of physician practices private sponsorship is more frequent than in the hospital sector but public sponsorship remains the more common form (*see also* Table 13.1). An array of private commercial initiatives has sprung up, as for example the physician rating websites in Germany (jameda.de), the Netherlands (independer.nl) and Austria (docfinder.at). Because of private, profit-oriented sponsorship, users have to accept – more or less health-related – advertisement, as these initiatives usually do not have access to other (public) funding sources. Public sponsorship exists in Denmark, Estonia, Germany, Norway, and the UK. In Germany, several sickness funds have set up their own physician rating websites by drawing on results of the weisse-liste.de, for example, the AOK *Gesundheitsnavigator*. The weisse-liste.de itself has been created by a private non-profit foundation in cooperation with three sickness funds as well as associations of patients and consumer organizations (Cacace et al., 2011). Weisse-liste.de allows members and co-insured family members of three large sickness funds to rate providers, and the entire population has access to the information (Emmert & Meszmer, 2018).

13.3.2 Quality indicators used in public reporting

Quality indicators used for public reporting are constantly changing, with new indicators being added and others being amended or dropped. Following Donabedian (1988), indicators included in existing initiatives can be classified into indicators of structure, process and outcome (*see also* Chapters 2 and 3). In addition, this chapter reports separately on indicators of patient satisfaction and patient experience to highlight the use of indicators for the evaluation of patient-centredness. An important challenge for public reporting of outcome indicators is risk-adjustment, which is needed to make comparisons across providers fair and meaningful (*see also* Chapter 3).

13.3.4 Indicators for the quality of hospital care

Table 13.2 provides an overview of indicators identified in public reporting initiatives in the area of ***hospital care***. The scope of reported indicators varies across initiatives from those providing basic information on availability of structures to those providing more detailed information on processes of care and outcomes. As public reporting in hospital care is often mandated by government, the initiatives usually cover a high proportion of hospitals and a broad range of structure, process and outcome indicators. As shown in Table 13.2, the majority of initiatives focuses on indicators related to structures, processes and clinical outcomes. The Swedish initiative vantetider.se ('Waiting time') is the only one to concentrate exclusively on just one indicator, i.e. waiting times. Outcome indicators are usually risk-adjusted using patients' age, gender and comorbidities, for which data are available in hospital databases. However, these adjustments never work perfectly and incentives to select healthier patients may remain, as we will discuss in more detail below.

Several systems provide also information on the patient perspective based on systematic surveys, including patients' experience and/or patient satisfaction (for example, nhs.uk in the UK, kiesbeter.nl in the Netherlands and sundhedskvalitet. dk in Denmark) while others (for example, QOF in England) dropped indicators related to the patient perspective in the data year 2014/2015 (Ashworth & Gulliford, 2016). Frequently, satisfaction and experience are measured on several dimensions covering, for example, satisfaction/experience with care, with the treating physician, cleanliness of wards, etc., optionally condensed into one (partial) composite index.

The overview also indicates whether systems use composite indices, such as star-ratings, in order to bundle overall or partial information and whether they provide options for open comments (for example, from patients about their individual experiences). While open comments fall outside our definition of public reporting (*see* above), we nevertheless decided to include this option in the overview tables, since three well-established initiatives (weisse-liste.de, independer.nl, nhs.uk) incorporated this option.

Table 13.2 *Publicly reported indicators on hospital care (2019)*

Country	Website	Indicators			Patient experience/ satisfaction	Composite indices	Open comments
		Structure	Process	Outcomes			
Austria	kliniksuche.at	✓	✓				
Germany	AOK Gesundheitsnavigator[a]	✓	✓	✓	✓	✓	
	deutsches-krankenhaus-verzeichnis.de	✓	✓	✓			
	g-ba-qualitaetsberichte.de	✓	✓	✓			
	qualitätskliniken.de	✓	✓	✓	✓	✓	
	weisse-liste.de	✓	✓	✓	✓	✓	✓
Denmark	sundhetskvalitet.dk		✓	✓	✓	✓	
	esundhed.dk	✓	✓	✓			
France	scopesante.fr	✓	✓	✓	✓	✓	
Italy	P.Re.Val.E[b]	✓	✓	✓			
Netherlands	independer.nl	✓	✓	✓	✓	✓	✓
	kiesbeter.nl	✓	✓	✓	✓	✓	
	ziekenhuischeck.nl	✓	✓	✓	✓	✓	
Norway	helsenorge.no[c]	✓	✓	✓	✓	✓	
Sweden	öppna jämforelser[d]	✓	✓	✓	✓		
	vantetider.se		✓				
UK	Hospital Scorecard Scotland[e]	✓	✓	✓	✓		
	nhs.uk[f]	✓	✓	✓	✓	✓	✓
	Quality and Outcomes Framework (QOF)[g]	✓	✓	✓	✓	✓	

Note: a: "AOK Health Navigator", one example of a sickness fund-led initiative based on results from weisse-liste.de;
b: for registered users only, website: https://bit.ly/2BtrebL;
c: patient perspective is separately presented from other quality indicators;
d: "open comparisons", website: socialstyrelsen.se/oppnajamforelser;
e: only in Scotland and only for NHS registered users, website: isdscotland.org;
f: former NHS Choices;
g: relaxed in Wales, dropped in Scotland, running in England and Northern Ireland, website: qof.digital.nhs.uk

Source: based on Cacace et al. 2011, updated in 2019

All public reporting initiatives included in Table 13.2 provide at least some guidance for users, for example through manuals opening up when scrolling over technical terms. Often interactive website tools allow users to perform one-to-one comparisons of a few hospitals, selected for example by entering a postal code search, often combined with a search according to body-parts or indications. Some public reporting initiatives provide a reference to national or regional averages to facilitate comparisons across hospitals. Another option is to set a reference threshold on the basis of scientific standards or clinical guidelines. For example, nhs.uk has defined, on the basis of clinical guidelines, that at least 95% of patients should be assessed for the risk of venous thromboembolism (blood clots). Kiesbeter.nl and weisse-liste.de indicate the deviation of indicators from averages and/or scientific standards using a flag system (green-yellow-red/green-red).

The German qualitaetskliniken.de used to have a somewhat different approach to presenting information on hospital quality. Here users were able to select hospitals by setting minimum performance thresholds for different criteria covering clinical quality, patient safety, patient perspective and/or satisfaction of referring physicians. However, Qualitaetskliniken.de discontinued this approach. Nevertheless, we find the idea of making information adaptable to users' needs by enabling them to prioritize search criteria quite remarkable.

13.3.5 Indicators on the quality of physician care

Table 13.3 provides examples of some public reporting systems on the quality of physician care at the *practice level*, covering general practitioners as well as specialists. In some countries, such as England, specialists work in hospitals and therefore are not included in reporting systems on physician practices.

Compared to the hospital sector, the number and diversity of quality indicators is less comprehensive in public reporting on physician practices. Most initiatives focus only on structures and patient experience/satisfaction. Only initiatives in Sweden and the UK include indicators for clinical processes and outcomes.

Measures of patient experience/satisfaction include satisfaction with waiting times, the premises (for example, cleanliness), care in general, the doctor or staff, and the service at the practice.

There are two fundamentally different ways of assessing the patient perspective with major consequences for the quality of data. One option is to invite patients to report their experience using the systems' website. This method is used by physician rating websites although it is prone to self-selection bias. The other option is to systematically collect patient views by using a validated survey instrument. This method is more costly, but supposedly leads to more representative results. Weisse-liste.de, as well as the English nhs.uk, use both methods of data collection. While weisse-liste.de combines the results into one database, nhs.uk reports the survey results separately from users' website ratings. As a means to improve reliability of reported information, weisse-liste.de does not publish scores based on fewer than five ratings per provider, and it reports average scores across providers as a reference. In the Austrian docfinder.at offensive comments are simply deleted in order to avoid a culture of "naming and blaming". Finally, there are also different ways to present patients' open comments to the user. Many systems endow all ratings and open comments with a calendar date in order to enable users to judge on the timeliness and thus relevance of data.

Major obstacles to the reporting of clinical outcome indicators at the level of physician practices are the comparably small numbers of cases and the lack of information in medical records to allow risk-adjustment. QOF reports on a comparatively large number of outcome indicators, although these are mostly "intermediate outcomes". Based on scientific evidence, these measures link specific processes to effective outcomes, such as rewarding GPs for the proportion of patients with hypertension whose last blood pressure reading was below 150/90, where there is evidence that lower blood pressure improves the odds for survival (Campbell & Lester, 2010). In order to enable fair comparisons, QOF relies mostly on exception reporting (and not on risk-adjustment), allowing physicians to exclude data from certain patients (for example, palliative patients), when calculating average scores (NHS Digital, 2019).

13.4 The effectiveness and cost-effectiveness of public reporting

The core question in the evaluation of the (cost-)effectiveness of public reporting is whether (and to what extent) public reporting influences health outcomes. However, measuring the impact of public reporting on health outcomes is difficult – just as for many other quality strategies – because of problems related to isolating its effect from other simultaneously implemented quality improvement strategies, such as improved documentation (Werner & Bradlow, 2010). In addition it seems to be useful to look for evidence on the effectiveness of public reporting systems in addressing potential users. These play a pivotal role in the processes of quality improvement, be it through the selection mechanism or by inducing providers to change behaviour.

Most evidence on the effectiveness of public reporting on quality of care is available from initiatives in the United States (Totten et al., 2012; Campanella et al., 2016; Metcalfe et al., 2018). However, some recent research is available from Europe, for example about the effects of public reporting of surgeons' outcomes in the UK (Behrendt & Groene, 2016; Vallance et al., 2018) or about

Table 13.3 *Publicly reported indicators on physician practices (2019)*

Country	Website	GPs	Specialists	Indicators Structure	Process	Outcome	Patient experience/ satisfaction	Composite indices	Open comments
Austria	docfinder.at[e]	✓	✓	✓			✓		✓
Denmark	sundhed.dk	✓	✓	✓					
Estonia	Quality Bonus Scheme (QBS)[d]	✓						✓	
Germany	AOK Gesundheitsnavigator[b]	✓	✓	✓			✓		
	weisse-liste.de	✓	✓	✓			✓	✓	
	jameda.de[c]	✓	✓	✓			✓	✓	✓
Netherlands	independer.nl	✓		✓			✓	✓	✓
	zorgkaartnederland.nl	✓	✓				✓	✓	✓
Norway	helsenorge.no	✓	✓	✓			(✓)[e]	✓	✓
Sweden	munin.vgregion.se[f]	✓		✓		✓	✓	✓	
UK	nhs.uk	✓		✓	✓	✓	✓	✓	✓
	cqc.org.uk	✓		✓	✓	✓	✓	✓	✓
	Quality and Outcomes Framework (QOF)[g]			✓	✓	✓		✓	

Note: a: negative commments are deleted; b: "AOK Health Navigator", one example of a sickness fund-led initiative based on results of weisse-liste.de; c: one example of an array of physician rating sites in Germany, *see* Emmert & Meszmer (2018) for more information; d: website: haigekassa.ee; e: planned; f: only in the region Vastra Götaland: the Quality Follow Up Programme for Primary Care (QFP); g: relaxed in Wales, dropped in Scotland, running in England and Northern Ireland, website: qof.digital.nhs.uk.

Source: authors' compilation

the effects of public reporting of hospital quality indicators in Germany (Kraska, Krummenauer & Geraedts, 2016).

In a recent Cochrane review including 12 studies from Canada, China, the Netherlands, South Korea and the US, the public release of performance data was shown to result in slightly improved processes. As to patient outcomes, the evidence on effectiveness was mixed with two studies reporting improvements and three studies reporting no differences (Metcalfe et al., 2018).

Another relatively recent review and meta-analysis of the effects of public reporting on clinical outcomes by Campanella et al. (2016) identified 27 studies that met the inclusion criteria. Almost all the studies (23) were from the United States, and only one study was from Europe (Italy). In general, studies were found to be of relatively low quality as almost all of them were observational studies. However, 14 of the studies included in the review reported positive results, and a further nine studies reported non-significant results. Three studies reported mixed results, where some indicators showed positive effects, while others indicated no or negative effects. One study indicated a negative effect of public reporting on clinical outcomes.

In addition, Campanella et al. (2016) performed a meta-analysis of data reported by 10 studies. In general, the meta-analysis found that public reporting was associated with lower mortality (risk ratio of 0.86, CI 0.80 to 0.92). However, the six studies without a control group reported (on average) slightly better results than the four studies, where mortality rates were compared between facilities with and without public reporting during the same period of time. Another subgroup analysis found that studies focusing on cardiovascular mortality found (on average) a slightly larger effect than studies assessing effects on mortality from a wider range of conditions. These findings confirm those of an earlier review by the Agency for Healthcare Research and Quality (AHRQ; Totten et al., 2012) that public reporting is associated with a small reduction in mortality.

Also a recent study on the effects of public reporting of surgeons' outcomes on mortality in colorectal cancer surgery in England found that the introduction of public reporting coincided with a significant reduction of mortality over and above the existing downward trend in mortality (Vallance et al., 2018). Similarly, the above-mentioned study by Kraska, Krummenauer & Geraedts (2016) found that publicly reported quality indicators of German hospitals improved more strongly than quality indicators that were not publicly reported. Another study suggested that the links between public reporting and quality improvement extend beyond improvements in the assessed measures (Giordano et al., 2010).

Numerous studies have found that public reporting leads to changes at provider or individual level, which will improve the quality of care (Totten et al., 2012;

Fung et al., 2008; Marshall et al., 2000; Hibbard, Stockard & Tusler, 2003; Werner & Bradlow, 2010). Totten et al. (2012) also found relatively robust evidence that the likeliness of quality improvement was greater for providers with low baseline performance.

Other reviews have focused on the unintended effects of public reporting. One relatively recent review investigated potential negative effects of public reporting of individual surgeons' outcomes, including 25 studies (22 from the US and three from the UK) (Behrendt & Groene, 2016). It found some evidence from the US that public reporting may lead to patient selection, although similar effects were not observed in the UK, where hospital care is provided mostly by public hospitals. However, another (narrative) review of negative effects resulting from performance measurement in the NHS identified several dysfunctional consequences, including measurement fixation, tunnel vision, gaming or increased inequality through patient selection (Mannion & Braithwaite, 2012). Also, the above-mentioned review by the AHRQ (Totten et al., 2012) found evidence of some unintended effects, such as changed coding and readmission practices.

Concerning the effect of public reporting on patients' choice of providers, the so-called selection pathway, there is relatively robust evidence that patients have – so far – not made much use of publicly reported quality information (Faber et al., 2009; de Cruppé & Geraedts, 2017). Patient surveys conducted in several European countries indicate that only 3% to 4% had looked at quality information before undergoing treatment (Kumpunen, Trigg & Rodrigues, 2014). One reason might be that they are not aware of publicly reported quality information (Hermeling & Geraedts, 2013; Patel et al., 2018).

Even if users are aware of publicly reported quality information, there is little evidence that they use this information to avoid low performers (Marshall et al., 2000; Fung et al., 2008; Victoor et al., 2012). Several studies have found that the sheer quantity of publicly released information on healthcare providers in terms of initiatives and the indicators can be overwhelming and confusing for users – especially when presented information is inconsistent (Boyce et al., 2010; Leonardi, McGory & Ko, 2007; Rothberg et al., 2008). As a consequence, the patient may seek information from other important sources of reference when it comes to provider choice, such as the referring physicians or family and friends (Victoor et al., 2012). In theory, physicians could use publicly reported information to counsel patients when choosing a provider. However, a recent study from Germany found that publicly reported quality information does not help physicians in counselling their patients (Geraedts et al., 2018).

There is moderate evidence that public reporting does not lead to increasing market shares for high-performing providers (Totten et al., 2012), implying that the selection pathway is not particularly relevant. These findings have been confirmed by the recent Cochrane Review (Metcalfe et al., 2018), where the authors concluded that the public disclosure of performance data may make little or no difference to healthcare utilization by consumers, except for certain subgroups of the population. In particular, it was shown that data may have a greater effect on provider choice among advantaged populations (Metcalfe et al., 2018). These results indicate that populations with lower socioeconomic status – just like older adults – may be disadvantaged because they are less likely to search for health information on the internet (Cacace et al., 2011; Kumpunen, Trigg & Rodrigues, 2014). This is of concern given that these groups generally tend to be in poorer health and therefore also in greater need of healthcare and of quality information.

Evidence on costs and cost-effectiveness of public reporting is missing. In fact, to our knowledge, even conceptual approaches to measuring costs and benefits of public reporting systematically are missing so far.

13.5 Organizational and institutional requirements for implementation

Considering the above-mentioned European examples of public reporting initiatives on the one hand and published evidence of the effects of public reporting on the other, there is obviously no easy answer to the question of which implementation strategy is most successful and which organizational and institutional requirements are essential for public reporting to have a positive impact on the quality of care.

Implementation strategies have to be adjusted to the respective circumstances, which include the configuration of the national health system and the aims of public reporting. If the principal aim is to enable informed decisions by users, the public reporting system will be different from a system that is primarily intended to motivate providers of care to change behaviour. Depending on the aim, the choice of the principal audience and indicators to be reported, data sources and media to be used will differ. Accordingly, the first step to successful implementation of a public reporting system is to clarify the aims of the system (Cacace et al., 2011).

When thinking about more specific organizational and institutional requirements for implementation, it is useful to consider the implications of a theoretical consumer choice model developed by Faber et al. (2009). Fig. 13.2 illustrates the different stages that, according to the model, are involved when consumers use quality of care information to select a healthcare provider. The figure shows that the intended audience must (1) be aware of the reports, (2) be able to interpret the information correctly and (3) trust the information before (4) switching or selecting a provider. The figure also shows that users in practice rarely meet the expectations of the theoretical model.

Fig. 13.2 *The consumer choice model*

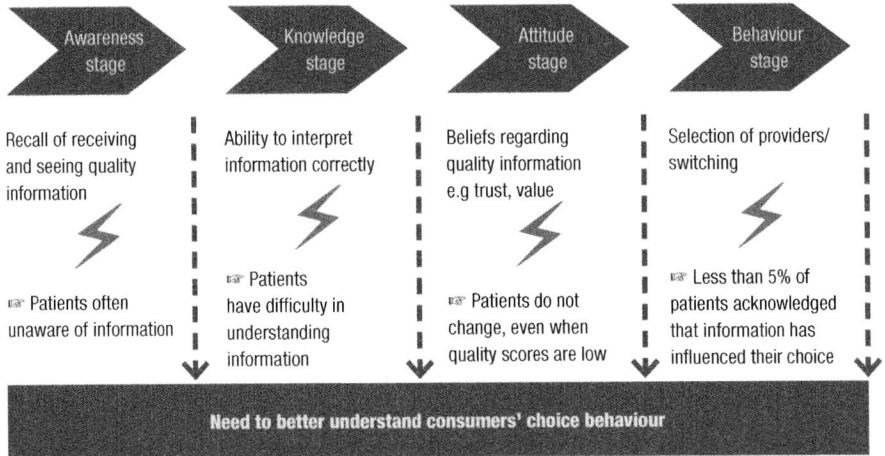

Source: based on Faber et al., 2009

Concerning the first point, i.e. to improve awareness, it is necessary to provide broad and easy access to public quality reports. Beyond accessibility, the information needs to be of interest and relevance to the user. In this context it may be worthwhile noting that most of the quality information publicly available in European countries is accessible exclusively through the internet. While interactive graphical interfaces provide unique opportunities to display complex data sets, inequitable access to the worldwide web is still a concern. While the percentage of households with internet access has increased in Europe over the last few years, there are still countries with less than 80% household coverage, for example, Bulgaria, Greece and Lithuania (Eurostat, 2019). In particular, people with lower levels of education and the elderly are less likely to search for information online, although the latter are catching up (Gilmour, 2007). According to Kurtzman & Greene (2016), effective presentation of performance information requires a reduction of complexity, for example by using non-technical language or symbols (such as traffic lights) as information processing capacity is limited. Another relevant aspect is that information needs are different among user groups, and might be different from those expected by the designers of public reporting.

Concerning the second point – to achieve knowledge of the public reports – sponsors have to give weight to the core attribute of public reporting, i.e. the general comprehensibility of the presented data. On the one hand, presented data should be easily interpretable, which is facilitated by displaying independent benchmarks and averages, as well as through the use of composite indicators and explanatory text (*see also* Chapter 3 concerning the advantages and disadvantages of composite indicators). On the other hand, many users desire more detailed information in order to better understand what lies behind the data. This is particularly true if the public reporting information aims to motivate providers to improve their practice. Therefore, it is useful to present data at different levels of aggregation and to allow users to expand the data and to see individual indicators. However, with a greater level of detail, explanatory notes become even more important because more specific (clinical) indicators are often more difficult to interpret for patients but they may also be more easily related to their particular health problem.

Concerning the third point – to enable a positive attitude towards the presented data – it is important that data are of high quality. In particular, they should be reliable, sensitive to change, consistent, valid and resistant to manipulation. In general, reporting strategies benefit from methods that safeguard the timeliness and completeness of data, for example through mandatory reporting or by using financial incentives (pay for reporting/pay for transparency). Furthermore, to generate trust, public reporting needs to provide information on whether and how outcome indicators are risk-adjusted and how composite indices are derived. In addition, sponsors must be aware of the fact that depending on the system, consumers will have more or less trust in different authors of public reports. German consumers, for example, express confidence in consumer protection organizations as authors of public reports whereas scientific societies, government agencies or other interest groups are less acknowledged (Geraedts, 2006). Other stakeholders, such as patient associations, self-help groups, the media, academic departments and GPs, could serve as information intermediaries who will help to interpret the information and test applicability to the patient's individual needs and preferences (Shaller, Kanouse & Schlesinger, 2014).

Finally, in order to be successful, implementation strategies will always have to consider that patient/user involvement is essential for public reporting initiatives that primarily aim to enable informed choice of providers. Ideally, reporting schemes are regularly re-evaluated and improved based on patient/user and patterns of information use (Pross et al., 2017). Also provider involvement is a prerequisite for public reporting to be successful in changing peer behaviour. To raise acceptance among providers, the achievements reported should be fully under the control of those being assessed, i.e. the issues reported addressable by providers' action (Campbell & Lester, 2010). Of course, this also recurs to the (necessarily) flawed risk-adjustment of outcome indicators, such as morbidity and mortality, which may potentially lead to unintended consequences, in particular for high-risk patients. As risk-adjustment is likely to be imperfect, some authors suggest abandoning the use of standardized mortality ratios completely from public reporting initiatives and using clinical audit data instead (Goodacre, Campbell & Carter, 2015; Lilford & Pronovost, 2010).

More generally, the implementation strategy has to be aligned with national traditions. In most European countries quality information systems have developed through a combination of bottom-up initiatives and top-down regulation (Cacace et al., 2011). It depends on the health system which of the two ways will be more successful in a specific country.

13.6 Conclusions for policy-makers

Many countries have made considerable investments in the design and implementation of public reporting systems. Our review of public reporting systems in European countries has found some differences across countries with regard to the number of initiatives and the degree of government involvement in the sponsorship and regulation of public reporting. There is a mix of public and private sponsors of public reporting initiatives. Public initiatives are dominant in the area of hospital care, while several private initiatives exist in the area of physician practices. This is related to the fact that regulation and oversight of public reporting through governments and other public actors is more pronounced in the area of hospital care than in the area of ambulatory care.

The scope of reporting systems ranges from single indicators, such as waiting times, to detailed information about structures, processes and outcomes of care. In general, public reporting is more detailed in the hospital sector, where structure, process and outcome indicators as well as patient experience/satisfaction are frequently reported. In comparison, public disclosure of quality information on physician practices is rather incomplete in most European countries. One possible explanation for this is that the state is directly involved in the provision of hospital services in all countries, while physician practices are mainly private. In addition, measuring the quality of care in physician practices raises additional practical difficulties, in particular when it comes to outcome indicators.

One of the most important challenges for public reporting initiatives is to achieve a high degree of coverage with regards to both the proportion of participating providers and the proportion of care covered by relevant indicators. Our review shows that strong government involvement in regulating public reporting is key to achieving high coverage of providers and high quality of data.

Many studies in Europe and overseas have investigated the effect of public reporting on effectiveness, safety and patient-centredness of care. The available evidence suggests that public reporting does reduce mortality and improve quality as measured through process indicators. However, available studies are often of relatively low quality.

Box 13.1 summarizes the implications of the chapter for policy-makers. First and foremost, an overarching strategy for public reporting is needed, which should include a clear definition of its goals and its target group(s). The strategy should also indicate the regulation and sponsorship of public reporting, for example if it is linked to external assessment (*see* Chapter 8) or financial incentives (*see* Chapter 14), and the role of governmental and private organizations should be defined. One critical question for policy-makers should be whether the expected benefits outweigh the administrative and financial costs of high-quality reporting initiatives. Clearly, a difficulty here is that approaches are missing so far to assess the cost-effectiveness of public reporting.

When implementing public reporting, it is important to systematically involve all relevant stakeholders, i.e. patients/patient organizations and providers and staff at all levels of the healthcare system (2). As described in Chapter 3, different stakeholders have different information needs. The designers of public reporting systems need to acknowledge, that "the typical user" is difficult to identify or does not even exist. As diverse as users are, so are their information requirements. Victoor et al. (2012) showed that the information needs of patients differ across primary and secondary care and that they vary by type of disease or treatment, by age group and by educational and socioeconomic background. Individual

---

Box 13.1 *Policy implications for successful public reporting*

(1) Clarify the aims as well as target groups and develop an overarching strategy.

(2) Systematically involve all relevant stakeholders.

(3) Display information on quality dimensions that are relevant for users.

(4) Design indicators that match the interest and skill levels of users.

(5) Improve presentation methods, in particular by reducing complexity.

(6) Present data at different levels of aggregation and allow users to expand the data to see individual indicators.

(7) Design decision aids and encourage their use.

(8) Educate patients and users about quality in healthcare and increase patient and user awareness of public reporting.

(9) Enlist professionals in supporting public reporting systems.

(10) Secure equitable access to quality information across the population.

(11) Take a long-term perspective and keep the system under constant review.

Sources: Cacace et al., 2011; Kumpunen, Trigg & Rodrigues, 2014

patients may consider a range of factors and may have different preferences as to their trade-offs. In line with the implications (3) to (5) in Box 13.1, we underline the importance of taking these aspects into account when developing a public-reporting system.

Continuous efforts are required to improve public reporting and to adapt it to the users' needs. These efforts should be made as we can take for granted that users want more information about the performance of their healthcare providers. Public reporting is widely accepted as a means to improve transparency and to involve the patient in decision-making. Although a considerable body of work intended exploring the benefits of public reporting, much less is known about the actual mechanisms behind these effects. One of the puzzles that remain is why utilization is low. Notoriously, patients are interested in receiving more information. More and more users are interested in sharing their experience with healthcare, as the growing quantity of provider ratings shows.

Quality information should be tailored to the information needs of the intended users. This concerns both the content of public reporting (i.e. the selection of indicators) and the methods of presentation, which should reduce complexity without losing important information. This can be achieved by displaying information using composite indicators, which can be expanded by users if they are interested to see the constituting indicators. It is also possible to sort information in such a way that users are pointed to the most important information (Kumpunen, Trigg & Rodrigues, 2014), although this is complicated by the fact that individual users have different preferences. An innovative approach could be to offer a range of both clinical and non-clinical indicators, and to let the users develop their own priorities and give them the opportunity of weighting results accordingly.

The provision of structured decision aids, such as evidence-based information and other tools that help patients to clarify their preferences, could support patients and users to make informed choices. Independently of the aspects mentioned above, education of patients and users about quality in healthcare and an increased awareness of public reporting are important. In addition, engaging professionals in supporting and using public reporting is essential to meet their own information needs and to support patients in better understanding information.

Furthermore, policy-makers should reflect how access to such reporting systems can be improved. The internet has turned out to be a smart way to present such comparative information on providers. However, the problem remains that access is not secured, in particular to the most vulnerable or less literate groups of the population. If policy-makers indeed favour equitable access to quality information across the population, more research is needed about how different target audiences can be reached. Should public reporting indeed enable better informed groups to receive higher-quality care, then everybody must have a fair chance to belong to that group.

Finally, "trial and error" experiences will be part of the process of developing public reporting systems, and international exchange may be a useful source for policy learning. As pointed out in Box 13.1, policy-makers should take a longer-term perspective and keep a public reporting system under constant review. Continuous efforts are required to find out what information users want and how information can be presented in an easily interpretable way.

References

Ashworth M, Gulliford M (2016). Funding for general practice in the next decade: life after QOF. *British Journal of General Practice*, 67(654): 4–5.

Behrendt K, Groene O (2016). Mechanisms and effects of public reporting of surgeon outcomes: a systematic review of the literature. *Health Policy*, 120(10):1151–61.

Berwick DM, James B, Coye MJ (2003). Connections between quality measurement and improvement. Health care consumers and quality in England and Germany. *Medical Care Research and Review*, 41(1): i30–i38.

Boyce T et al. (2010). Choosing a high-quality hospital: the role of nudges, scorecard design and information. London: The King's Fund.

Cacace M et al. (2011). How health systems make available information on service providers: Experience in seven countries. RAND Europe and London School of Hygiene & Tropical Medicine. Available at: http://www.rand.org/pubs/technical_reports/TR887.html, accessed 11 February 2019.

Campanella P et al. (2016). The impact of Public Reporting on clinical outcomes: a systematic review and meta-analysis. *BMC Health Services Research*, 16:296.

Campbell S, Lester H (2010). Developing indicators and the concept of QOFability. In: Gillam SA, Siriwardena N (eds.). The Quality and Outcomes Framework: QOF – transforming general practice. Abingdon: Ratcliffe Publishing, 16–27.

de Cruppé W, Geraedts M (2017). Hospital choice in Germany from the patient's perspective: a cross-sectional study. *BMC Health Services Research*, 17:720.

Dixon A, Robertson R, Bal R (2010). The experience of implementing choice at point of referral: a comparison of the Netherlands and England. *Health Economics, Policy and Law*, 5:295–317.

Donabedian A (1988). The quality of care: How can it be assessed? *Journal of the American Medical Association*, 260:1743–8.

Emmert M, Meszmer N (2018). Eine Dekade Arztbewertungsportale in Deutschland: Eine Zwischenbilanz zum aktuellen Entwicklungsstand. *Das Gesundheitswesen*, 80(10):851–8. doi: 10.1055/s-0043-114002.

Emmert M et al. (2016). Internetportale für die Krankenhauswahl in Deutschland: Eine leistungsbereichsspezifische Betrachtung. *Das Gesundheitswesen*, 78(11):721–34.

Eurostat (2019). Broadband and connectivity. Available at: http://appsso.eurostat.ec.europa.eu/nui/show.do?dataset=isoc_bde15b_h&lang=en, accessed 9 February 2019.

Faber M et al. (2009). Public reporting in health care: how do consumers use quality-of-care information? A systematic review. *Medical Care*, 47(1):1–8.

Fung CH et al. (2008). Systematic review: the evidence that publishing patient care performance data improves quality of care. *Annals of Internal Medicine*, 148(2):111–23.

Geraedts M (2006). Gesundheitsversorgung und Gestaltungsoptionen aus der Perspektive von Bevölkerung und Ärzten. In: Böcken J et al. (eds.). Gesundheitsmonitor 2006. Gütersloh: Bertelsmann, 154–70.

Geraedts M et al. (2018). Public reporting of hospital quality data: What do referring physicians want to know? *Health Policy*, 122:1177–82. doi: 10.1016/j.healthpol.2018.09.010

Gilmour JA (2007). Reducing disparities in the access and use of Internet health information. A discussion paper. *International Journal of Nursing Studies*, 44(7):1270–8.

Giordano L et al. (2010). Development, implementation, and public reporting of the HCAHPS survey. *Medical Care Research and Review*, 67(1):27–37.

Goodacre S, Campbell M, Carter A (2015). What do hospital mortality rates tell us about quality of care? *Emergency Medicine Journal*, 32:244–7.

Haggerty JL (2010). Are measures of patient satisfaction hopelessly flawed? *BMJ*, 341:c4783.

Hamblin R (2008). Regulation, measurements and incentives. The experience in the US and UK: does context matter? *Journal of the Royal Society for the Promotion of Health*, 128(6):291–8.

Hermeling P, Geraedts M (2013). Kennen und nutzen Ärzte den strukturierten Qualitätsbericht? *Das Gesundheitswesen*, 75:155–9. doi: 10.1055/s-0032-1321744.

Hibbard JH, Stockard J, Tusler M (2003). Does Publicizing Hospital Performance Stimulate Quality Improvement Efforts? *Health Affairs*, 22(2):84–94.

Hirschman AO (1970). Exit, voice, and loyalty. Responses to decline in firms, organizations, and states. Cambridge, Mass.: Harvard University Press.

Kraska RA, Krummenauer F, Geraedts M (2016). Impact of public reporting on the quality of hospital care in Germany: a controlled before-after analysis based on secondary data. *Health Policy*, 120(7):770–9.

Kumpunen S, Trigg L, Rodrigues R (2014). Public reporting in health and long-term care to facilitate provider choice. Policy Summary 13. Copenhagen: WHO Regional Office for Europe and European Observatory on Health Systems and Policies.

Kurtzman ET, Greene J (2016). Effective presentation of health care performance information for consumer decision making: a systematic review. *Patient Education and Counseling*, 99:36–43.

Leonardi MJ, McGory ML, Ko CY (2007). Publicly available hospital comparison websites: determination of useful, valid, and appropriate information for comparing surgical quality. *Archives of Surgery*, 142(9):863–8.

Lilford R, Pronovost P (2010). Using hospital mortality rates to judge hospital performance: a bad idea that just won't go away. *BMJ*, 340:c2016.

Mannion R, Braithwaite J (2012). Unintended consequences of performance measurement in healthcare: 20 salutary lessons from the English National Health Service. *Internal Medicine Journal*, 42(5):569–74. doi: 10.1111/j.1445-5994.2012.02766.x.

Marshall MN, Romano PS, Davies HTO (2004). How do we maximize the impact of the public reporting of quality of care? *International Journal for Quality in Health Care*, 16(suppl1):i57–i63.

Marshall MN et al. (2000). The public release of performance data: What do we expect to gain? A review of the evidence. *Journal of the American Medical Association*, 283(14):1866–74.

Metcalfe D et al. (2018). Impact of public release of performance data on the behaviour of healthcare consumers and providers. *Cochrane Database of Systematic Reviews* 9:CD004538. doi: 10.1002/14651858.CD004538.pub3.

NHS Digital (2019). Quality and Outcomes Framework. Search for practice results: http://qof.digital.nhs.uk/search/index.asp, accessed 8 February 2019.

OECD (2018). Reviews of Health Systems. Lithuania. Available at: https://www.oecd.org/health/health-systems/OECD-Reviews-of-Health-Systems-Lithuania-2018-Assessment-and-Recommendations.pdf, accessed 7 February 2019.

OECD (2019). Health System Characteristics Survey. 2016 wave. Available at: https://qdd.oecd.org/subject.aspx?Subject=hsc, accessed 25 February 2019.

Patel S et al. (2018). Public Awareness, Usage, and Predictors for the Use of Doctor Rating Websites: Cross-Sectional Study in England. *Journal of Medical Internet Research*, 20(7):e243. doi:10.2196/jmir.9523.

PNE (Programma Nazionale Esiti) (2019). Website. Available at: http://95.110.213.190/PNEedizione16_p/spe/spe_prog_reg.php?spe, accessed 10 February 2019.

Pross C et al. (2017). Health care public reporting utilization – user clusters, web trails, and usage barriers on Germany's public reporting portal Weisse-Liste.de. *BMC Medical Informatics and Decision Making*, 17(1):48.

Rodrigues R et al. (2014). The public gets what the public wants: experiences of public reporting in long-term care in Europe. *Health Policy*, 116(1):84–94.

Rothberg MB et al. (2008). Choosing the best hospital: the limitations of public quality reporting. *Health Affairs*, 27(6):1680–7.

Schlesinger M (2010). Choice cuts: parsing policymakers' pursuit of patient empowerment from an individual perspective. *Health Economics, Policy and Law*, 5:365–87.

Shaller D, Kanouse DE, Schlesinger M (2014). Context-based Strategies for Engaging Consumers with Public Reports about Health Care Providers. *Medical Care Research and Review*, 71(5 Suppl):17S–37S.

Shekelle PG (2009). Public performance reporting on quality information. In: Smith PC et al. (eds). Performance measurement for health system improvement. Cambridge: Cambridge University Press, 537–51.

Totten A et al. (2012) Closing the quality gap series: public reporting as a quality improvement strategy (No. 208). Evidence Report. Agency for Healthcare Research and Quality (AHRQ). Available at: https://effectivehealthcare.ahrq.gov/sites/default/files/pdf/public-reporting-quality-improvement_research.pdf, accessed 5 December 2018.

Vallance AE et al. (2018). Effect of public reporting of surgeons' outcomes on patient selection, "gaming," and mortality in colorectal cancer surgery in England: population-based cohort study. *BMJ*, 361:k1581.

Van den Hurk J, Buil C, Bex P (2015). Tussentijdse evaluatie Kwaliteitsinstituut. De ontwikkeling van regeldruk van transparantie door de komst van het Kwaliteitsinstituut. Available at: https://www.siracompanies.com/wp-content/uploads/tussentijdse-evaluatie-kwaliteitsinstituut.pdf, accessed 8 February 2019.

Victoor A et al. (2012). Determinants of patient choice of healthcare providers: a scoping review. *BMC Health Services Research*, 12:272.

Werner RM, Asch DA (2005). The unintended consequences of publicly reporting quality information. *Journal of the American Medical Association*, 239(10):1239–44.

Werner RM, Bradlow ET (2010). Public reporting on hospital process improvements is linked to better patient outcomes. *Health Affairs*, 29(7):1319–24.

Zorginstituut (2019). Transparantiekalender. Available at: https://www.zorginzicht.nl/bibliotheek/Paginas/transparantiekalender.aspx?p=1563, accessed 08 February 2019.

Chapter 14

Pay for Quality: using financial incentives to improve quality of care

Helene Eckhardt, Peter Smith, Wilm Quentin

Summary

What are the characteristics of the strategy?

The main attribute of Pay for Quality (P4Q) is that a financial incentive is paid to a provider or professional for achieving a quality-related target within a specific time-frame. P4Q can be implemented in various healthcare settings, targeting a range of healthcare providers or professionals. P4Q schemes can reward high quality measured in terms of structures, processes and/or outcomes, and/or penalize low quality. P4Q schemes can be implemented in line with other quality improvement interventions.

What is being done in European countries?

The implementation of P4Q schemes began in the late 1990s. A total of 14 primary care P4Q programmes and 13 hospital P4Q programmes were identified in a total of 16 European countries. P4Q schemes in primary care incentivize mostly process and structural quality with respect to prevention and chronic care. P4Q schemes in hospital care incentivize more often improvements in health outcomes and patient safety. The size of financial incentives varies between 0.1% and 30% of total provider income in primary care (individual physicians or primary care practices) and between 0.5% and 10% of total provider income in hospital care.

What do we know about the effectiveness and cost-effectiveness of the strategy?

Overall, the effectiveness and cost-effectiveness of P4Q schemes remains unclear. The most reliable studies of P4Q in primary care suggest small positive effects on process-of-care (POC) indicators, while in-hospital care schemes appear to be ineffective with respect to POC measures. For both settings the evidence on effectiveness with respect to improving health outcomes and patient safety indicators is inconclusive. Patient experience and patient satisfaction were rarely evaluated and if they were, they usually did not improve. In fact, in some primary care programmes chronically ill patients experienced worsened continuity of care. Furthermore, a few studies suggest that P4Q schemes are less effective than other quality improvement initiatives, such as public reporting or audit and feedback.

How can the strategy be implemented?

P4Q schemes are more effective when the focus of a scheme is on areas of quality where change is needed and if the scheme embraces a more comprehensive approach, covering many different areas of care. Quality measures should be developed in collaboration with relevant healthcare professionals and reinforce professional norms and beliefs. Payment mechanisms have to be codified very clearly, with statements of entitlements, conditions, time horizons and criteria for receipt of funds.

Conclusions for policy-makers

While reliable evidence on the effectiveness of P4Q programmes is scarce, there is a broad consensus that such programmes are technically and politically difficult to implement. All relevant stakeholders should be involved in the process of scheme development. The contents and structure of the scheme have to be kept under review and regularly updated, and adverse behavioural responses need to be monitored. More evidence is needed on the comparative effectiveness of P4Q schemes in comparison to other quality improvement initiatives.

14.1 Introduction: the characteristics of pay for quality

Pay for quality (P4Q) initiatives are increasingly used in healthcare systems in Europe and beyond. Interest in P4Q by researchers and policy-makers has seen an incredible growth since the late 1990s, when the first programmes started to emerge in Europe and the USA (Cashin, 2014). However, despite the growth in P4Q programmes, P4Q remains highly controversial for a wide range of conceptual, practical and ethical reasons (Roland & Dudley, 2015; Wharam et al., 2009). In fact, there is no universally accepted definition of P4Q, and the term is often used interchangeably with "pay for performance" (P4P). Yet the term P4Q is more precise, as it makes clear that payment depends on the quality of care – and not on other dimensions of health system performance (*see also* Chapter 1).

The two characteristic features of P4Q programmes are that (1) performance of providers is monitored in relation to pre-specified quality indicators and (2) a monetary transfer is made conditional on the (achievement or improvement of) measured quality of care. In theory, as discussed in Chapter 3, quality can be measured by use of structure, process or outcome indicators of quality – and this is true also for P4Q programmes. In addition, P4Q programmes can, in theory, aim at assuring or improving quality in different areas of care (preventive, acute, chronic or long-term care), and target different types of professional (for example, physicians, nurses or social workers) and providers (for example, primary care practices, hospital departments or hospitals). Furthermore, quality may be incentivized with the aim of assuring or improving quality in terms of effectiveness, safety and/or responsiveness. Nevertheless, despite the potentially very large variation of different characteristics of P4Q programmes, this chapter shows that most existing programmes target a more narrow set of providers (namely primary care providers and hospitals), and that certain characteristics are much more common in P4Q programmes in primary care than in P4Q programmes in hospital care.

P4Q can be implemented together with other quality improvement strategies, such as audit and feedback (*see* Chapter 10) and public reporting (*see* Chapter 13). In fact, by design, a P4Q programme includes elements of audit and reporting, since the performance has to be monitored and performance data have to be transmitted to the programme administrators.

The chapter follows the standard structure of chapters in Part 2 of this book. The next section explains why P4Q is expected to contribute to healthcare quality. The following section provides an overview of a selection of existing national and regional P4Q programmes in Europe based on a rapid review (*see* Box 14.1 for a summary of the methods). The next section summarizes the available evidence on the effectiveness and cost-effectiveness of existing P4Q programmes in Europe and other high-income countries based on a review of reviews, followed by a discussion of the organizational and institutional requirements for the implementation of P4Q programmes, before we draw together the conclusions of the chapter for policy-makers.

Box 14.1 *Review methods used to inform the content of this chapter*

In order to identify existing P4Q schemes in Europe, we searched the European Observatory on Health Systems and Policies' Health Systems in Transition (HiT) reviews of all 28 EU countries. In addition, we extracted information from the OECD Health Systems Characteristics Survey database and searched the OECDiLibrary. The list of identified initiatives was complemented by initiatives identified during a systematic review of reviews (next paragraph). Information on the characteristics of the identified P4Q initiatives was drawn from HiT reviews, OECD reports, studies identified during the systematic review of reviews and websites of relevant national institutions.

In order to assess the effectiveness and cost-effectiveness of P4Q programmes, we performed a systematic review of reviews between August 2016 and May 2017. A broad search strategy was used to identify all potentially relevant publications in several electronic databases (including amongst others Pubmed, the Cochrane library and Business Source Complete). The review protocol "Effectiveness and cost-effectiveness of pay for quality initiatives in high-income countries: a systematic review of reviews" has been published in PROSPERO (Eckhardt et al., 2016). We included 31 reviews published between 1999 and 2016 in our final analysis.

14.2 Why should pay for quality contribute to healthcare quality?

The incentives of provider payment systems are known to have a profound impact on the volume and quality of care (Busse & Blümel, 2015; Conrad & Christianson, 2004; Dudley et al., 1998). However, under traditional payment mechanisms, the incentives for the provision of high or better quality of care are indirect and often incidental. For example, fee-for-service payment creates incentives for high levels of provision, and thus might indirectly lead to higher levels of quality. However, fee-for-service may also lead to overprovision of unnecessary, inappropriate and potentially unsafe services, and potentially may pose a barrier to quality improvement if this leads to lower numbers of services being delivered. In contrast, capitation payments eliminate incentives for overprovision and facilitate expenditure control. However, they do not create incentives for quality – and may even be a barrier for quality improvement – because providers have incentives to skimp on necessary services in order to achieve lower costs. Similar problems arise with two common payment methods in the hospital sector – global budgets and Diagnosis Related Group (DRG)-based case payments (Busse & Blümel, 2015) – as neither provides incentives for quality and instead may even pose barriers to quality improvement.

In this context, the idea of P4Q programmes is to change the incentives for providers (professionals and organizations) and to explicitly reward the provision of high or better quality of care – or to penalize poor quality. The assumption is that providers (professionals and/or organizations) will improve the quality of care – through whatever mechanism – if they have a direct financial interest to do so. However, this assumption is highly controversial (Kronick, Casalino & Bindman, 2015). Proponents of P4Q (and P4P more generally) believe that quality improvement strategies relying exclusively on intrinsic motivation of providers (for example, audit and feedback; *see* Chapter 10) or on non-financial incentives (for example public reporting; *see* Chapter 13) are insufficient to motivate quality improvements (Rosenthal et al., 2004). Opponents believe that financial incentives could crowd out the intrinsic motivation of physicians to provide high-quality care and could potentially have adverse consequences, such as an exclusive focus on incentivized quality measures while disregarding other potentially important areas of quality (Kronick, Casalino & Bindman, 2015).

The theory underlying many P4Q programmes can be traced to the economic principal/agent literature (Christianson, Knutson & Mazze, 2006; Conrad, 2015; Robinson, 2001). According to the theory, a principal (usually a strategic purchaser) wishes to structure the contractual relationship with the agent (either an individual practitioner or an organization) to secure high-quality health services. It is assumed that increasing quality requires "effort" on the part of the agent, who must therefore be compensated with a financial reward if improvements are to be secured. The agent will then assess how much effort to exert by comparing the expected financial benefits to the effort required. In the simplest form of this model, the principal then sets the financial rewards for the agent knowing how the agent will respond to the incentives, in terms of exerting increased effort, and thereby delivering improved quality. In setting the incentive regime, the principal must of course balance the expected costs of the rewards against the expected improvements in quality.

As set out by Cashin (2014) there are several elements in this model that require more detailed scrutiny. First, measurement plays a key role. Effort cannot usually be observed and measured, so instead there must be some way of explicitly measuring the quality attained. Quality indicators therefore play a key role in any P4Q programme. Ideally these should be accurate and timely indicators of the desired quality criterion, sensitive to variations in provider effort, and resistant to manipulation or fraud. In examining the programmes described in this chapter, it is important to assess the strengths and limitations of the quality metrics being used (*see also* below).

Second, design of the financial reward mechanism requires numerous judgements, such as the magnitude of the rewards, how they increase with increased quality, whether or not the rewards are based on performance relative to other providers, whether rewards are based on individual aspects of performance or on an aggregate measure of organizational attainment, and whether they are based on absolute levels of attainment or on improvements from previous levels (Eijkenaar, 2013). These design considerations are a central concern of all P4Q programmes, and are likely to play a crucial role in their effectiveness. They are described in Box 14.2 and discussed in more detail later in this chapter.

Third, the effect of any P4Q scheme depends crucially on the intrinsic motivation of the professionals and organizations at whom the programme is directed. If the desired improvements in quality are aligned with professional objectives, and the programme serves to offer focus and encouragement to professionals and organizations seeking to secure such improvements, then it may indeed contribute to the desired outcomes. However, if the P4Q programme contradicts or undermines professional motivation, it may prove ineffective or even lead to adverse outcomes.

More generally, it is likely that contextual factors play a key role in the success or otherwise of P4Q programmes. Some aspects of health services are more amenable to P4Q than others, for example those for which reliable performance metrics can be developed. Furthermore, professionals and provider organizations may require a long-term commitment from payers to the P4Q before they are prepared to commit resources to quality improvement efforts. Finally, a persistent theme found throughout the P4Q literature (for example, Damberg et al., 2014; Kane et al., 2004; Kondo et al., 2016; Milstein & Schreyoegg, 2016; Scott et al., 2011) is that effective governance arrangements are an essential prerequisite for the success of any scheme. These have to ensure that information is reliable, that providers are not "cherry-picking" patients who are expected to secure high-quality outcomes, and that non-incentivized aspects of care remain satisfactory.

14.3 What is being done in Europe?

Our review (*see* Box 14.1) identified a total of 27 P4Q programmes that have been implemented in 16 European countries in both primary and hospital care (Tables 14.1 and 14.2). To our knowledge, the first nationwide P4Q programme introduced in Europe was the *Incitant Qualité*, implemented in Luxembourg in 1998 (FHL, 2012). We did not identify any P4Q programmes focusing on palliative care.

14.3.1 Primary care

Table 14.1 provides an overview of the most important characteristics of 14 P4Q programmes in primary care in 13 European countries (Croatia, the Czech Republic, Estonia, France, Germany, Italy, Latvia, Lithuania, Poland, the Republic of Moldova, Portugal, Sweden and the United Kingdom (UK)). The first P4Q programme in primary care was introduced in 2001 in the context of

---

Box 14.2 *Structures of financial incentives within P4Q*

Types of incentive

Bonus	is a monetary reward for achievement or improvement of performance (predominantly paid by "new money")
Penalty	is a reduction of usual payment for poor performance
Withhold	is a combination of bonuses and penalties, where an amount of usual payment is withheld and redistributed according to the performance of the participating healthcare providers (paid by "old money")

Types of measurement

Absolute measurement	When measuring performance, there is no ranking of performance of different providers or time-points in place; the reward is linked to the achievement of a pre-specified target (for example, 95% vaccination coverage of children on the list of a primary care physician)
Relative measurement	When measuring performance, ranking of performance can concern different time- points, different providers or a combination of both; based on this, the incentive can feature different structures – the reward can address the best 20% of all participants, there can be a reward for best performance improvement in place, or a penalty can apply to the worst 20% of all participants.

Source: authors' compilation based on Eijkenaar, 2013

---

disease management programmes in Germany, while the last was introduced in 2016 in Poland (*see* Table 14.1). Most P4Q programmes are implemented at the national level, but Germany, Italy and Sweden have regional P4Q programmes. About half of all programmes are mandatory, while the other half are voluntary.

All programmes have a strong focus on incentivizing quality in chronic and preventive care – with the exception of the one known programme in Italy, which only focuses on chronic care. All programmes include indicators that target improved effectiveness of care (for example, provision of certain services, compliance with guidelines, improved coordination and achievement of certain health outcomes). Only four programmes also include indicators that aim at improved responsiveness of care in terms of patient experience or patient satisfaction.

Quality indicators in most programmes focus on structures and processes of care but five countries also measure quality in terms of intermediate or final outcomes. Intermediate health outcomes, such as the achievement of a certain blood-pressure or a certain blood-glucose level in a pre-defined proportion of a

Table 14.1 *Identified P4Q programmes in primary care in eleven EU countries*

Country	Programme (nationwide/regional, voluntary/mandatory)	Start	Care area	Quality dimensions	Type and number of indicators	Area of activity	Incentive structure	Size of FI as % of total income	Type and number of provider
CZ	(NW, V)	-	PC, CC	EFFS	P, S	Disease management and provision of services; IT services	B, AM	-	IND
DE	DMP (R, V)	2001	PC, CC	EFFS	P, S	Disease management and provision of services	B, AM	-	IND, ORG
EE	PHC QBS (NW, M since 2015)	2006	PC, CC	EFFS	P, S – change annually	Disease management (esp. diabetes) and provision of (preventive) services, coordination; Appropriate prescription; Paediatric care; Pregnancy and maternity care; Surgical services	B, AM, A+I	≤5 %	IND
FR	ENMR (NW, V)	2009	PC, CC	EFFS	S	Multiprofessional cooperation; Practice organization; Educational activities; Access	B, W (since 2014)	5%, 40% (since 2014)	ORG (MPMH, MPMF, HS – 300)
FR	ROSP – CAPI until 2012 (NW, V – opt out)	2009	PC, CC	EFFS	O, P, S – 29	Disease management (esp. diabetes) and provision of services; Efficient prescribing; Practice organization	B, AM, A+I	≤11%	IND (c. 97% of all GPs)
HR	(NW, V)	2013	PC, CC	EFFS, RESP	P, S	Disease management and provision of services; Effective prescribing (polypharmacy, antibiotics); Paediatric care; Pregnancy care; Patient satisfaction	B, AM	≤30%	IND
IT	Diabetes care programme (Emilia-Romagna, M)	2003	CC	EEFS	P, S	Diabetes management	B, AM, A	0.1–6%	IND (GPs – 2 938)
LT	(NW, V)	2005	PC, CC	EFFS	O, P – 22	Disease management and provision of services; Access	B, AM	-	ORG (PCPs)
LV	(NW, M)	2013	PC, CC	EFFS	O, P, S – change annually	Disease management and provision of services; Paediatric care; Access	B, AM	≤5%	ORG (PCPs)

MD	NHIC quality indicators	2013	PC, CC	EFFS	O, P – 20	Disease management (cardiovascular diseases, diabetes, TB); Cancer screening; Pregnancy and maternity care; Paediatric care	B, AM	–	IND, ORG
PL	(NW, M)	2016	PC, CC	EFFS	P	Prevention/surveillance (correct and timely diagnosis of 15 diagnoses in cancer patients, timely initiation of treatment)	B, AM	–	IND, ORG (PCPs)
PT	Model B (NW, V)	2006	PC, CC	EFFS, RESP	O, P, S – 22	Disease management (esp. diabetes) and provision of services; Paediatric care; Pregnancy and maternity care; Patient satisfaction	B, AM, A	GPs: ≤30%, nurses: ≤10%	IND (FHU – 181)
SE	VGR – P4P (Västra Götaland, M, P4Q schemes in 20 out of the 21 regions; very first programme implemented in 2002)	2011	PC, CC	EFFS, RESP	O, P, S – 40 (other regions 1–17)	Disease management; Practice organization; Computer-based services; Patient satisfaction; Patient experience (other regions – Coordination; Paediatric care; Mental care; Rehabilitation care, etc.)	B, AM, A (certain regions – PN, RR)	≤4% (certain regions – 1–6%)	ORG (PCPs – 200)
UK (ENG)	QOF (NW, V)	2004	PC, CC	EFFS, RESP	O, P, S – 148 in 2012/13 and 77 in 2015/16	Disease management and provision of services; Practice organization; Patient experience	B, AM, A	≤15% (2013)	ORG (96–99% of all PCPs)

Abbreviations: **Countries:** CZ = Czech Republic; DE = Germany; EE = Estonia; ENG = England; FR = France; IT = Italy; LV = Larvia; LT = Lithuania; MD = Republic of Moldova; PL = Poland; PT = Portugal; SE = Sweden; UK = United Kingdom

Programmes: CAPI = Contracts for Improved Individual Practice; DMP = Disease Management Programmes; ENMR = Expérimentations de nouveaux modes de rémunération (Experimentation of new modes of remuneration); NHIC = National Health Insurance Company; QBS = PHC Quality Bonus System; QOF = Quality and Outcomes Framework; ROSP = Rémunération sur objectifs de santé publique (Payment for Public Health Objectives); VGR = Västra Götaland Region

Diffusion/participation: NW = nationwide; R = regional; M = mandatory; V= voluntary **Quality dimension:** EFFS = effectiveness; EFFY = efficiency; RESP = responsiveness

Care area: CC = chronic care; PC = preventive care **Type of Outcome:** O = outcomes; P = processes; S = structures

Incentive structure: A = achievement; AM = absolute measure; B = bonus; I = improvement; PN = penalty; RR = relative ranking

Type and number of provider: GP = general practitioner; IND = individual providers; ORG = organizations (for example, practices, primary clinics, etc.); MPMH = "maisons de santé" (multiprofessional medical home); MPMF = "pôles de santé" (multiprofessional medical facilities); HS = "centre de santé" (traditional health centre); PCP = primary care practice; FHU = Family Health Units

Source: authors' compilation

patient population, have been the target of programmes in France, Latvia and the UK. In addition, a final outcome – i.e. reduced hospitalization in patients with chronic diseases – is included as an indicator in P4Q programmes in Latvia and Lithuania (Mitenbergs et al., 2012; Murauskiene et al., 2013). Furthermore, programmes in Portugal, Sweden and the UK reward outcomes of patient satisfaction or patient experience of care. The programme in Poland is the only known programme rewarding correct and timely diagnosis and timely treatment of cancer (OECD, 2016). Coordination efforts are rewarded in French, German, Italian and Swedish P4Q programmes, while practice organization and implementation of information technology and provision of other computer-based services are incentivized in at least seven countries, namely the Czech Republic, France, the Netherlands, Portugal, Spain, Sweden and the UK (Anell, Nylinder & Glenngård, 2012; OECD, 2016; Srivastava, Mueller & Hewlett, 2016). Finally, some programmes also reward improved access to care (for example, the scheme in the Czech Republic) – but this goes beyond the narrow definition of quality adopted by this book (*see* Chapter 1).

In all programmes, providers are rewarded with a bonus payment in relation to the measured quality of care – there are no penalties in any of the countries, except in certain regions of Sweden. The bonus is usually relatively small (<5% of total income) and is paid in relation to absolute performance. This means that the bonus of an individual provider is independent from the performance of other providers, except in certain regions of Sweden (Lindgren, 2014), where relative achievement compared to peers is rewarded. Only four programmes (in Croatia, France, Portugal and the UK) pay a bonus of more than 10%.

In Portugal bonuses are paid to physicians (up to 30% of income) and nurses (up to 10% of income) working in organizationally mature Family Health Units (FHU) that have gained greater autonomy from public administration (Biscaia & Heleno, 2017). Bonuses depend on achievements related to preventive and monitoring services in vulnerable populations (pregnant women, children, patients with diabetes or high blood-pressure) and in women of reproductive age (Almeida Simoes et al., 2017; Srivastava, Mueller & Hewlett, 2016).

Under the Quality and Outcomes Framework (QOF), implemented in the UK in 2004, practices could originally receive a bonus of up to 25% of income until 2013, when this share was reduced to 15% (Roland & Guthrie, 2016). The bonus comprises an up-front payment at the beginning of the year and achievement payments at the end. Points are awarded for the achievement of each incentivized indicator, and total payment depends on the monetary value of a QOF point, practice list size and prevalence data (NHS Digital, 2016). Indicators and the value of QOF points differ between England, Northern Ireland, Scotland and Wales. Initially, the scheme in England comprised 146 incentivized indicators from clinical, public health, organizational and patient experience domains (Doran et al., 2006; Gillam & Steel, 2013). However, in 2015 the number of indicators was reduced to 77; while many indicators were retired, some other indicators, such as smoking cessation and osteoporosis, were newly introduced (NHS Digital, 2016; NHS Employers, 2011). Even though the QOF has been implemented as a voluntary programme, participation rates have been very high, ranging from 96% to 99% (around 7 600 to 8 000) of eligible practices in England.

The French programme *Rémunération sur objectifs de santé publique* (ROSP) provides an incentive of up to 11% of the usual income to primary care physicians and in some cases to specialists (Cashin, 2014). The second programme in France, *Expérimentations de nouveaux modes de remuneration* (ENMR) applies a different incentive structure from other identified schemes in Europe. The scheme is comprised of basic and optional requirements, while the payment for each type of requirement consists of fixed and variable payment. In order to be able to participate in the programme, a provider has to fulfil basic requirements (Minister of Finance and Public Accounts/Minister of Social Affairs, Health and Women's Rights, 2015). Overall, the payment depends on the achievements in three categories – access to healthcare, work in multiprofessional teams (which aims at better coordination of care), and implementation of computerized information systems. The scheme provides a bonus of up to 5% of the provider's income, 60% of which can be paid in advance at the beginning of a period (Srivastava, Mueller & Hewlett, 2016).

14.3.2 Hospital care

Table 14.2 provides an overview of 13 P4Q programmes in nine European countries. The first P4Q programme in hospital care was introduced in Luxembourg in 1998 and the last of the included programmes was implemented in Norway in 2014 (*see* Table 14.2). Identified programmes are typically mandatory, implemented at the national level mainly in western European countries.

The focus of all programmes in hospitals is on acute care. The majority of programmes includes indicators that either target improved effectiveness of care (for example, performing surgery or initiating treatment within a pre-specified period of time) or patient safety (for example, avoidance of 30-day readmissions, wrong-side surgery and hospital-acquired conditions). Responsiveness in terms of patient experience or in terms of patient satisfaction is part of programmes in Denmark, Norway, Sweden, and the UK's Advancing Quality (AQ) and Commissioning for Quality and Innovation (CQUIN).

Table 14.2 A selection of P4Q programmes in hospital care in Europe

Country	Programme (nationwide/regional, voluntary/mandatory)	Start	Care area	Quality dimensions	Type and number of indicators	Area of activity	Incentive structure	Size of FI as % of total income	Type and number of provider
DK	Journalauditindikatoren (NW, M)	2009	AC	EFFS RESP	O, P, S	Proportion of patients with a case manager; Patient satisfaction	B, PN, AM	<1%	IND (departments in four hospitals)
FR	IFAQ (NW, M+V)	2012	AC	EFFS	P, S	Disease management (AMI, acute stroke, renal failure); Prevention and management of postpartum haemorrhage; Documentation	B, RR, TOP20P	0.4–0.6% – V; 0.2–0.5% – M; (€15t–500t)	ORG (hospital) – 460 in 2014–2015
HR	(NW, M)	2015	AC	EFFS	O, P, S	All-cause mortality; % of day-hospital cases; % of treatment by reserve antibiotics in the total number of cases	W, AM (RR)	10%	ORG (hospital)
IT	PAFF (Lazio, M)	2009	AC	EFFS	P – 1	Hip-fracture surgery within 48 hours of admission	PN, AM	Reduced reimbursement	ORG (hospital)
LU	Incitants qualité (NW, V)	1998	AC	EFFS, SFTY	O, P, S	Change annually	B, AM	≤2.00%	ORG (hospital)
NO	QBF (NW, V)	2014	AC	EFFS, RESP, SFTY	O, P – 33	Clinical outcomes (five-year survival rates in cancer, 30-day survival for hip fracture, AMI, stroke and all admissions), management of diseases (treatment of hip fractures within 48 hours, cancer treatment initiation within 20 days, waiting time, etc.); Waiting times; Patient satisfaction	W, RR	Redistribution of NOK 500M	ORG (hospitals in four regions)
PT	Hospital contract (NW, M)	2002	AC	EFFS, SFTY	O, P – 12	LOS; 30 days ER; Hip-fracture surgery within 48 hours of admission; Waiting times; Day case surgeries; Generics prescription; Use of Surgical Safety Checklist	B, PN, RR	≤5%	ORG (hospital)
SE	R, M (in 10 out of the 21 regions)	2004	AC	EFFS, RESP	O, P, S	Compliance with guidelines (AMI, diabetes, hip fracture, renal failure – within 48 hours, stroke); Patient satisfaction	W, AM	2–4%	ORG (hospital)

UK (ENG)	Advancing Quality (NW, V)	2008	AC	EFFS, RESP	O, P – 52	Disease management (AKI, AMI, ARLD, CABG, COPD, diabetes, dementia, HKRS, hip-fracture, heart failure, pneumonia, psychosis, sepsis, stroke); Patient-reported outcomes; Patient experience	B, AM	2–4%	IND (clinical teams), ORG (hospital – 24)
UK (ENG)	CQUIN (NW, M)	2009	AC	EFFS, RESP, SFTY	O, P – depends on agreement	PSIs and process quality; Patient experience	PN, AM	0.5–2.5% of the contract	ORG (hospital)
UK (ENG)	BPT (NW, M+V)	2010	AC	EFFS, SFTY	P – 65	Avoiding unnecessary admissions (day case surgeries); Delivering care in appropriate settings; Promoting provider quality accreditation; Improving quality of care	B, W, AM	<1% (5–43% of tariff)	ORG (hospital)
UK (ENG)	Non-payment for never events (NW, M)	2009	AC	SFTY	O – 14	PSIs – reduce 14 never events	PN, AM	No reimbursement	ORG (hospital)
UK (ENG)	Non-payment for ER (NW, M)	2011	AC	SFTY	O – 1	PSIs – 30 days ER	PN, AM	No reimbursement	ORG (hospital)

Abbreviations: **Countries:** DK = Denmark; ENG = England; FR = France; IT = Italy; LU = Luxembourg; NO = Norway; PT = Portugal; SE = Sweden; UK = United Kingdom

Programmes: BPT = Best Practice Tariffs; CQUIN = Commissioning for Quality and Innovation; ER = emergency readmission; IFAQ = Incitation financière à l'amélioration de la qualité; PAFF = Applicazione del percorso assistenziale nei pazienti ultrasessantacinquenni con fratture di femore; QBF = Kvalitetsbaserat finansiering (Quality-based financing)

Diffusion/participation: NW = nationwide; R = regional; M = mandatory; V= voluntary

Quality dimension: EFFS = effectiveness; RESP = responsiveness; SFTY = safety **Care area:** AC = acute care; PC = preventive care

Area of activity: AKI = Acute Kidney Injury; AMI = Acute Myocardial Infarction; ARLD = Alcohol-Related Liver Disease; CABG = Coronary Artery Bypass Graft; COPD = Chronic Obstructive Pulmonary Disease; HKRS = Hip and Knee Replacement Surgery Hip Fracture; PSIs = patient safety indicators

Type of indicators: O = outcomes; P = processes; S = structures

Incentive structure: A = achievement; AM = absolute measure; B = bonus; I = improvement; PN = penalty; RR = relative ranking; TOP20P = reward of the upper 20% of all performers; W = withhold **Type and number of provider:** IND = individual providers; ORG = organizations

Source: authors' compilation

Most P4Q programmes for hospitals have a stronger focus on outcomes and/or processes than P4Q programmes in primary care (where the focus is on structures). Only P4Q programmes for hospitals in Croatia, Denmark, France and Luxembourg include indicators for structures. Final health outcomes are only measured in Norway (for example, five-year survival rate for different cancer types, 30-day survival rates after hospital admission for hip fracture, AMI and stroke) and in Croatia (all-cause-mortality). Patient-reported health outcomes are measured in Advancing Quality (AQ) in the north-west of England (for example, quality of life), while patient safety outcomes are measured in the English "Non-payment for never-events" programme in terms of reduction of 14 never-events including wrong-side surgery, wrong implant/prosthesis, and retained foreign object post procedure (AQuA, 2017; NHS England Patient Safety Domain, 2015). Outcomes in terms of patient experience and patient satisfaction (for example, experience or satisfaction with waiting times) are rewarded by programmes in Denmark, Norway, Sweden and England (within AQ and CQUIN) (Anell, 2013; AQuA, 2017; Olsen & Brandborg, 2016).

Acute myocardial infarction (AMI), acute stroke, renal failure, hip fracture, and hip and knee replacement surgery are the main medical conditions targeted by programmes in France, Italy, Norway, Portugal, Sweden and the UK for process quality improvement. A few countries target additional conditions, such as cancer (Norway), diabetes (Sweden, UK), postpartum haemorrhage (France) and a few more in the UK. Indicators concern timely treatment (for example, surgical treatment of hip-fracture within 48 hours of admission, initiation of cancer treatment within 20 days), appropriate disease management (for example, medication at admission, discharge and during the stay, disease monitoring and diagnostic activities), and care coordination (for example, referrals to rehabilitation and primary care, plans for disease management, discharge summary sent within seven days).

Nine of the 13 identified programmes have penalties – either as a withhold of reimbursement (for example, non-payment schemes in the UK), as a payment adjustment of usual payment depending on performance (for example, CQUIN in the UK, programmes in Italy, Norway, Portugal and Sweden), or as a predefined fine if the targets are not met (for example, *Journalauditindikatoren* in Denmark) (Kristensen, Bech & Lauridsen, 2016). Some of the programmes have both penalties and bonuses (for example, schemes in Denmark, Portugal and CQUIN in the UK). In France, Luxembourg and the AQ scheme in the UK programmes rewarded providers with a bonus payment. The size of bonus payments or penalties is usually relatively small (<2% of total hospital income) and the payment is almost always made in relation to absolute performance. Only in France, Norway and Portugal does the payment depend on relative performance of providers compared to their peers. In most countries the bonus or penalty amounts to less than 2% of the total hospital budget. The scheme in Croatia is the only one where as much as 10% of a hospital's revenue depends on a broader measure of performance including activity- and quality-based indicators (MSPY, 2016).

The earliest programme, the *Incitant Qualité* (IQ) in Luxembourg, was established with the aim to improve patient-centredness, and the sensibility of actors for quality of care. In the first four years the programme targeted prevention of nosocomial infections, implementation of electronic health records, preventive care and pain management, as well as the technical quality of mammography. The financial incentive currently amounts to up to 2% of the annual budget. The reward depends on the number of achieved points on a scale of 0 to 100 and the corresponding percentage with respect to all the available points (i.e. 0% for 0–10 points, 10% for 10–20 points and so on) (Sante.lu, 2015).

The Norwegian Quality-Based Financing (QBF) programme was introduced as a pilot among four regions in Norway and covers all public secondary care providers and also private hospitals with a contract with the Regional Health Authority (RHA) in Norway in January 2014. The rewards are paid to the four RHAs according to their performance and the performance of hospitals in the region measured by process, outcome and patient satisfaction indicators. While most indicators are measured on the hospital level, the five-year survival rates for cancer are measured on the regional level. The patient satisfaction results came from the National Patient Satisfaction Survey. The QBF rewards four types of performance: reporting quality, minimum performance level, best performance and best relative improvement in performance of RHA. The rewards are based on achieved points for the reporting quality and the three indicator types (outcome indicators – 50 000 points, process indicators – 20 000 points and indicators of patient satisfaction – 30 000 points). The fulfilment of reporting requirements is the prerequisite for the possibility to generate indicator-based points. QBF redistributes around 500 million Norwegian crones to RHAs according to the weighted performance of the regions and the regions' hospitals. However, the RHAs have no fixed requirements regarding how to distribute the QBF rewards among regional hospitals (Olsen & Brandborg, 2016).

The French programme *Incitation financière à l'amélioration de la qualité* (IFAQ) was introduced as an experiment in 2012 and became a nationwide programme in 2016. The aim of the programme is to improve management of myocardial infarction, acute stroke, renal failure, the prevention and management of post-partum haemorrhage, documentation and efficient medication prescription. Only the upper 20% of the providers with the highest performance receive a bonus between 0.2 and 0.6% of total income. The total remuneration of the scheme amounts to between €15 000 and €500 000 (Minister of Social Affairs and Health, 2016).

14.4 The effectiveness and cost-effectiveness of pay for quality initiatives

The available evidence about the effectiveness of P4Q programmes has been summarized in 31 reviews published between 1999 and 2016. Tables 14.3, 14.4 and 14.5 provide an overview of the characteristics, methods and results of the included reviews. Most reviews were performed in the US and the UK. Seven reviews were conducted in non-English-speaking countries, and one review was in Portuguese. Nineteen reviews evaluated P4Q programmes in primary care (Table 14.3), nine[1] reviews investigated effects in both primary and hospital care (Table 14.4) and only three reviews had an exclusive focus on hospital care (Table 14.5).

Five reviews focused solely on preventive care, while another three focused only on chronic care. Three reviews evaluated the effectiveness of P4Q in comparison to other interventions, with one review focusing on audit and feedback (Ivers et al., 2012), one review focusing on different interventions that can improve the appropriate use of imaging (French et al., 2010), and one review focusing on financial incentives (not only P4Q) for prescribers (Rashidian et al., 2015). In addition, two out of the three reviews reported by Damberg et al. (2014) evaluated accountable care organization models (ACOs) and bundled payment (BP) programmes, which aimed to improve quality and to simultaneously reduce costs of care.

The number of studies included in each review varies from two studies included by Giuffrida et al. (2000) to 128 studies included by van Herck et al. (2010). The original studies (around 400) included in the 31 reviews were conducted between the "early 1980s" (Armour et al., 2001) and 2013 (Milstein & Schreyoegg, 2016 suppl.), and reported between 1991 and 2015. Overall, reviews found the quality of included studies to be low to moderate. Most evidence stems from studies without a control group, i.e. studies of observational (for example, cross-sectional, longitudinal studies) and quasi-experimental nature (for example, uncontrolled before-after studies – UBA, time-series analyses). Even the relatively few available studies with a control group (approx. n = ≤100), such as randomized controlled trials (RCTs, n = ≤10), controlled before-after studies (CBA) and interrupted time-series (ITS) and other quasi-experimental designs with a control group, exhibit a number of biases.

---

1 The review by Kondo et al. (2015) evaluated effects of both primary and hospital care but the presentation of the results was split between Table 14.3 and Table 14.5.

With the exception of the reviews by Huang et al. (2013) and Ogundeji, Bland & Sheldon (2016), all the included systematic reviews synthesized included studies in a narrative manner. Ogundeji, Bland & Sheldon (2016) conducted a meta-analysis and a meta-regression, while Huang et al. (2013) only performed a meta-analysis.

14.4.1 Effectiveness of P4Q in primary care

The most frequently evaluated programme in primary care was QOF but most reviews evaluated a range of P4Q programmes in the US. Programmes in other European countries and in the Asia-Pacific region were evaluated only by individual studies included in the reviews (*see* Table 14.3).

The effectiveness of QOF has been evaluated by seven reviews in total, summarizing evidence from a total of 71 individual studies (Christianson, Leatherman & Sutherland, 2007, 2008; Gillam, Siriwardena & Steel, 2012; Hamilton et al., 2013; Houle et al., 2012; Kondo et al., 2015; Langdown & Peckham, 2014; Lin et al., 2015). The best evidence is available from five reviews that included studies evaluating at least four programme years after the start of the programme in 2004 and using results of ITS and other studies that accounted for secular trends (Gillam, Siriwardena & Steel, 2012; Houle et al., 2012; Kondo et al., 2015; Langdown & Peckham, 2014; Lin et al., 2015). Based on this body of evidence, review authors concluded that performance of primary care providers significantly improved in almost all process-of-care indicators (for example, smoking cessation activities, diabetes management activities) during the first year of the programme, with some improvements greater than 30 percentage points, while intermediate health outcomes (for example, blood pressure, cholesterol and blood glucose level under control) showed less improvement.

In subsequent years (2005 to 2007) performance reached a plateau but continued to slowly improve for process-of-care indicators in both chronic and preventive care (Gillam, Siriwardena & Steel, 2012; Houle et al., 2012; Kondo et al., 2015). However, this slow improvement was, in fact, very similar to the underlying trend before the implementation of QOF, and for some health outcomes (for example, blood pressure, cholesterol and blood glucose level under control), the observed improvement was even below the pre-QOF trend (Damberg et al., 2014; Houle et al., 2012; Kondo et al., 2015; Langdown & Peckham, 2014). In addition, no effect was observed on final health outcomes such as incidence of AMI, stroke, renal failure and all-cause mortality (Damberg et al., 2014; Kondo et al., 2015). In general, positive effects of QOF on process-of-care indicators were more often reported by observational studies and studies without a control group (Gillam, Siriwardena & Steel, 2012; Houle et al., 2012; Kondo et al., 2015), while effects on health outcomes were mixed and inconclusive.

Table 14.3 *Overview of systematic reviews evaluating P4Q schemes in primary care*

Review	Review focus	Care area	Quality aim of review	Included studies			Study type	Study quality	Results
				No.	Country of origin	Date range			
Lin et al., 2016	Effect of P4Q on healthcare quality	AC, CC, PC	EFFS	44	FR, NL, TW, UK, US	1998–2013	RCT = 1, CBA = 17, ITS = 18, OS = 8	M/H	POC measures showed higher rates of improvement than health outcomes; overall positive effect on disease management varied by baseline performance and practice size; no separation of effects of concurrent QIs
Kondo et al., 2015	Effect of P4Q on healthcare quality (an ambulatory setting)	AC, CC, PC	EFFS	41	CA, FR, NL, TW, US, UK, TW	2006–2014	ITS = 17, UBA+OS = 24	NR	In general, UBA and OS short-term studies reported more often positive results in POCs compared to long-term ITS analyses; there is no clear, consistent evidence of the QOF's effect on patient outcomes; internationally: little or no effect on disease-related hospitalizations and complications
Rashidian et al., 2015	Effects of FI-based drug policies on drug use, healthcare utilization, health outcomes and costs	CC	EFFS	3 (18)	UK, NL	2007–2011	ITS = 2, CBA = 1	L	Uncertain effects of P4Q policies on health outcomes due to low quality of evidence
Damberg et al., 2014	Shared savings models (linked to quality of care)	CC, PC	EFFS	6 (45)	US	2009–2013	QE = 6, OS = 11	L	Some but not all POC measures within ACOs improved more than in controls; due to limited available evidence and methodological limitations, improvement cannot be clearly attributed to ACOs
Langdown & Peckham 2014	Efficacy of the QOF in improving health outcomes, its impact on non-incentivized activities and the robustness of the clinical targets adopted in the scheme	CC	EFFS	10 (11)	UK	2007–2012	RCT = 1, UBA = 4, ITS = 2, TS = 1, OS = 3	L/M	Strong evidence of initially improved health outcomes for a limited number of conditions and subsequent fall to the pre-existing trend; limited impact on non-incentivized activities with adverse effects for some subpopulations and on health outcomes due to programme's focus on POC indicators and the indicators' ceiling thresholds
Hamilton et al., 2013	Effectiveness of FI in provision of smoking cessation interventions and in health outcomes	CC, PC	EFFS	18	UK, US, DE, TW	2003–2010	C/RCT = 3, UBA = 13, OS = 2	M	Most UBAs showed improvements in recording the smoking status (RSS) and providing smoking cessation advice (SCA); RCTs showed mixed effects on RSS and SCA, and no effect on quit rates and long-term abstinence; authors found no sufficient evidence that reductions of smoking rates are attributed to the introduction of P4Q programmes

Table 14.3 Overview of systematic reviews evaluating P4Q schemes in primary care [continued]

Review	Review focus	Care area	Quality aim of review	Included studies		Date range	Study type	Study quality	Results
				No.	Country of origin				
Huang et al., 2013	Effects of P4Q on management of diabetes (a meta-analysis)	CC	EFFS	11 MA (21)	UK, US	2003–2010	CBA = 4, ITS = 6, OS = 1	L/M	Generally positive effects in most indicators; higher rates of improvement in POC indicators than in outcomes; inconsistent results in health outcomes
Houle et al., 2012	Effect of P4Q on healthcare quality	CC, PC	EFFS	30	UK	1995–2012	RCT = 4, N-RCT = 1, ITS/CBA = 5/3, OS/UBA = 2/15	L/M	Uncontrolled studies (UBA+OS) suggested that P4Q improved quality of care, but higher-quality studies with adequate controls failed to confirm these findings
Gillam, Siriwardena & Steel, 2012	Impact of QOF on the quality of UK's primary care	CC	EFFS, RESP, C-EFFS	53 (94)	US, TW	2004–2011	OS+QE = 83, IW+S = 11	L	Greater improvement of quality of care in the first year of QOF compared to the pre-intervention trend and subsequent return to prior rates in later years; modest cost-effective reductions in mortality and hospital admissions in some medical conditions; negative effects on person-centredness of consultations, continuity and patient satisfaction
Ivers et al., 2012	Effectiveness of audit and feedback	–	EFFS	3 (111)	US	1980–1999	RCT = 3	L/M	All three studies showed a positive impact of audit and feedback compared to groups applying FI alone or supplementary to audit and feedback
Scott et al., 2011	Effect of changes in the method and level of payment on the quality of care	CC, PC	EFFS	6 (7)	UK, US, DE	2003–2009	C-RCT = 3, CBA = 1, ITS = 2	L	Modest effects on some process measures (RSS, SCA, cervical screening rates and eye examinations for diabetes), but not on outcomes (quit rates, long-term abstinence); all studies have several methodological limitations
De Bruin et al., 2011	Effects of P4Q on healthcare quality and costs of chronic care through disease management	CC	EFFS	5 (18)	US, AU	2003–2010	CBA = 1, OS = 2, S = 2	NA	Four out of five studies showed positive effects on POCs; a limited number of studies and differences between schemes hinder comparability of their effects and from drawing conclusions on the effectiveness; studies did not adjust effects for concurrent QIs

Table 14.3 *Overview of systematic reviews evaluating P4Q schemes in primary care [continued]*

Review	Review focus	Care area	Quality aim of review	Included studies No.	Country of origin	Date range	Study type	Study quality	Results
French et al., 2010	Effects of interventions that aim to improve the appropriate use of imaging for people with musculoskeletal conditions	CC	EFFS	1 (28)	US	2007	ITS = 1	M	The study evaluated a multifaceted intervention consisting of an organizational and reminder intervention in Phase 1 and FI in Phase 2 with the aim to improve osteoporosis management after a fracture. The likelihood of receiving osteoporosis management did not change stat. significantly in Phase 2 of the intervention
Sabatino et al., 2008	Effectiveness of audit and feedback, and FI on cancer screening	PC	EFFS	3 (12)	US	1991–1998	RCT = 2, UBA = 1	M	Due to a low number of qualifying studies and inconsistent results authors could not determine the effectiveness of provider incentives in increasing use of screening for breast, cervical or colorectal cancers
Petersen et al., 2006	Effect of explicit FI on healthcare quality	CC, PC	EFFS	16 (17)	US	1992–2005	RCT = 9, CBA = 4, OS = 2	L/M	13 out of 16 studies found partial or positive effects on POC measures at the physician level and the provider group level; most of the measures were for preventive services
Sorbero et al., 2006	Effect of P4Q on healthcare quality	AC, CC, PC	EFFS	15	US	1995–2006	RCT = 7, UBA = 6, QE=2	NA	RCTs and QE analyses found no or only small effects on preventive activities in intervention group, while the UBAs tended to report positive results for at least one aspect of a programme under examination
Dudley et al., 2004	EFFS and potential of P4Q schemes to improve quality of care	PC	EFFS	9	US	1987–2003	RCT = 9	NA	The results are mixed – among the 11 POC indicators evaluated, seven showed a statistically significant response to P4Q strategies while four did not
Kane et al., 2004	Effects of FI on preventive care delivery	PC	EFFS	10 (66)	UK, US	1992–2001	RCT = 6, UBA = 2, OS = 1	L/M	Only one out of eight interventions led to a significantly greater provision of preventive services; rewards offered in these studies tend to be small; authors conclude that small rewards hinder increase in doctors' motivation to change their preventive care routines

Table 14.3 Overview of systematic reviews evaluating P4Q schemes in primary care [continued]

Review	Care area	Quality aim of review	Included studies			Study type	Study quality	Results
			No.	Country of origin	Date range			
Giuffrida et al., 2000	PC	EFFS	2	UK, US	1992–1998	RCT = 1, QE = 1	M	P4Q was associated with improvements in immunization rates (statistically significant increase in only one of the two studies)
Achat, McIntyre & Burgess, 1999	PC	EFFS	3(8)	UK, US	1992-1996	QE=2, S=1	NA	Groups receiving the incentives were up to 3x more likely to be immunized and had overall immunization rates of up to 17% higher than comparison groups.

Abbreviations: NR = not reported; f.i. = from inception   **Country codes:** AU = Australia; CA = Canada; DE = Germany; ES = Spain; FR = France; IT = Italy; JP = Japan; KR = Republic of Korea (South); NL = The Netherlands; SE = Sweden; TR = Turkey; TW = Taiwan; UK = United Kingdom; US = United States

Review objectives: ACO = accountable care organization; BP = bundled payment; HQID = Premier Hospital Quality Incentive Demonstration project by Centers for Medicare and Medicaid Services; FI = financial incentives; P4Q = pay for quality; PCP = primary care physicians; QOF = Quality and Outcomes Framework

Included studies: CBA = controlled before-after; C-RCT = cluster randomized controlled trial; ITS = interrupted time-series; MA = meta-analysis; MR = meta-regression; N-RCT = non-randomized controlled trial; OS = observational studies; QE = quasi-experimental; RCT = randomized controlled trial; S = survey; IW = interview; UBA = uncontrolled before-after studies

Study quality: L = low; L/M = low to moderate; M = moderate; M/H = moderate to high   **Results:** MCO = managed care organization; OR = odds ratio; RSS = recording the smoking status; SCA = smoking cessation advice; SMD = standardized mean difference

* 9(66) = 9 out of the 66 references evaluate effectiveness or cost-effectiveness of P4Q schemes for healthcare providers in high-income countries. Remaining studies do not meet the criteria.

Table 14.4 *Overview of systematic reviews evaluating P4Q schemes in both primary and hospital care*

Review	Review focus	Care area	Quality aim of review	Included studies No.	Country of origin	Date range	Study type	Study quality	Results
Korenstein et al., 2016	Impact of system-level interventions on the value of US healthcare, defined as the balance between quality and cost	AC, CC, PC	EFFS, C-EFFS	30	US	2009–2015	RCT = 1, CBA = 27, CS = 1, QE = 1	M	Quality, cost and utilization outcomes varied widely: quality improved in 17 reports; many improvements were small, POC measures predominated; the value improved in 23 reports; all studies have several methodological limitations
Ogundeji, Bland & Sheldon, 2016	To explore systematically the extent and sources of heterogeneity in the results of evaluations of P4Q schemes with the aim to identify features associated with success in P4Q schemes	AC, CC, PC	EFFS	37 MA, Div. 96 MR	—	1998–2014	RCT = 6, QE = 11, UBA = 20	NA	Estimates of effect of P4Q schemes: lowest effect in schemes measuring outcomes (SMD = 0.0), and highest in schemes measuring POCs (SMD = 0.18). Other design features and evaluation methods: the odds of showing a positive effect was three times higher in schemes with larger incentives (>5% of usual budget; OR = 3.38), less rigorous evaluation designs were 24 times more likely to have positive estimates of effect than RCTs (OR = 24).
Barreto, 2015	Effect of P4Q on healthcare quality	AC, CC, PC	EFFS	25 (27)	US, UK, SE, TW, IT	1991–2011	C/RCT=7OS = 20	NR	Less frequently reported positive effects of P4Q schemes in RCTs compared to OS, due to methodological limitations of OS and the heterogeneity (with respect to conceptual and contextual aspects) of P4Q schemes
Damberg et al., 2014	Effects of P4Q on quality and resource use, efficiency and costs	AC, CC, PC	EFFS, RESP	58 (89)	UK, US	2001–2013	C/RCT = 6, ITS = 2, CBA = 19, UBA = 7, QE = 11, OS = 13	L/M	Studies with stronger methodological designs were less likely to identify significant improvements associated with scheme – any identified effects were relatively small; studies with weaker study designs reported more often a significant association between P4Q and higher levels of quality, with large effect sizes
Emmert et al., 2012	Analyse the existing literature regarding economic evaluation of P4Q	CC, PC	C-EFFS	9	UK, US, DE	1992–2010	RCT = 3, CBA = 3, UBA = 3	L	Authors concluded that based on the full economic evaluations, P4Q efficiency could not be demonstrated; several methodological limitations undermine the importance of positive results of the partial economic evaluations; ranges of costs and consequences were typically narrow, and programmes differed considerably in design

Table 14.4 Overview of systematic reviews evaluating P4Q schemes in both primary and hospital care [continued]

Review	Review focus	Care area	Quality aim of review	Included studies No.	Country of origin	Date range	Study type	Study quality	Results
Van Herck et al., 2010	Effect of P4Q on healthcare quality	AC, CC, PC	EFFS, RESP, C-EFFS	51 (128)	AU, DE, ES, IT, UK, US	1992–2009	RCT/N-RCT = 9/3, ITS = 20, QE = 37, OS/EM = 51/8	M	Mixed results depending on the primary objectives of the scheme; the effects varied according to design choices and characteristics of the context; authors found less evidence on the impact on coordination, continuity, patient-centredness and cost-effectiveness.
Christianson, Leatherman & Sunderland, 2007, 2008	Effect of P4Q on healthcare quality	AC, CC, PC	EFFS, RESP	37	UK, US, TW, ES	1992–2007	RCT = 7, CBA = 7, ITS = 2, QE = 16, OS+S=5	NA	Mixed findings – few significant impacts reported; authors complain published research on hospital payments was too limited to draw conclusions with confidence; small, if any, effects on preventive care by RCTs; no separation of effects of concurrent QIs
Armour et al., 2001	Effects of FI on physician resource use and the quality of medical care	AC, PC	EFFS	5(7)	UK, US	1994–1998	RCT = 2, OS = 3	NA	Mixed results; authors conclude lack of knowledge of the relationship between the MCO, the physician and the FI complicates the prediction of the effectiveness

Abbreviations: NR = not reported; f.i. = from inception

Country codes: AU = Australia; CA = Canada; DE =Germany; ES =Spain; FR = France; IT = Italy; JP = Japan; KR = Republic of Korea (South); NL = The Netherlands; SE = Sweden; TR = Turkey; TW =Taiwan; UK = United Kingdom; US = United States

Review objectives: ACO = accountable care organization; BP = bundled payment; HQID = Premier Hospital Quality Incentive Demonstration project by Centers for Medicare and Medicaid Services; FI = financial incentives; P4Q = pay for quality; PCP = primary care physicians; QOF = Quality and Outcomes Framework

Included studies: CBA = controlled before-after; C-RCT = cluster randomized controlled trial; ITS = interrupted time-series; MA - meta-analysis; MR = meta-regression; N-RCT = non-randomized controlled trial; OS = observational studies; QE = quasi-experimental; RCT = randomized controlled trial; S = survey; IW = interview; UBA = uncontrolled before-after studies

Study quality: L = low; L/M = low to moderate; M = moderate; M/H = moderate to high

Results: MCO = managed care organization; OR = odds ratio; RSS = recording the smoking status; SCA = smoking cessation advice; SMD = standardized mean difference

* 9(66) – 9 out of the 66 references evaluate effectiveness or cost-effectiveness of P4Q schemes for healthcare providers in high-income countries. Remaining studies do not meet the criteria

Table 14.5 Overview of systematic reviews evaluating P4Q schemes in hospital care

Review	Review focus	Quality Care area	Quality aim of review	Included studies No.	Included studies Country of origin	Date range	Study type	Study quality	Results
Milstein and Schreyoegg, 2016	Impact of P4Q programmes in the inpatient sector	AC	EFFS	46	DK, CA, IT, KR, JP, TR, UK, US	2006–2015	QE = 30, OS = 16	NA	Modest, short-term improvements – possibly attributed to concurrent QIs and increased awareness of data recording
Kondo et al., 2015	Effect of P4Q on healthcare quality (hospital setting)	AC, CC, PC	EFFS, RESP	7	IT, TW, UK, US	2010–2014	CBA = 2, UBA = 2, OS = 3	NR	In US: limited effect on both POCs and patient outcomes, only one OS reported positive results on POCs. In TW and IT: generally positive effects on POCs and patient outcomes. In UK (AQ): slowing down improvements, which reached a plateau over time, or returned to pre-intervention levels
Damberg et al., 2014	Bundled payments (linked to quality)	AC	EFFS	1(3)	US	2007–2011	UBA = 1, OS = 1	L	Adherence to 40 POC measures increased from 59% to 100%; generalizability is difficult due to unique characteristics
Damberg et al., 2007 ; Mehrotra et al., 2009	Impact of P4Q in inpatient or outpatient hospital services	AC	EFFS	9	US	2004–2007	QE = 3, IW = 1, OS = 5	L	The three QE studies with a control group evaluated effects of HQID and focused on POC measures; improvement in HQID-hospitals 2–4% greater than in control group; effectiveness without public reporting remains unclear

Abbreviations: NR = not reported; f.i. = from inception   **Country codes:** AU = Australia; CA = Canada; DE = Germany; ES = Spain; FR = France; IT = Italy; JP = Japan; KR = Republic of Korea (South); NL = The Netherlands; SE = Sweden; TR = Turkey; TW = Taiwan; UK = United Kingdom; US = United States   **Review objectives:** ACO = accountable care organization; BP = bundled payment; HQID = Premier Hospital Quality Incentive Demonstration project by Centers for Medicare and Medicaid Services; FI = financial incentives; P4Q = pay for quality; PCP = primary care physicians; QOF = Quality and Outcomes Framework   **Included studies:** CBA = controlled before-after; C-RCT = cluster randomized controlled trial; ITS = interrupted time-series; MA = meta-analysis; MR = meta-regression; N-RCT = non-randomized controlled trial; OS = observational studies; QE = quasi-experimental; RCT = randomized controlled trial; S = survey; IW = interview; UBA = uncontrolled before-after studies   **Study quality:** L = low; L/M = low to moderate; M = moderate; M/H = moderate to high   **Results:** MCO = managed care organization; OR = odds ratio; RSS = recording the smoking status; SCA = smoking cessation advice; SMD = standardized mean difference

* 9(66) – 9 out of the 66 references evaluate effectiveness or cost-effectiveness of P4Q schemes for healthcare providers in high-income countries. Remaining studies do not meet the criteria

Reported results of P4Q programmes in non-European countries are somewhat similar to those of QOF. Reviews identified 124 studies evaluating effects of P4Q programmes in primary care for chronic conditions. In general, short-term and observational or uncontrolled quasi-experimental studies frequently reported large positive effect sizes for process-of-care indicators in chronic care patients independent of the disease (Damberg et al., 2014; Houle et al., 2012; Kondo et al., 2015). Better designed studies, such as ITS, CBAs and other quasi-experimental designs with a comparison group, examining data over a longer time period (for example, several years before and several years after the implementation of a P4Q programme), found no effect or a slightly positive effect (Damberg et al., 2014; Houle et al., 2012; Kondo et al., 2015). Only small positive effects on chronic care management could be found in the networks within the ACOs (Damberg et al., 2014).

Reviews investigating effects of P4Q schemes on preventive care did not find convincing evidence for the effectiveness of P4Q interventions on preventive services (87 studies). Again, higher quality studies, i.e. those with an intervention and a control group, reported positive results only for individual process-of-care measures. For example, positive effects were found on colorectal and cervical cancer screening rates, on influenza immunization rates and on smoking cessation activities (for example, recording of smoking status and provision of cessation advice) (Damberg et al., 2014; Giuffrida et al., 2000; Hamilton et al., 2013; Houle et al., 2012; Kondo et al., 2015; Sabatino et al., 2008; Scott et al., 2011; Town et al., 2005; van Herck et al., 2010). However, no effects were found on screening rates for other cancer types, on screening referrals, as well as on adherence to cancer screening guidelines, and on paediatric immunization (Armour et al., 2001; Damberg et al., 2014; Sabatino et al., 2008; Town et al., 2005). Hamilton et al. (2013) identified seven studies which investigated effects of P4Q interventions on quit rates and smoking prevalence. One RCT and one cluster RCT found no superiority of interventions which applied a financial incentive for a healthcare provider over a control group or over other types of intervention on quit rates (Roski et al., 2003; Salize et al., 2009). In addition, the identified decrease of smoking prevalence could not be attributed to the P4Q intervention in the United Kingdom (QOF), nor in Taiwan (Hamilton et al., 2013).

Two reviews reported results of 11 studies that had investigated effects of P4Q on final health outcomes in non-European countries (Damberg et al., 2014; Kondo et al., 2015); seven of the 11 studies were of low quality and found positive effects on diabetes-related hospitalization and complications in the long-term, on reduced emergency department visits, on depression treatment response and on neonatal intensive care unit admissions. Two studies, one of good and one of low quality, found no effect on 30-day mortality, readmission, hospitalization and emergency department visits related to diabetes, AMI, heart failure and pneumonia (Damberg et al., 2014). For the remaining two studies, reviews reported detrimental effects on acute emergency department visits related to asthma, diabetes and heart failure (Kondo et al., 2015).

Effects of P4Q on responsiveness of care are reported in five reviews. Gillam, Siriwardena & Steel (2012) found on the basis of six observational studies of patient experience in QOF that no statistically significant changes in communication, nursing care, coordination or overall satisfaction were reported by patients between 2003 and 2007. However, the same six original studies found that timely access to chronic care worsened in terms of continuity of care and visits to the usual physician, but not in terms of urgent appointments, which actually improved statistically significantly. In general, and especially for older patients, access to care in QOF worsened. Christianson, Leatherman & Sutherland (2007) and van Herck et al. (2010) reported for several international P4Q programmes that patient satisfaction with care did not change. Two other reviews highlighted that positive effects on patient experience reported by original studies could not be clearly attributed to a P4Q programme, either because of structural changes implemented as part of the programme (for example, implementation of electronic reminder and prescribing systems) or because other quality improvement interventions were implemented simultaneously with the P4Q programme (Damberg et al., 2014; Kondo et al., 2015).

Finally, one cluster-RCT identified by Ivers et al. (2012) evaluated the effects of financial incentives compared to audit and feedback on test-ordering. The financial incentives turned out to be less effective than audit and feedback in reducing test ordering.

14.4.2 Effectiveness of P4Q in hospital care

Reviews that evaluated programmes in hospital care (Tables 14.4 and 14.5) identified 30 studies of 15 P4Q programmes, most of which were located in the US and incentivized primarily process-of-care measures (Armour et al., 2001; Barreto, 2015; Christianson, Leatherman & Sutherland, 2007, 2008; Damberg et al., 2007, 2014; Kondo et al., 2015; Korenstein et al., 2016; Mehrotra et al., 2009; Milstein & Schreyoegg, 2016). P4Q programme effects on health outcomes were evaluated by 13 studies. Only few programmes were evaluated exhaustively – such programmes are "Advancing Quality" in the UK evaluated by four studies and the discontinued HQID (2003–2009) in the US evaluated by 17 studies.

Reviews reported that studies with a comparison group found predominantly small short-term and often statistically non-significant positive effects on a composite score that combined several process-of-care measures, or positive effects on individual process-of-care indicators (Damberg et al., 2007, 2014; Kondo et al., 2015; Mehrotra et al., 2009; Milstein & Schreyoegg, 2016). Highly positive effects were identified in the initial phase of HQID, while in the long term the effects were not sustained (Damberg et al., 2014; Mehrotra et al., 2009; Milstein & Schreyoegg, 2016). In contrast, the positive effects of the initial phase of the more recent Hospital Value-Based purchasing incentive Payment programme (HVBP) were not statistically significant (Kondo et al., 2015; Milstein & Schreyoegg, 2016). In three US programmes (MassHealth, Non-payment for HACs and Baylor Healthcare System) evaluated by three studies with relatively strong designs (i.e. with a comparison group or with time-trend adjustment), positive programme effects were observed only on individual process-of-care measures related to pneumonia, AMI and CHF management (for example, influenza vaccination in pneumonia patients – one out of the 19 pneumonia measures) (Damberg et al., 2014; Kondo et al., 2015). Six studies with no comparison group found positive effects on breast cancer, AMI and CHF management, on obstetric services and common surgeries (Armour et al., 2001; Damberg et al., 2007, 2014; Kondo et al., 2015; Mehrotra et al., 2009). One UBA evaluation of a P4Q programme in Taiwan found no effect on tuberculosis treatment length (Kondo et al., 2015).

Similar results were also found with respect to health outcomes. The rate of decrease of risk-adjusted mortality associated with AMI, heart failure or pneumonia was larger in the initial phase of Advancing Quality than in the long term. That is, 42 months after the introduction of the programme, no further improvements in mortality rates were observed and hospitals in other regions of England showed greater reductions in mortality (Damberg et al., 2014; Kondo et al., 2015; Milstein & Schreyoegg, 2016). The effects of other P4Q programmes were mixed. Positive effects were identified for different types of health outcomes: five-year breast cancer survival, negative surgical margins and breast cancer recurrence rate in the Taiwanese Breast Cancer Pay for Performance programme (BC-P4P), nine-months tuberculosis cure rate in the Taiwanese Tuberculosis Pay for Performance (TB-P4P) programme and on quality-adjusted life-years (QALYs) associated with AMI and CHF in the Blue Cross Blue Shield Michigan P4P (BCBS-P4P) programme (Christianson, Leatherman & Sutherland, 2007, 2008; Damberg et al., 2007, 2014; Kondo et al., 2015; Mehrotra et al., 2009; Milstein & Schreyoegg, 2016; van Herck et al., 2010). However, in the original Taiwanese studies, no information on study design was provided, while other studies either lacked a comparison group (for example, BCBS-P4P), or lacked adjustment for time-trend and the coincident public-reporting effects (for example, the Italian DRG-P4P) (Kondo et al., 2015; Mehrotra et al., 2009). In three studies Damberg et al. (2014) and Mehrotra et al. (2009) found no difference between HQID hospitals and the comparison group in mortality rates associated with AMI, CHF and pneumonia.

Patient safety or utilization outcomes were evaluated by seven studies included in six reviews with respect to readmissions, length-of-stay (LOS), surgery-related complications or infections, blood catheter-associated infections and other hospital acquired conditions (HACs) in seven programmes –Advancing Quality; Hawaii Medical Service Association Hospital Pay for Performance (HMSA-P4P); HQID; HVBP; Non-payment for HACs by the US Centers for Medicare and Medicaid Services; Geisinger ProvenCareSM integrated delivery system; and MassHealth P4Q. Positive and statistically significant effects on preventable conditions or LOS were only identified by two studies in HMSA-P4P and in Non-payment for HACs, while in four studies positive effects were small and statistically not significant (Christianson, Leatherman & Sutherland, 2008; Damberg et al., 2014; Korenstein et al., 2016; Mehrotra et al., 2009; Milstein & Schreyoegg, 2016).

Responsiveness in terms of patient experience was evaluated by four studies in five reviews. The reviews by Kondo et al. (2015) and Milstein & Schreyoegg (2016) did not find evidence for improved patient experience of care after the introduction of HVBP but rather found a statistically non-significant worsening of care. Patient satisfaction with inpatient care in HMSA-P4P hospitals improved by a few percentage points. However, the evaluation did not involve a control group and the statistical significance was not calculated either (Christianson, Leatherman & Sutherland, 2008; Damberg et al., 2014; Mehrotra et al., 2009).

14.4.3 Cost-effectiveness

Emmert et al. (2012) is the only review that examined economic evaluations of P4Q programmes. It identified only three full economic evaluations. Six studies were partial economic evaluations, which evaluated costs and consequences separately or assessed only the impact on costs. The reviews by Christianson, Leatherman & Sutherland (2007), van Herck et al. (2010), Gillam, Siriwardena & Steel (2012), Hamilton et al. (2013) and Kondo et al. (2015) identified three other studies with partial economic evaluations.

All full economic evaluations included in the review by Emmert et al. (2012) reported positive cost-effectiveness. All three studies evaluated the effects of financial incentives on processes of care in primary or hospital care in the US. The RCTs by Kouides et al. (1998) evaluated effects of additional bonuses on influenza immunization coverage. The study found additional costs of $4 362 and $1 443 for additional immunizations. Overall, in the intervention group median improvement of coverage was 10.3% compared to the pre-intervention period, while in the control group median improvement was only 3.5%. The RCT by An et al. (2008) evaluated effects of incentives on referrals and enrolment in a quit smoking programme. The programme resulted in 1 483 total referrals and $95 733 total costs ($64 per referral) in the intervention group and 441 total referrals and $8937 total costs in the control ($20 per referral) group. The referrals in the intervention group resulted in 289 additional enrolees in the quit smoking programme and $300 per additional enrolee. The study by Nahra et al. (2006) evaluated the hospital BCBS-P4P programme, focusing on effects for AMI and CHF patients, and estimated costs per QALYs gained of between $12 967 and $30 081.

Most partial economic evaluations also reported positive results (Emmert et al., 2012; van Herck et al., 2010). Only one cost-effectiveness study conducted by Salize et al. (2009) evaluated the effects side using a health outcome, i.e. smoking abstinence. The RCT compared three arms with different combinations of interventions – physician training, financial incentive and free medication prescription – to usual care. In contrast to the two arms containing free medication prescription, the combination of physician training and financial incentive turned out to be not cost-effective when comparing the intervention costs per smoking-abstinent patient to the usual treatment. Even the third arm, which contained training, free medication prescription and financial incentive, did not dominate over the arm containing only training and free medication prescription (Hamilton et al., 2013; Scott et al., 2011; van Herck et al., 2010).

In general, the economic evaluations included in identified reviews have a number of weaknesses: included analyses predominantly considered process-of-care indicators on the effects side and costs from the third-party-payer's perspective on the costs side. Costs from the provider's perspective, such as administrative costs or costs for participating in other quality improvement initiatives, were not taken into account, and the costs were rarely described in detail (Emmert et al., 2012). In addition, designs of the included analyses have several limitations (for example, lack of separation of the effects generated by public reporting, small sample sizes, unit-of-analysis errors, etc.), which restrict the reliability of their conclusions on cost-effectiveness (Emmert et al., 2012; Mehrotra et al., 2009). Furthermore, a number of evaluated programmes (for example, HQID, QOF and HVBP) has been found to be ineffective in the long term (Gillam, Siriwardena & Steel, 2012; Houle et al., 2012; Kondo et al., 2015). Therefore, cost-effectiveness, if any, could have only been achieved in the programme's short term, when the combination of health gain and the sum of additional costs (administrative and reward costs) of the programme did not exceed a pre-specified amount. For many P4Q programmes, reviews found no positive effects which means that these programmes could not be cost-effective because they required additional financial resources.

14.5 How can pay for quality programmes be implemented? What are the organizational and institutional requirements?

The implementation of P4Q schemes is quite complex as many strategic and technical questions need to be addressed. Eijkenaar (2013) has proposed three broad strategic questions that need to be considered and we have added another two:

1. What to incentivize?

2. How to measure quality?

3. Whom to incentivize?

4. How to incentivize? and

5. How to implement and administer a P4Q programme?

14.5.1 What to incentivize?

The question of "what to incentivize?" requires scrutiny of the quality objectives that the payer wishes to prioritize. It is important that programmes focus on areas of quality where change is needed, rather than on areas where performance is already widely embedded in clinical practice (Lin et al., 2015; van Herck et al., 2010). Piecemeal attention to only some aspects of quality might encourage neglect of non-incentivized aspects. Therefore, P4Q should likely embrace a comprehensive approach and aim at covering most (or many) relevant areas of care (for example, Milstein & Schreyoegg, 2016).

Furthermore, a common theme in the literature (for example, Doran, Maurer & Ryan, 2017; Roland & Dudley, 2015; van Herck et al., 2010) is that incentivized activities should be aligned with widely held professional principles. This is one of the reasons why P4Q schemes should be developed in collaboration with healthcare professionals. Schemes are unlikely to be effective unless they reinforce professional norms and beliefs. In fact, the principles of P4Q can be considered to be somewhat antithetic to the principles of professional practice, which imply doing the best for patients irrespective of financial reward. Therefore, the very existence of a P4Q scheme may be a signal that some aspects of current professional practice are unacceptable.

14.5.2 How to measure quality?

Indicators and metrics to be used as the basis of reward should be reliable and timely, and not vulnerable to distortion (such as the provision of high-quality care only to healthier patients) or mis-reporting (such as only reporting values desired by the scheme). Indicators may reflect the structures, processes or outcomes of quality, and the choice of indicators will involve a trade-off between on the one hand the simplicity and practicality of structural and process metrics, and on the other hand the greater relevance but also greater complexity of outcome measures (*see also* Chapter 3).

While the *structures* of care reflect provider characteristics, such as the qualifications or accreditation of staff, the link of such structures to the eventual desired quality outcomes is often quite remote. Structural indicators can be considered in P4Q programmes when other data collection is infeasible, or there is a clear link from the structure to eventual quality.

Rewarding the *processes* of care is a more direct approach towards promoting quality, so long as the incentivized metrics are known to be associated with the desired quality outcomes. Process-based schemes are the most practical approach towards P4Q in many circumstances, as they obviate the need to directly measure outcomes. They can be aligned with clinical guidelines to motivate professionals to adopt best practices (*see also* Chapter 9), especially if this requires changes to existing methods and investments such as retraining. In principle, it should be unnecessary to reward processes that are already embedded in good professional practice.

Rewarding the *outcomes* of care seeks to directly reward the desired results of high-quality care. Examples might include future health status, or health service utilization metrics, such as hospital readmission. However, although directly addressing health system objectives, outcome-related P4Q is also the most challenging type of scheme. Levels of quality attained may be highly dependent on the characteristics of the patients treated, so some sort of casemix adjustment to the performance metrics is essential in order to avoid cherry-picking of healthier patients (*see* Chapter 3). Methods of risk-adjustment can vary from crude approaches (for example, excluding "complex" patients from the calculations) to statistically sophisticated methods. Many authors argue that statistical risk-adjustment is preferable because excluding complex patients from the calculation means that quality of care for these patients will not be incentivized by the P4Q scheme (Christianson, Leatherman & Sutherland, 2007, 2008; Gillam, Siriwardena & Steel, 2012; Houle et al., 2012; Kondo et al., 2015; Langdown & Peckham, 2014). Another approach to deal with the potential risk for risk-selection can be to pay more for target achievement amongst patients with comorbidities, for example, achievement of blood pressure control in diabetic patients or among patients with chronic kidney disease, because these targets are more difficult to achieve (Roland & Dudley, 2015). Such stronger incentives would be desirable also from a societal perspective since they may prevent costly disease-related complications in the long term.

Another challenge for outcome-based metrics is that some aspects of high-quality care may take a long time to materialize, rendering them infeasible as a basis for measurement and reward. Therefore, although they offer the most direct link to desired objectives, the outcome-focused approach towards P4Q is likely to have limited applicability in practice.

14.5.3 Who to incentivize?

The question of "who to incentivize?" is often a finely balanced decision (Conrad, 2015; Kondo et al., 2015, 2016; Rynes, Gerhart & Parks, 2005). It is generally easiest administratively for the payer to target entire provider organizations. However, this requires that the organizations have some leverage over the practitioners on whom most aspects of quality ultimately depend. In contrast, targeting clinical teams or individual practitioners may sacrifice the collective responsibility and peer pressure needed to improve some aspects of quality, and the associated metrics may be less reliable and vulnerable to random fluctuation.

It is usually preferable to make participation in a P4Q scheme compulsory, especially as providers with unsatisfactory performance are the target of many schemes. Voluntary participation may result in a joining-in of already high-performing providers, which leads to a reward of the historical and not the improvement of performance (Christianson, Leatherman & Sutherland, 2007; Mehrotra et al., 2009). Secondly, depending on the scheme design, voluntary participation may prevent poorly performing providers from joining and may allow premature cancellation of participation in the programme (Scott et al., 2011). However, there may be circumstances when voluntary participation is needed to secure acceptance of the principle of P4Q, and if necessary the rewards can be designed to encourage high levels of participation.

14.5.4 How to incentivize?

A great variety of approaches towards incentivizing mechanisms have been tested and discussed in the literature (for example, Conrad, 2015; Doran, Maurer & Ryan, 2017; Kondo et al., 2015; Milstein & Schreyoegg, 2016; Roland & Dudley, 2015). Decisions must be taken on a wide range of characteristics of the quality-related payments, which are listed in Box 14.3. Choices will depend on criteria such as the disease area, the information available, administrative feasibility, the funds available, and the capacity of the payer and providers. Each of the decisions taken may influence the effects of the programme.

Box 14.3 *Aspects of financial incentives that must be considered when planning a P4Q programme*

1. How much reimbursement is "at risk" due to the P4Q scheme?
2. Is P4Q reimbursement formulated as a (positive) reward, or a (negative) penalty?
3. Is payment based on "old" or "new" money?
4. Is payment based on absolute attainment or is it relative to others in the scheme?
5. Is payment based on absolute levels of attainment or on improvement from previous levels?
6. Is P4Q separate for each element of performance, or is it based on a single composite measure of performance?
7. What is the relationship arithmetically between P4Q reimbursement and performance – for example, is it directly increasing, is there an upper or lower limit, or is it simply conditional on reaching a performance threshold?
8. What is the time period for the scheme?
9. How strong is the relationship between reimbursement and performance?

Source: authors' compilation based on Eijkenaar, 2013

When deciding about the size of the financial incentive, prospective expected incremental costs of the quality improvement and the share of total provider's income affected should be taken into account. If incentives are too small, they are likely to be ineffective, while very large incentives are unlikely to be cost-effective. For instance, Ogundeji, Bland & Sheldon (2016) showed in a meta-regression that the positive effects of a programme tend to be higher in programmes applying larger incentives ($\geq$ 5% of annual income).

The decisions on the structure of the financial incentive (for example, reward vs. penalty), the source of the payment (for example, "old" money – withholding part of the annual payment at the start of a period and redistributing it according to performance at the end of the period, or "new" money – payment of additional bonuses), the payment basis (for example, absolute vs. relative measurement, attainment vs. improvement) and performance targets (for example, single elements vs. composite score, availability of a threshold) influence the reaction of providers to the financial incentive. Each of these elements considered individually has various advantages and disadvantages.

Rewards of absolute performance measures are easy to manage and they provide some certainty of payment to providers. However, evidence from many programmes shows that absolute performance rewards often do not lead to the desired effects in the long term. The predetermined absolute performance thresholds hamper continuous incentives for further improvement of quality in healthcare if the targets are not revised on a regular basis (Langdown & Peckham, 2014).

There are also numerous negative aspects of penalties and relative performance measurements (Arnold, 2017; Conrad, 2015). They may lead to discrimination and unfairness and result in low acceptance and negative (unintended) behavioural reactions of providers or professionals. However, relative measures can incentivize continuous improvement and penalties usually have a stronger influence on performance due to the loss aversion of individuals (Emanuel et al., 2016). Individuals will make more effort to protect their revenues rather than to earn an uncertain reward. Furthermore, redistribution of "old" money can be perceived as unfair by providers (Milstein & Schreyoegg, 2016), which may again result in negative reactions (Eijkenaar, 2013; Kahneman, Knetsch & Thaler, 1986).

There is no clear evidence that would support the superiority of one incentive structure over another. However, blended payment systems, combining various characteristics, can reduce the unintended consequences. For example, the combination of "old" and "new" money, as well as of rewards, penalties and relative performance measures, can exploit the advantages of these elements, while avoiding some of the disadvantages. Loss aversion of individuals can be exploited by rewarding P4Q participants with part of a quality-related payment at the beginning of a period, which will be adjusted for performance at the end of the period. Another approach can be to fine providers who are not achieving quality aims, while a bonus is paid if further performance goals are reached.

In general, the emphasis of P4Q programmes should be to reward improvement of individual performance from previous levels, especially compared to the previous period. Highly competitive approaches that reward only the top 20% of providers with the highest performance or the largest improvement should rather be avoided because of the aforementioned potential negative consequences. However, whichever choices are made, it is important that they are codified very clearly, with statements of entitlements, conditions, time horizons and criteria for receipt of funds.

14.5.5 How to implement and administer?

In order to increase acceptance of a P4Q programme, all relevant stakeholders (providers, patients and payers) should be involved from the beginning of programme development, through implementation and evaluation (Damberg et al., 2014; van Herck et al., 2010). When implementing a programme, participating providers have to be trained about involved measures and about the relationship between the measures and the financial incentives (Kane et al., 2004; Kondo et al., 2015; Milstein & Schreyoegg, 2016; Sorbero et al., 2006). Time horizons of financial incentives should be clearly communicated, and allocation of rewards within an institution should be clear, too. Commissioners of a programme should assume that all participating providers can achieve the pre-specified targets in a short period of time and calculate funds accordingly. Furthermore, it is important that all relevant aspects of quality are monitored – not only incentivized aspects – even if they are not included in the P4Q scheme.

Finally, implemented programmes have to be monitored and evaluated on a regular basis. A number of recommendations for P4Q evaluations emerge from the available literature (for example, Damberg et al., 2014; Kondo et al., 2015; Mehrotra et al., 2009; Milstein & Schreyoegg, 2016). Evaluations should usually be planned before a P4Q programme starts and an appropriate evaluation design selected, depending on the number of participating providers and the time horizon of the programme. For programmes with high participation rates (for example, almost all hospitals), it is appropriate to apply an interrupted time-series design when assessing programme effectiveness. In doing so, performance and quality data should be collected for several years before and after the implementation of the programme. However, because studies without a comparison group systematically over-estimate the positive effects of P4Q programmes (Ogundeji, Bland & Sheldon, 2016), evaluation designs should, ideally, contain a comparison group, adjust for baseline performance of participating and non-participating providers, and account for secular trends. Furthermore, an evaluation should account for the implementation of concurrent quality improvement interventions, such as audit and feedback and public reporting, and also for the – often – frequent changes in programme design.

14.6 Conclusions for policy-makers

For obvious reasons, P4Q is not a panacea for solving a health system's quality problems. Despite the many implemented programmes in Europe, and even more programmes in the United States, the effectiveness and cost-effectiveness of P4Q programmes remain unclear. However, implementing P4Q programmes is complex and the main lessons concerning the design of P4Q programmes are summarized in Box 14.4.

Our review of existing P4Q schemes in Europe found 27 programmes in 16 European countries, with 14 programmes in primary care and 13 programmes in hospital care. Most P4Q programmes in primary care focus on quality in terms of structures and processes. Programmes for hospitals also focus on quality of processes but they focus just as often on quality of outcomes. Regardless of the increasing number of programmes in Europe, available evidence about the effectiveness of P4Q mostly stems from the United States or from England. P4Q programmes in other European countries have rarely been evaluated.

Box 14.4 *Conclusions with respect to P4Q programme design*

What to incentivize?

- Performance is ideally defined broadly, provided that the set of measures remains comprehensible
- Concerns that P4Q encourages risk selection and "teaching to the test" should not be dismissed.
- P4Q incentives should be aligned with professional norms and values; it is vital that providers are actively involved in programme design and in the selection of performance measures

How to measure quality?

- Outcome measures should be included provided that risk-adjustment is sophisticated and sample size is sufficient. Other strategies to minimize incentives for risk selection may still be necessary.
- Measure sets should at least incorporate "high-impact" measures; the more indeterminate aspects of care such as patient satisfaction and continuity of care are ideally also included or monitored

Who to incentivize?

- On balance, group incentives are preferred over individual incentives, mainly because performance profiles are then more likely to be reliable
- Individual or small-group incentives, as well as using measures with small sample size, will become increasingly feasible as methods for constructing composite scores evolve
- Caution should be upheld in applying hybrid schemes (for example,, using both group and individual incentives for a team with high interdependence among team members)
- Participation is ideally voluntary provided that broad participation among eligible providers can be realized

How to incentivize?

- Whether rewards or penalties should be used is context-dependent
- Offering providers a choice among schemes also including penalties may be considered
- Increasing the size of the incentive increases their strength up to a certain point. Yet relatively low-powered payments are preferred, provided that providers' costs of improving performance are covered
- Differentiated absolute targets across groups and/or a tiered series of absolute targets, possibly combined with additional "piece-rates" for each appropriately managed patient, are preferred over single targets and schemes using relative targets
- The time-lag between care delivery and payment should be minimized

> - P4P should be a permanent component of compensation and is ideally decoupled from base payments. Measures should be re-evaluated periodically and replaced or updated as necessary
>
> *How to implement and administer?*
>
> - Involving all relevant stakeholders, including providers, patients and payers, right from the start of the programme development is key to its success
> - Monitoring, structured feedback and sophisticated information technology will remain important in preventing undesired provider behaviour
>
> *Source:* authors' compilation based on Eijkenaar (2013), with modifications

Reviews of P4Q programmes in primary care showed that incentivizing process quality more often had a positive effect than incentivizing intermediate health outcomes. In contrast, P4Q programmes in hospital care appeared to be ineffective with respect to process quality, while the evidence on their effectiveness with regard to final health outcomes and patient safety indicators was inconclusive. Effects on final health outcomes were rarely evaluated in primary care and available results were partly contradictory. The relationship between intermediate and final health outcomes also remains unclear for evaluated P4Q programmes. Patient satisfaction and patient experience in primary care did not improve and sometimes deteriorated with respect to continuity of care, communication, nursing care, coordination and overall care satisfaction. The effect of hospital P4Q programmes on patient experience and patient satisfaction was rarely evaluated and showed only minor changes. However, patient satisfaction and patient experience are important indicators that should not be disregarded.

A few evaluations showed that P4Q programmes were less effective compared to other quality improvement interventions, such as public reporting, and audit and feedback. Cost-effectiveness of P4Q was rarely evaluated. Two studies were found that show P4Q interventions to be cost-effective from a third-party-payer perspective. However, these results need to be viewed in the context of the larger body of literature that found no or minor effects on improved quality of care. As programmes certainly entail additional costs, it is rather unlikely that these programmes are cost-effective.

Even if there is limited evidence about the effectiveness of P4Q programmes, there is substantial evidence from various countries that implementing such programmes is complex. A number of important governance issues must be resolved for any P4Q scheme to function properly. The most basic is that arrangements must be put in place to develop the content and structures of the scheme, and to review and update the quality metrics. Involvement of relevant professionals and patients is important, but the interests of payers must also be protected.

A fundamental element of any P4Q scheme is the information on which its payments are based, including any information used for risk-adjustment. Furthermore, proper monitoring requires information on certain non-incentivized aspects of care, to ensure that they have not been harmed by the P4Q scheme. It is likely that receipt of funds should be conditional on timely provision of relevant data by the providers involved, and that the quality of the data should be properly monitored and validated. More generally, the payer should have the capacity to monitor adverse behavioural responses on the part of providers, such as "cream-skimming" healthier patients.

Finally, any P4Q scheme should be subjected to routine monitoring and evaluation. This should seek to identify the benefits of the scheme and any adverse consequences. Payers may consider some sort of phased introduction, so that the scheme can be properly evaluated. The contents of the scheme should be regularly reviewed and refreshed, as certain elements are likely to become redundant (for example if variations in performance are reduced) and new concerns arise.

References

Achat H, McIntyre P, Burgess M (1999). Health care incentives in immunisation. *Australian and New Zealand Journal of Public Health*, 23(3):285.

Almeida Simoes J de et al. (2017). Portugal: Health System Review. *Health Systems in Transition*, 19:(2).

An LC et al. (2008). A randomized trial of a pay-for-performance program targeting clinician referral to a state tobacco quitline. *Archives of Internal Medicine*, 168(18):1993.

Anell A (2013). Vårdval i specialistvården: Utveckling och utmaningar. Stockholm: Sveriges kommuner och landsting.

Anell A, Nylinder P, Glenngård AH (2012). Vårdval i primärvården: Jämförelse av uppdrag, ersättningsprinciper och kostnadsansvar. Stockholm: Sveriges kommuner och landsting.

AQuA (2017). About Us: How does Advancing Quality measure performance? Available at: http://www.advancingqualitynw.nhs.uk/about-us/, accessed 26 October 2017.

Armour BS et al. (2001). The effect of explicit financial incentives on physician behavior. *Archives of Internal Medicine*, 161(10):1261.

Arnold DR (2017). Countervailing incentives in value-based payment. *Healthcare* (Amsterdam, Netherlands), 5(3):125.

Barreto JO (2015). [Pay-for-performance in health care services: a review of the best evidence available]. *Cien Saude Colet*, 20(5):1497.

Biscaia AR, Heleno LCV (2017). A Reforma dos Cuidados de Saúde Primários em Portugal: portuguesa, moderna e inovadora. *Ciencia & saude coletiva*, 22(3):701.

Busse R, Blümel M (2015). Payment systems to improve quality, efficiency and care coordination for chronically ill patients – a framework and country examples. In: Mas N, Wisbaum W (eds.). The "Triple Aim" for the future of health care. Madrid: Spanish Savings Banks Foundation (FUNCAS).

Cashin C (2014). Paying for performance in health care: Implications for health system performance and accountability. European Observatory on Health Systems and Policies series. Maidenhead, England: Open University Press, McGraw-Hill Education.

Christianson JB, Knutson DJ, Mazze RS (2006). Physician pay-for-performance. Implementation and research issues. *Journal of General Internal Medicine*, 21(Suppl 2):S9–S13.

Christianson JB, Leatherman S, Sutherland K (2007). Financial incentives, healthcare providers and quality improvements: a review of the evidence. London: Health Foundation.

Christianson JB, Leatherman S, Sutherland K (2008). Lessons from evaluations of purchaser pay-for-performance programs: a review of the evidence. *Medical Care Research and Review*, 65(6 Suppl):5S–35S.

Conrad DA (2015). The Theory of Value-Based Payment Incentives and Their Application to Health Care. *Health Services Research*, 50(Suppl 2):2057.

Conrad DA, Christianson JB (2004). Penetrating the "black box": financial incentives for enhancing the quality of physician services. *Medical Care Research and Review*, 61(3 Suppl):37S–68S.

Damberg CL et al. (2007). An Environmental Scan of Pay for Performance in the Hospital Setting: Final Report. Washington, DC: RAND Corporation.

Damberg CL et al. (2014). Measuring Success in Health Care Value-Based Purchasing Programs: Findings from an Environmental Scan, Literature Review, and Expert Panel Discussions. Washington, DC: RAND Corporation.

De Bruin SR, Baan CA, Struijs JN (2011). Pay-for-performance in disease management: a systematic review of the literature. *BMC Health Services Research*, 11:272.

Doran T, Maurer KA, Ryan AM (2017). Impact of Provider Incentives on Quality and Value of Health Care. *Annual Review of Public Health*, 38:449.

Doran T et al. (2006). Pay-for-performance programs in family practices in the United Kingdom. *New England Journal of Medicine*, 355(4):375.

Dudley RA et al. (1998). The Impact of Financial Incentives on Quality of Health Care. *Milbank Quarterly*, 76(4):649.

Dudley RA et al. (2004). Strategies To Support Quality-based Purchasing: A Review of the Evidence. AHRQ Publication, No. 04-0057. Rockville MD: Agency for Healthcare Research and Quality.

Eckhardt H et al. (2016). Effectiveness and cost-effectiveness of pay for quality initiatives in high-income countries: a systematic review of reviews. PROSPERO 2016: CRD42016043043. Available at: http://www.crd.york.ac.uk/PROSPERO/display_record. asp?ID=CRD42016043043, accessed 17 May 2019.

Eijkenaar F (2013). Key issues in the design of pay for performance programs. *European Journal of Health Economics*, 14(1):117.

Emanuel EJ et al. (2016). Using Behavioral Economics to Design Physician Incentives That Deliver High-Value Care. *Annals of Internal Medicine*, 164(2):114.

Emmert M et al. (2012). Economic evaluation of pay-for-performance in health care: a systematic review. *European Journal of Health Economics*, 13(6):755.

FHL (2012). Le modèle des Incitants Qualité – Bilan des démarches communes EHL – CNS et perspectives. Fédération des Hôpitaux Luxembourgeois.

French SD et al. (2010). Interventions for improving the appropriate use of imaging in people with musculoskeletal conditions. *Cochrane Database of Systematic Reviews*, (1):CD006094. West Sussex: John Wiley & Sons, Ltd.

Gillam S, Siriwardena AN, Steel N (2012). Pay-for-performance in the United Kingdom: impact of the quality and outcomes framework: a systematic review. *Annals of Family Medicine*, 10(5):461.

Gillam S, Steel N (2013). The Quality and Outcomes Framework – where next? *BMJ*, 346(2):f659.

Giuffrida A et al. (2000). Target payments in primary care: effects on professional practice and health care outcomes. *Cochrane Database of Systematic Reviews*, (3):CD000531.

Hamilton FL et al. (2013). Effectiveness of providing financial incentives to healthcare professionals for smoking cessation activities: systematic review. *Tobacco Control*, 22(1):3.

Houle SK et al. (2012). Does performance-based remuneration for individual health care practitioners affect patient care? A systematic review. *Annals of Internal Medicine*, 157(12):889.

Huang J et al. (2013). Impact of pay-for-performance on management of diabetes: a systematic review. *Journal of Evidence-Based Medicine*, 6(3):173.

Ivers N et al. (2012). Audit and feedback: effects on professional practice and healthcare outcomes. *Cochrane Database of Systematic Reviews*, (6):CD000259.

Kahneman D, Knetsch JL, Thaler R (1986). Fairness as a Constraint on Profit Seeking: Entitlements in the Market. *American Economic Review*, 76(4):728.

Kane RL et al. (2004). Economic incentives for preventive care. *Evidence Report/Technology Assessment (Summary)*, (101):1.

Kondo K et al. (2015). Understanding the Intervention and Implementation Factors Associated with Benefits and Harms of Pay for Performance Programs in Healthcare. Washington, DC: Department of Veterans Affairs.

Kondo KK et al. (2016). Implementation Processes and Pay for Performance in Healthcare: A Systematic Review. *Journal of General Internal Medicine*, 31(Suppl 1):61.

Korenstein D et al. (2016). Do Health Care Delivery System Reforms Improve Value? The Jury Is Still Out. *Medical Care*, 54(1):55.

Kouides RW et al. (1998). Performance-based physician reimbursement and influenza immunization rates in the elderly. The Primary-Care Physicians of Monroe County. *American Journal of Preventive Medicine*, 14(2):89.

Kristensen SR, Bech M, Lauridsen JT (2016). Who to pay for performance? The choice of organisational level for hospital performance incentives. *European Journal of Health Economics*, 17(4):435–42.

Kronick R, Casalino LP, Bindman AB (2015). Introduction. Apple Pickers or Federal Judges: Strong versus Weak Incentives in Physician Payment. *Health Services Research*, 50(Suppl 2):2049.

Langdown C, Peckham S (2014). The use of financial incentives to help improve health outcomes: is the quality and outcomes framework fit for purpose? A systematic review. *Journal of Public Health* (Oxford, England), 36(2):251.

Lin Y et al. (2015). Impact of Pay for performance on Behavior of Primary Care Physicians and Patient Outcomes. *Journal of Evidence-Based Medicine*, 9(1):8–23.

Lindgren P (2014). Ersättning i sjukvården: Modeller, effekter, rekommendationer. Stockholm: SNS Förl.

Mehrotra A et al. (2009). Pay for performance in the hospital setting: what is the state of the evidence? *American Journal of Medical Quality*, 24(1):19.

Milstein R, Schreyoegg J (2016). Pay for performance in the inpatient sector: a review of 34 P4P programs in 14 OECD countries. *Health policy* (Amsterdam, Netherlands), 120(10):1125–40.

Minister of Finance and Public Accounts/Minister of Social Affairs, Health and Women's Rights (2015). Arrêté du 23 février 2015 portant approbation du règlement arbitral applicable aux structures de santé pluri-professionnelles de proximité, 49.

Minister of Social Affairs and Health (2016). Arrêté du 5 août 2016 fixant les modalités de calcul du montant de la dotation allouée aux établissements de santé en application de l'article L. 162-22-20.

Mitenbergs U et al. (2012). Latvia: Health system review. *Health Systems in Transition*, 14(8).

MSPY (2016). National social report of Republic of Croatia. Ministry of Social Policy and Youth.

Murauskiene L et al. (2013). Lithuania: Health System Review. *Health Systems in Transition*, 15(2).

Nahra TA et al. (2006). Cost-effectiveness of hospital pay-for-performance incentives. *Medical Care Research and Review*, 63(1 Suppl):49S–72S.

NHS Digital (2016). Quality and Outcomes Framework – Prevalence, Achievements and Exceptions Report: England, 2015–2016. Available at: http://www.content.digital.nhs.uk/catalogue/PUB22266/qof-1516-rep-v2.pdf, accessed 13 March 2017.

NHS Employers (2011). Quality and Outcomes Framework for 2012/13: Guidance for PCOs and practices. Available at: http://www.nhsemployers.org/your-workforce/primary-care-contacts/

general-medical-services/quality-and-outcomes-framework/changes-to-qof-2012-13, accessed 13 March 2017.

NHS England Patient Safety Domain (2015). Revised Never Events Policy and Framework.

OECD (2016). OECD Health Systems Characteristics Survey: Section 10: Pay-for-performance and other financial incentives for providers. Available at: https://qdd.oecd.org/subject. aspx?Subject=hsc.

Ogundeji YK, Bland JM, Sheldon TA (2016). The effectiveness of payment for performance in health care: a meta-analysis and exploration of variation in outcomes. *Health Policy*, 120(10):1141–50.

Olsen CB, Brandborg G (2016). Quality Based Financing in Norway: Country Background Note: Norway. Norwegian Directorate of Health.

Petersen LA et al. (2006). Does Pay-for-Performance Improve the Quality of Health Care? *Annals of Internal Medicine*, 145(4):265.

Rashidian A et al. (2015). Pharmaceutical policies: effects of financial incentives for prescribers. *Cochrane Database of Systematic Reviews*, (8):CD006731.

Robinson JC (2001). Theory and Practice in the Design of Physician Payment Incentives. *Milbank Quarterly*, 79(2):149.

Roland M, Dudley RA (2015). How Financial and Reputational Incentives Can Be Used to Improve Medical Care. *Health Services Research*, 50(Suppl 2):2090.

Roland M, Guthrie B (2016). Quality and Outcomes Framework: what have we learnt? *BMJ (Clinical Research edition)*, 354:i4060.

Rosenthal MB et al. (2004). Paying For Quality: Providers' Incentives For Quality Improvement. *Health Affairs*, 23(2):127.

Roski J et al. (2003). The impact of financial incentives and a patient registry on preventive care quality: increasing provider adherence to evidence-based smoking cessation practice guidelines? Surveys available upon request from corresponding author. *Preventive Medicine*, 36(3):291.

Rynes SL, Gerhart B, Parks L (2005). Personnel psychology: performance evaluation and pay for performance. *Annual Review of Psychology*, 56:571.

Sabatino SA et al. (2008). Interventions to increase recommendation and delivery of screening for breast, cervical, and colorectal cancers by healthcare providers systematic reviews of provider assessment and feedback and provider incentives. *American Journal of Preventive Medicine*, 35(1 Suppl):S67–74.

Salize HJ et al. (2009). Cost-effective primary care-based strategies to improve smoking cessation: more value for money. *Archives of Internal Medicine*, 169(3):230–5 [discussion 235–6].

Sante.lu (2015). Incitants Qualité. Available at: http://www.sante.public.lu/fr/politique-sante/ systeme/financement/budget-hospitalier/incitants-qualite/index.html, accessed 4 July 2017.

Scott A et al. (2011). The effect of financial incentives on the quality of health care provided by primary care physicians. *Cochrane Database of Systematic Reviews*, (9):CD008451.

Sorbero ME et al. (2006). Assessment of Pay-for-Performance Options for Medicare Physician Services: Final Report. Washington, DC: RAND Corporation.

Srivastava D, Mueller M, Hewlett E (2016). Better Ways to Pay for Health Care. Paris: OECD Publishing.

Town R et al. (2005). Economic incentives and physicians' delivery of preventive care: a systematic review. *American Journal of Preventive Medicine*, 28(2):234.

van Herck P et al. (2010). Systematic review: effects, design choices, and context of pay-for-performance in health care. *BMC Health Services Research*, 10:247.

Walker S et al. (2010). Value for money and the Quality and Outcomes Framework in primary care in the UK NHS. *British Journal of General Practice*, 60(574):e213–20.

Wharam JF et al. (2009). High quality care and ethical pay-for-performance: a Society of General Internal Medicine policy analysis. *Journal of General Internal Medicine*, 24(7):854.

Part III

Chapter 15

Assuring and improving quality of care in Europe: conclusions and recommendations

Wilm Quentin, Dimitra Panteli, Niek Klazinga, Reinhard Busse

15.1 Introduction

Part I of this book started with the observation that quality is one of the most often-quoted principles of health policy – but that the understanding of the term and what it encompasses varies. Therefore, Part I provided a definition of the concept of quality (Chapter 1) before developing a comprehensive framework for understanding and describing the characteristic features of different quality strategies in Europe (Chapter 2). This was followed by an introduction to the conceptual and methodological complexities of measuring the quality of care (Chapter 3) and an analysis of the influence of international and European actors in governing and guiding the development of quality assurance and improvement strategies in Europe (Chapter 4).

Part II of this book provided an overview on the implementation of ten selected quality strategies across European countries and assessed the evidence on their effectiveness and, where possible, cost-effectiveness, before distilling recommendations that are useful for policy-makers interested in prioritizing, developing and implementing strategies to assure and improve the quality of care. The term "strategy" is used here in a relatively narrow sense to describe certain activities geared towards achieving selected quality assurance or improvement goals by targeting specific health system actors (for example, health professionals, provider organizations or patients). Elsewhere, these activities may be described as "quality interventions", "quality initiatives", or "quality improvement tools" (WHO, 2018). Together, these two parts of the book illustrate the high level of interest and activity in the field of quality assurance and improvement – and at the same time the lack of consensus about basic definitions and concepts, as well as the limitations of the evidence about how best to assure and improve quality of care.

This chapter draws together the main findings from Parts I and II in order to address the main question reflected in the title of this book, namely what we know about the characteristics, the effectiveness and the implementation of different quality strategies in Europe, and to make recommendations for policy-makers interested in comprehensive approaches for improving quality of care in their countries. The next section summarizes the main lessons from Part I of the book, clarifying key terms and concepts that enable a systematic assessment of the characteristics, the effectiveness and the implementation of the ten selected strategies discussed in the subsequent section. The final section concludes with policy recommendations on how to bring together the individual strategies into a coherent approach for assuring and improving the quality of care.

15.2 Defining, understanding and measuring quality of care within the international context

Quality is multidimensional, as explained in the first two chapters of this book and demonstrated throughout the volume. Many definitions take a very broad perspective on quality, including not only effectiveness, safety and patient-centredness, but often also efficiency, access, equity, appropriateness and timeliness. Common language constructs like "quality of care", "quality of health professionals", "quality of healthcare services" and "quality of healthcare systems" relate the concept of quality to a magnitude of subjects. This is, in fact, not surprising because quality – in general terms – is broadly understood as the ability to achieve desirable objectives using legitimate means (Donabedian, 1980). However, as highlighted in Chapter 1, it is important to have a clear and focused understanding of what we mean when we speak about the quality of healthcare. Otherwise, it becomes impossible to measure, to assure or to improve it.

To facilitate understanding of what quality entails, it is useful to distinguish between two levels: the first is the level of healthcare services, which may include preventive, acute, chronic and palliative care. When using the term quality in relation to healthcare services, there seems to be an emerging consensus that quality of care can be defined as the degree to which health services for individuals and populations are effective, safe and people-centred. The second is the level of the healthcare system as a whole. Internationally, healthcare systems have been conceptualized as having to assure access and quality (as intermediate goals) in order to achieve the overall goals of improved health, responsiveness, financial protection and efficiency (WHO, 2007).

In line with Donabedian's general definition of quality mentioned above, health-care systems can be considered to be of "high quality" when they achieve these goals. However, Chapter 1 argues that using the term quality at the health system level may create confusion. Instead, it proposes using the term "health system performance" for the degree to which health systems achieve their goals, thus distinguishing it from the concept of quality, which should be reserved for the healthcare services level. Such a narrow definition of quality is useful because it allows for a conceptual distinction between the concepts of access and quality. This is important because strategies aiming to improve access (for example, improving financial protection, assuring geographic availability of resources) often differ from the ones needed to improve quality of care.

Existing frameworks for understanding healthcare quality and describing quality strategies have traditionally focused on specific aspects of quality or on particular quality improvement strategies, for instance classifying different types of indicators (Donabedian, 1966) or describing the different steps needed to achieve quality improvements (Juran & Godfrey, 1999). However, there was no single, unifying framework for a systematic comparison of the wide range of different quality strategies discussed in the literature (Slawomirksi, Aaureen & Klazinga, 2017; WHO, 2018), which include those analysed in Part II of this book. Therefore, Chapter 2 develops a comprehensive framework that facilitates a better understanding of the characteristics of these strategies, and of how they can contribute to assessing, assuring or improving quality of care.

The resulting five-lens framework draws on existing concepts and approaches for thinking about quality assessment and implementation of change. The five lenses of the framework are meant to be complementary conceptual perspectives and include:

1. the three core dimensions of quality: safety, effectiveness and patient-centredness;

2. the four functions of healthcare: primary prevention, acute care, chronic care and palliative care;

3. the three main activities of quality strategies: setting standards, monitoring and assuring improvements;

4. Donabedian's triad: structures, processes and outcomes; and

5. the five main targets of quality strategies: health professionals, technologies, provider organizations, patients and payers.

Using the five lenses in combination can provide a more complete and more actionable picture of different quality strategies. For example, it is useful to characterize quality strategies according to their main target(s) (professionals, technologies, provider organizations, patients or payers – lens 5) and their main activity (setting standards, monitoring or assuring improvements – lens 3) to better understand the essence of the strategy. At the same time, the underlying rationale of why a strategy should contribute to healthcare quality can be understood by examining its effects on safety, effectiveness and/or patient-centredness (lens 1) through changes of structures, processes and/or outcomes (lens 4). Furthermore, it is possible to identify care areas missed by existing quality strategies using lens 2, i.e. examining whether strategies target preventive care, acute care, chronic care or palliative care.

In addition, the five-lens framework may help policy-makers decide where to focus their efforts by enabling a systematic assessment of different aspects of healthcare quality in their country: Which dimensions of quality need improvement (effectiveness, safety, patient-centredness)? Which functions of healthcare have received relatively limited attention (primary prevention, acute care, chronic care, palliative care)? Which activities have been neglected (standard setting, monitoring, assuring improvements)? Which part(s) of Donabedian's triad is problematic (structures, processes or outcomes)? And who could be targeted to achieve the greatest level of improvement (health professionals, technologies, provider organizations, patients and/or payers)?

A prerequisite for numerous quality assurance and improvement strategies discussed in Part II of this book is the availability of reliable information about the quality of care provided by different professionals and/or providers. For example, audit and feedback (*see* Chapter 10), public reporting (*see* Chapter 13), and pay for quality (*see* Chapter 14) rely heavily on indicators that measure quality of care. Moreover, without robust measurement of quality, it is unclear whether new regulations and/or quality assurance and improvement strategies actually work as expected and/or if there are adverse effects related to these changes. In light of the importance of quality measurement and the increasing interest of policy-makers, researchers and the general public, there is surprisingly little comprehensive guidance about how best to approach the conceptual and methodological challenges related to quality measurement.

Chapter 3 presents different approaches, frameworks and data sources used in quality measurement. It also highlights methodological challenges that need to be considered when making decisions on the basis of measured quality of care, such as risk-adjustment. As quality cannot be measured directly, most quality measurement initiatives are concerned with the development and assessment of quality indicators, which have been defined as quantitative measures that provide information about the effectiveness, safety and/or people-centredness of care. It is useful to distinguish between two main purposes of quality measurement: (1)

quality assurance, i.e. using reliable quality information for external account-ability and verification, and (2) quality improvement, i.e. using and interpreting information about quality differences to motivate change in provider behaviour. Depending on the purpose, quality measurement systems face different challenges with regard to indicators, data sources and the level of precision required.

More generally, the development of quality measurement systems should always take into account the purpose of measurement and different stakeholders' needs. Depending on the purpose and the concerned stakeholders, it may be useful to focus on indicators of structures (for example, for governments concerned about the availability of appropriate facilities, technologies or personnel), processes (for example, for professionals interested in quality improvement), or outcomes (for example, for citizens or policy-makers interested in international comparisons). Also, the appropriate level of aggregation of indicators into summary (composite) measures depends on the intended users of the information. For example, professionals will be interested mostly in detailed process indicators, which enable the identification of areas for improvement, while policy-makers and patients may be more interested in composite measures that help identify good (or best) providers. However, the wide range of methodological choices that determine the results of composite measures create uncertainty about the reliability of their results (*see* Chapter 3). Therefore, it is useful to present composite measures in a way that enables the user to disaggregate the information and see the individual indicators that went into the construction of the composite. Furthermore, methods should always be presented transparently to allow users to assess the quality of indicators and data sources (for example, using the criteria listed in Chapter 3), as well as the methods of measurement.

Existing conceptual frameworks and available approaches for measurement and assessment, as well as national policies for quality assurance and improvement, have been strongly influenced by WHO, the EU and other international actors. The influence of these international actors on quality policies and strategies has been explored in more detail in Chapter 4. The international influence is evident through a range of different (legally binding or non-binding) mechanisms in four main areas:

1. raising political awareness for quality and creating a common vision on how to improve it;

2. providing frameworks for implementation and sharing experiences across countries;

3. developing and providing standards and models that can be transposed into national policy; and

4. measuring, assessing and comparing quality.

WHO and the EU have been instrumental in raising political awareness through a range of declarations and strategies (for example, Health 21 or the 2006 Council Conclusions on Common Values and Principles in EU Health Systems), which contributed to putting quality of care on the agenda of national governments. They both also actively promote the exchange of experience between countries, helping governments to translate political awareness into concrete policy action, for example, by mapping the various approaches taken by different countries in designing quality improvement strategies and organizing quality structures. WHO also supported the development of common indicators in several areas of healthcare and of benchmarking tools to support national quality improvement efforts.

Common quality standards have been developed most importantly by the Council of Europe and the EU. On the one hand, the Council of Europe has promoted quality through legally non-binding recommendations, for example, on the development and implementation of quality improvement systems (No. R(97)17) and on evidence-based clinical practice guidelines (No. R(2001)13). On the other hand, it has provided compulsory standards for the production and quality control of medicines (through the European Pharmacopoeia) and legally binding international instruments of criminal law to fight against the production and distribution of counterfeit medicines (through the Medicrime Convention). Also the European Foundation for Quality Management, the International Organization for Standardization (ISO) and the European Committee for Standardization (CEN) provide standards that contribute to assuring the quality of care and facilitating the free movement of services and goods. These standards are particularly important for external institutional strategies, such as accreditation or certification of providers (*see* Chapter 8).

However, even more important in terms of assuring the safety of available products and services are the legally binding EU standards under the internal market legislation for pharmaceuticals, medical devices and other healthcare products, health professionals and health services (*see* Chapter 4), which have a direct influence on the regulation of professionals (*see* Chapter 5), medical technologies (*see* Chapter 6), and facilities (*see* Chapter 7) in countries in Europe.

With regard to measuring, assessing and comparing quality of health service provision in different countries, the Organisation for Economic Co-operation and Development (OECD) has played an important role in complementing and coordinating the efforts of national and other international bodies. It developed specific indicators for measuring quality in several disease areas (for example, cancer, cardiovascular diseases) and for measuring patient safety and patient experience, which have been widely adopted in Europe (*see also* related discussions in Chapter 1 and the rationale behind the two first lenses of the five-lens framework in Chapter 2). More recently, the EU has also increased its role in monitoring quality as part of the broader monitoring process of financial sustainability, which has led to increasing activity in health system performance assessment, as illustrated (amongst others) by the Expert Group on Health System Performance Assessment (2016) report on quality.

15.3 Characteristics, effectiveness and implementation of different quality strategies in Europe

The discussion of the ten selected quality strategies in Part II of the book was guided by the five-lens framework developed in Chapter 2. Each chapter provided a definition of the discussed strategy, and sometimes also of different substrategies that were included within one chapter (for example, accreditation, certification and supervision in Chapter 8 on external institutional strategies). Several lenses of the five-lens framework guided the ordering of chapters in Part II: Donabedian's triad, i.e. structures, processes and outcomes of care (lens 4), the primary target groups of quality strategies (lens 5), and the main activities of different strategies, i.e. standard setting, monitoring and/or assuring improvements (lens 3).

Fig. 15.1 illustrates how the different strategies discussed in Part II can be classified into three main groups defined on the basis of these three lenses of the framework:

- The first group consists of strategies that are mostly concerned with healthcare structures and inputs, mainly by setting standards: the regulation of health professionals (Chapter 5), of technologies through Health Technology Assessment (Chapter 6), and of healthcare facilities (Chapter 7). In addition, this group includes external institutional strategies, such as accreditation, certification and supervision (Chapter 8). However, these strategies mark the transition towards the second group of strategies because they set standards also for processes and they are also concerned – to a considerable degree – with monitoring compliance with these standards in order to assure improvements.

- The second group consists of strategies that steer and monitor quality of healthcare processes. This group includes two strategies, which are focused on setting standards for processes, i.e. clinical guidelines for professionals (Chapter 9) and clinical pathways for provider institutions (Chapter 12), and two strategies that focus on monitoring processes and assuring improvements, i.e. audit and feedback directed primarily at professionals (Chapter 10), and patient safety strategies (Chapter 11).

- The third group consists of two strategies that are concerned with leveraging processes and outcomes; i.e. they use information about quality of processes and outcomes to assure improvements in the quality of care. This group includes public reporting (Chapter 13) and pay-for-quality (Chapter 14).

Fig. 15.1 *The complementarity of different quality strategies included in this book*

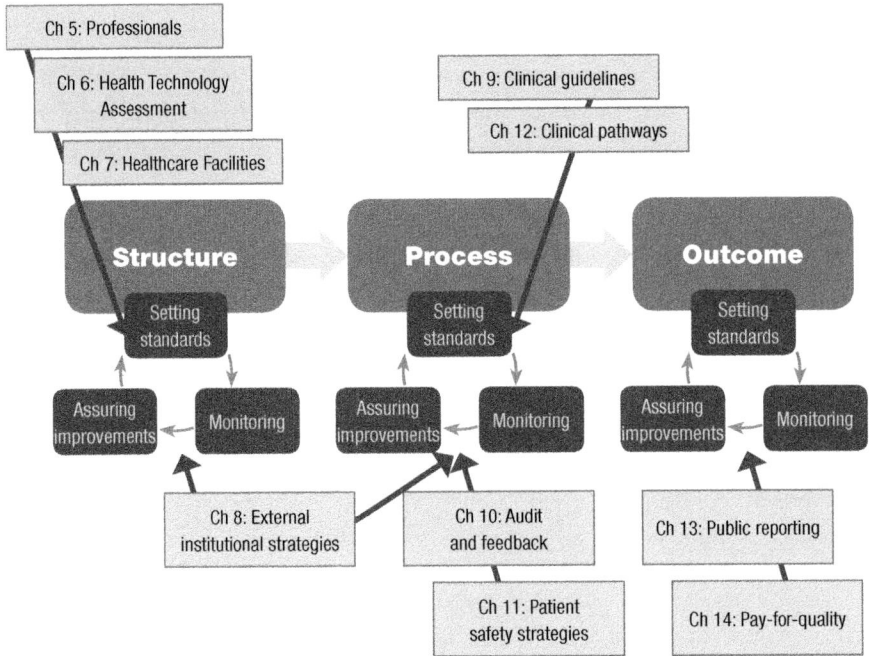

Source: authors' compilation

Of course, this classification ignores several details of individual strategies, for example, audit and feedback may be concerned also with structures and outcomes, and public reporting may also report on structures. Nevertheless, it is useful as it underlines the characteristic features of each strategy.

Fig. 15.1 also highlights the complementarity of the discussed strategies in assuring and improving different aspects of healthcare quality. This means that each of these strategies has its place in the overall mission of assuring and improving quality of care, and the same effects are unlikely to be achieved through implementation of another strategy. In addition, Fig. 15.1 may support policy-makers in identifying the most important areas of work, where additional strategies are needed to assure and improve the quality of care. For example, in the figure no strategy contributes to assuring improvements of structures. Yet other strategies are available (*see* Chapter 1) which could be implemented, such as training and supervision of the workforce.

The next subsections discuss the main findings of Chapters 5 to 14 separately for the three groups of strategies.

15.3.1 Setting standards for healthcare structures and inputs

Table 15.1 summarizes information about the characteristics, effectiveness and implementation of the four strategies primarily aimed at setting standards for healthcare structures and inputs based on Chapters 5 to 8. In general, there is a range of different standards for health professionals, technologies and facilities in every country. However, the level of detail of regulation and the maturity of programmes for Health Technology Assessment and/or accreditation vary widely. The available evidence on the effectiveness of different strategies is surprisingly limited and often inconclusive.

For professionals, the most important standards concern educational require-ments for entering the profession and requirements for continuous professional development. These standards exist in most countries of the EU for both physi-cians and nurses, and the necessary educational attainment for achieving profes-sional qualification is largely influenced by the relevant European directives (*see* Chapter 4). There has been very little research investigating different parts of professional requirements, and evidence on the effects of specific standards for entry requirements or continuous education is almost non-existent.

Standards for health technologies, including pharmaceuticals, medical devices and other medical products, are often directly determined by EU regulations, as discussed in Chapter 4. However, the purpose of most EU regulations is only to assure the safety of different technologies and conformity with certain mini-mum standards. EU regulations rarely concern effectiveness or cost-effectiveness of different technologies. More detailed regulation is (still) left to the national level, where most countries have implemented a system of Health Technology Assessment (HTA). As discussed in Chapter 6, HTA is a process that systemati-cally reviews the evidence base to select safe, effective technologies that provide value for money in healthcare. In most countries the focus of HTA is on assessing pharmaceuticals but increasingly HTA is also performed to assess medical devices.

Different countries have to deal with different challenges, depending on the maturity of their HTA programmes as these differ considerably concerning the size of institutions and the robustness of the assessment, as well as the uptake of HTA results in decision-making. However, the effectiveness of HTA at assuring or improving quality of care depends on the rigour of its methods and the influ-ence of HTA on decision-making. No research is available that has systematically

Table 15.1 *Characteristics, effectiveness and implementation of strategies setting standards for healthcare structures and inputs*

	Characteristics	Implementation in Europe	Effectiveness
Regulating the input – professionals (Chapter 5)	A wide range of standards for professionals, including regulating (educational) requirements for entering the profession, continuous professional development, etc.	Most countries have entry requirements and professional development requirements (for physicians and nurses); these are strongly influenced by EU regulations	Very limited evidence on effectiveness of different parts of the strategy
Regulating the input: Health Technology Assessment (HTA) (Chapter 6)	HTA provides the evidence base for decision-making on (cost-)effective and safe technologies	Established frameworks for HTA are in place in most Member States, usually focusing on pharmaceuticals and increasingly also on medical devices. HTA programme structures, processes and methodologies vary by country but have been influenced by cross-country collaboration	Effectiveness depends on rigour of applied methods and the implementation of HTA results. Very little evidence on (cost)-effectiveness.
Regulating the input: facilities (Chapter 7)	Setting standards for the structures of care that will lead to improved effectiveness, safety and patient-centredness.	Some European-wide standards for buildings and construction materials apply. Most countries have general building standards, some have healthcare-specific standards. Integration of "evidence-based design" elements is variable and requires strong leadership	Evidence on the effectiveness and cost-effectiveness of different design elements in the context of quality ("evidence-based design") is expansive but largely inconclusive
External assessment strategies (Chapter 8)	Accreditation, certification and supervision encourage the compliance of healthcare organizations with published standards through monitoring.	Widely implemented in Europe. Most countries have market entry requirements (supervision), coupled with certification and accreditation strategies. There is no overview of certified/accredited institutions in different countries. Increasing involvement of the EU in standardizing standards	Most research available on effectiveness of accreditation. Little robust evidence available that supports effectiveness of the three substrategies, no evidence on cost-effectiveness

assessed the effect of introducing a national HTA programme on assuring or improving quality of care in a country. In the upcoming years changes in HTA programmes at country level will likely be influenced by European developments, and it is clear that the potential for synergies is immense.

Potentially, standards for healthcare facilities that would take into account the available evidence about the effect of certain features, such as single-bed rooms, good acoustic environment, etc., could have an important impact on quality of care (*see* Chapter 7). However, most countries have only general building standards for healthcare infrastructure, which are influenced by EU standards for buildings and construction materials. Some countries, like the UK, have more specific healthcare-related standards, while other countries with a more market-oriented healthcare system, like the Netherlands, make fewer requirements for healthcare facilities. The evidence on the effectiveness and cost-effectiveness of different design elements in the context of quality (so-called "evidence-based design") is expansive but largely inconclusive. Fostering the creation of a robust evidence base that informs and is informed by new projects seems necessary.

In order to assure compliance with defined standards, all countries need to have a monitoring process in place. Depending on the country, (regular) monitoring of compliance with standards is sometimes called (re)licensing, (re)certification, or (re-)accreditation – and the use of these terms may further differ depending on whether monitoring concerns organizations, technologies and/or professionals. In the context of external institutional strategies (Chapter 8), the monitoring of compliance with government (minimum) standards for provider organizations was defined as "supervision", while the monitoring of standards that go beyond minimum standards was defined as "accreditation" (if standards come from independent bodies) or "certification" (if standards come from the International Standardization Organization).

External institutional strategies are widely implemented in Europe. Most countries have in place market entry requirements (licensing strategies) for healthcare providers, coupled with certification or accreditation strategies to ensure and improve the quality of care. The scope of these strategies differs substantially between and sometimes within countries. Despite the widespread uptake of external institutional strategies, there is little robust evidence to support their effectiveness and no evidence on cost-effectiveness. In light of the widespread implementation of, often expensive, external assessment strategies and the lack of conclusive evidence of what is (cost-)effective and how it can be implemented, decision-makers should further support research into the relative effectiveness of (a) the strategies themselves (accreditation, certification and supervision), (b) the key components of each strategy, and (c) their impact on patients and workforce.

15.3.2 Steering and monitoring quality of healthcare processes

Table 15.2 provides an overview of the characteristics, effectiveness and implementation of the four strategies with a focus on steering and monitoring quality of healthcare processes based on Chapters 9 to 12. Again, most countries in Europe have implemented all of the strategies included in the table. However, implementation varies even more strongly than for strategies concerned with setting standards for healthcare structures, which is related to the fact that EU regulations play only a minor role with regard to steering and monitoring the quality of healthcare processes. Often Germany, the Netherlands and the UK are amongst those countries that have relatively strong programmes. There is much more research available on strategies concerned with healthcare processes than on strategies concerned with structures, but results are mixed for clinical guidelines (Chapter 9) and several patient safety strategies (Chapter 11). The most reliable evidence is available for the effectiveness of audit and feedback (Chapter 10) and clinical pathways (Chapter 12), although effects were often relatively small and mostly related to process quality.

As discussed in Chapter 9, clinical guidelines inform clinical practice to facilitate evidence-based healthcare processes. However, as guidelines need to be adapted to the national context, they cannot be based exclusively on evidence from the global scientific literature but have to consider the regulatory context as well as empirical data, for example, about the availability of equipment and pharmaceuticals in the specific country and context. Clinical guidelines are being used in many countries as a quality strategy, albeit usually without a legal basis. Country practices in Europe are diverse, ranging from well established, broad and prolific systems to nascent utilization with cross-country borrowing. The rigour of guideline development, mode of implementation and evaluation of impact can be improved in many settings to enable their goal of achieving "best practice" in healthcare.

There is mixed evidence about the effectiveness of guidelines at improving patient outcomes but a clear link has been established between effects and the modalities of guideline implementation. In particular, user experience should be taken into account, which is already attempted to varying degrees by means of stakeholder involvement in guideline development. There is currently no discussion about a concerted centralization of the dissemination, let alone the development, of guidelines at EU level (although umbrella organizations of different professional associations produce European guidelines for their specialties). Persisting challenges for guideline implementation include up-to-dateness and inclusion of new evidence; another issue that should receive sufficient consideration is the issue of multimorbidity, which will need to be better addressed in guideline development.

Audit and feedback strategies may support the implementation of clinical guidelines by monitoring compliance, and they may provide professionals with information about their performance and the existence of best practices (*see* Chapter 10). An audit is a systematic review of professional performance, based on explicit criteria or standards. Often audits are based on a broad set of indicators, including mostly process indicators (but sometimes also indicators of structures and outcomes) that are mostly focused on the effectiveness and/

Table 15.2   *Characteristics, effectiveness and implementation of quality strategies steering and monitoring healthcare processes*

	Characteristics	Implementation in Europe	Effectiveness
Clinical practice guidelines (Chapter 9)	Guidelines mainly support clinical decision-making in order to reduce unwarranted variation of healthcare processes, mostly in order to improve effectiveness and safety. They increasingly account for patient-centredness by fostering shared decision-making.	Systematically developed, evidence-based clinical guidelines are being used in many countries as a quality strategy, albeit usually without a legal basis. Country practices in Europe are diverse, ranging from well established, broad and prolific systems to nascent utilization with cross-country borrowing.	Studies show mixed results regarding the effect of guidelines on outcomes, but a clear link with implementation modalities.
Audit and feedback (Chapter 10)	Audit and feedback reviews professional performance based on explicit criteria of standards of care, with the aim to improve healthcare processes, thus leading to better effectiveness and safety.	The UK and the Netherlands are the countries in Europe that have the longest history of audit and feedback, but other countries have become increasingly active since the late 1990s, with prominent programmes existing in Finland, Germany, Ireland, Italy, the Netherlands and the UK.	Numerous robust studies on the effects of audit and feedback show a small to moderate effect on professional compliance with desired clinical practice. Effect on patient outcomes is less clear, although several studies indicate positive results.
Patient safety culture (Chapter 11)	A broad range of initiatives and interventions that foster safety of care exist at system, organization and clinical levels, using a range of different strategies. The contribution of developing a culture conducive to safety to anchor individual interventions is considered critical.	In 2014, 26 EU countries had patient safety strategies or programmes, and patient safety standards were mandatory in 20 countries. In addition, 27 countries had adverse event reporting and learning systems, mostly at national and provider levels. However, only four countries had targeted patient safety education and training of health workers, highlighting the need for a stronger focus on safety culture. Certain countries, like the Netherlands, are pioneers in this respect.	Empirical research on the link between safety culture and patient outcomes is inconclusive. Evidence suggests that the relationship between culture, behaviours and clinical outcomes could be circular, with changes in behaviours and outcomes also improving safety culture.
Clinical pathways (CPWs) (Chapter 12)	Pathways focus on standardizing healthcare processes to align clinical practice with guideline recommendations in order to provide high-quality care within institutions (mostly hospitals).	The use of CPWs has been growing in Europe since the 1990s, beginning in the UK. Clinical pathways are currently being used in most EU and other European countries. The European Pathways Association has more than 50 national members. Increasing use of pathways was found in Belgium, England, Germany and the Netherlands.	Available research found significantly improved clinical documentation and reduced hospital complications, while reductions in hospital mortality and readmissions were not significant. Most available studies found reductions in costs of hospital stays.

or safety domains, as these are usually easiest to measure using administrative databases and/or electronic medical records. In some countries/regions patient surveys are also used to add indicators of patient-centredness to measurement systems. This information is subsequently fed back to professionals in a structured manner, with the goal of behavioural change.

The UK and the Netherlands are the countries in Europe that have the longest history of audit and feedback, but other countries have become increasingly active since the late 1990s. There are numerous robust studies on the effects of audit and feedback on patient care. Generally they show a small to moderate effect on professional compliance with desired clinical practice. The available evidence on effects on patient outcomes is less clear, although several studies indicate positive results. The effectiveness of audit and feedback compared to other quality improvement interventions has not been evaluated, nor has its cost-effectiveness compared to usual care. As a strategy, audit and feedback is more effective when focusing on providers with poor performance at baseline. Audit and feedback schemes should always include clear targets and an action plan specifying the steps necessary to achieve them. Organizational commitment to a constructive (i.e., non-punitive) approach to continuous quality improvement is essential and the availability of reliable, routinely collected data (which impact the costs of an intervention) should be taken into account when considering audit and feedback interventions.

Monitoring and improving processes of care is also at the heart of most patient safety strategies (*see* Chapter 11). However, to achieve improvements in patient safety the implementation of a (non-punitive) patient safety culture is essential, allowing blame-free reporting of adverse events and promoting an organizational environment that is open to change and continuous learning. Almost all countries (26 in 2014) have patient safety strategies or programmes, and these are mostly mandatory (*see* Table 15.2). Almost all countries also have adverse event reporting and learning systems, mostly at national and provider levels. However, cultivating a safety culture is crucial for the success of safety interventions. The Netherlands has been a pioneer in this regard.

Evidence on the effectiveness of patient safety strategies and in particular on the effectiveness of having a patient safety culture is inconclusive. This is also related to the wide range of different strategies, and some are considered to be cost-effective by many experts. Different patient safety strategies should be coordinated, and a patient safety culture should already start at the policy level. Professional education, clear evidence-based safety standards and the possibility for blame-free reporting of adverse events are indispensable in this respect. To effectively, sustainably and adaptively address patient safety issues, leadership across all levels of the healthcare systems will be of the utmost importance.

Still concerning healthcare processes, clinical pathways provide practical standards that provide guidance to professionals concerning the treatment of particular groups of patients with regard to the use of technologies within the context of a specific organization (*see* Chapter 12). Clinical pathways usually aim at both improving quality and increasing efficiency of care. The main difference between clinical guidelines and clinical pathways is that guidelines are focused on supporting the decisions of health professionals in the treatment of patients (based on the best available evidence), while clinical pathways are focused on describing the successive steps in the diagnosis and treatment of a specific patient group in a particular organization.

In a number of countries, such as the UK but increasingly also Belgium, Germany and the Netherlands, clinical pathways have been implemented in healthcare organizations, often based on decentralized decisions of hospital managers. It is likely that pathways will become increasingly used also in many other countries in Europe in an attempt to further standardize care processes and to increase efficiency. Overall, clinical pathways have been shown to be associated with improved patient safety and better documentation. Also, most studies found reductions in hospital costs related to implementation. Engagement of both clinical and management staff in the development and adoption of clinical pathways is required. Since developing pathways can be resource-intensive, for local healthcare providers and policy-makers the choice of implementing clinical pathway strategies should be based upon considerations of their likely costs and benefits.

15.3.3 Leveraging processes and outcomes

Table 15.3 draws together the findings of Chapters 13 and 14, summarizing the characteristics, effectiveness and implementation of public reporting and pay for quality (P4Q) strategies. In general, fewer countries have implemented P4Q and public reporting than the other strategies but they are still found in many countries in Europe (*see* Table 15.3). The two strategies are probably the most controversial ones discussed in the book as there has been considerable debate about the potential unintended consequences of both strategies. There have been a lot of studies investigating the effectiveness of public reporting and P4Q in improving quality of care but the available evidence remains inconclusive because studies are often of poor to moderate quality.

Public reporting uses systematically collected information about quality of care measured in terms of structure, process or outcome indicators and reports this information to the general public, enabling evaluation of the quality of healthcare services provided by specific organizations and professionals. Public reporting is expected to contribute to improvements in effectiveness, safety and/

or responsiveness (depending on the measured and reported indicators) by enabling patients to select high-quality providers. The strategy provides incentives to providers to improve their quality of care because patients may, in theory, choose those providers that provide better quality of care. However, in practice, patients have been found to make relatively limited use of publicly reported information about quality.

An increasing number of countries in Europe uses public reporting of quality indicators by hospitals, GPs or specialists. Relatively elaborated public reporting initiatives have been implemented in the United Kingdom (NHS Choices), the Netherlands (KiesBeter, "Make better Choices"), Germany (Weisse Liste, "White List") and Denmark (sundhed.dk, "Health"). Studies have shown that public reporting is associated with a small reduction in mortality, although the quality of the available evidence is moderate or low. Public reporting seems to be more effective in competitive markets and if baseline performance is low. However, there has been substantial debate about potential unintended consequences, such as an exclusive focus on measured and reported quality indicators with the risk that quality in other areas receives less attention or that providers may select healthier patients to look better on reported quality of care – although evidence for the existence of these unintended consequences is limited. Involving all relevant stakeholders (patients/patient organizations and staff at all levels of organization) is paramount for the implementation of public reporting initiatives. Both clinical outcomes and patient satisfaction should be reported, and information should be available at different levels of aggregation. Of course, the effectiveness of public reporting depends strongly on the quality of quality measurement (*see* Chapter 3).

P4Q initiatives provide direct financial incentives to providers and/or professionals related to the measured quality of care. As financial incentives are a powerful tool to change the behaviour of providers, P4Q could potentially have an important effect on assuring improvements. P4Q can be implemented in various healthcare settings and in combination with other quality improvement strategies and can concern different types of healthcare providers and professionals. P4Q schemes can reward desired outcomes, processes and structures, or penalize poor performance. The implementation of P4Q schemes began in the late 1990s. P4Q programmes for primary and/or hospital care exist in at least 16 European countries. The size of the financial incentives varies between 0.1% and 30% of total provider income in primary care and between 0.5% and 10% of total provider income in hospital care.

Overall, the effectiveness and cost-effectiveness of P4Q schemes remain unclear. The best available evidence suggests small positive effects on process-of-care (POC) indicators in primary care, but not in hospitals. Evidence remains inconclusive regarding health outcomes and patient safety. Patient experience and satisfaction were rarely evaluated and usually did not improve. It is clear that P4Q programmes are technically and politically difficult to implement. They seem to be more effective when the focus of a scheme is on areas of quality where change is needed and if the scheme embraces a more comprehensive approach, covering many different areas of care. Again, all relevant stakeholders should be involved in the process of scheme development and schemes should reinforce professional norms and beliefs. The contents and structure of the scheme have to be regularly reviewed and updated, and adverse behavioural responses need to be monitored in order to avoid unintended consequences. More evidence is needed on the comparative effectiveness of P4Q schemes in comparison to other quality improvement initiatives.

Table 15.3 *Characteristics, effectiveness and implementation of quality strategies leveraging processes and especially outcomes of care*

	Characteristics	Implementation in Europe	Effectiveness
Public reporting (Chapter 13)	Public reporting is characterized by the reporting of quality-related information to the general public about non-anonymous, identifiable professionals and providers, using systematically gathered comparative data.	At least 10 countries in Europe publicly report quality at provider level. Relatively elaborated public reporting initiatives have been implemented in the United Kingdom, the Netherlands, Germany and Denmark.	Several reviews found that public reporting is associated with improved care processes and a reduction of mortality, although the quality of available evidence is moderate or low. Public reporting has been found to be more effective if baseline performance is low.
Pay for Quality (Chapter 14)	Pay for Quality (P4Q) consists of a financial incentive being paid to a provider or professional for achieving a quality-related target within a specific time-frame.	Since the late 1990s 14 primary care P4Q programmes and 13 hospital P4Q programmes were identified in a total of 16 European countries. P4Q schemes in primary care incentivize mostly process and structural quality with respect to prevention and chronic care. P4Q schemes in hospital care prioritize improvements in health outcomes and patient safety.	Studies suggest small positive effects on process-of-care (POC) indicators in primary care but not in hospital care. Evidence on health outcomes and patient safety indicators is inconclusive. Cost-effectiveness is unlikely because of lacking effectiveness.

15.4 A coherent approach for assuring and improving quality of care

The previous section brought together the quality strategies discussed individually in Part II of this book. It highlighted that many countries in Europe have implemented several of those strategies, and that although several of them are effective (primarily regarding process indicators), the size of these effects is generally modest and data on relative effectiveness and cost-effectiveness are often inconclusive or unavailable. What is more, while the volume of evidence on some of the discussed strategies is considerable, the overall quality of evidence is low.

In general, political activities related to the quality strategies discussed in this book are increasing, albeit with unsurprising variability across countries. At first sight, this increase in activity might be surprising given the limitations of the available evidence. However, from a policy-maker's perspective, implementation of quality strategies may be warranted even if evidence is limited because several of the strategies respond to important needs of patients and politicians. For example, external institutional strategies may assure the population (and the politicians) that quality is under control. Public reporting responds to the desire of patients to have information about the quality of care (even if they do not use it) and to increase transparency and accountability of providers. Similarly, the need for continuous improvement in professional practice may warrant the implementation of strategies such as audit and feedback.

Despite the increased political attention, quality strategies are often not coordinated or placed within a coherent policy or overall strategic framework. Thus, from a policy-maker's perspective, the goal becomes understanding the potential for best practice, the possibility for synergies between strategies and the meaningfulness of investing in different elements given existing practices and identified areas where action is needed. Fig. 15.1 in this chapter provides a visual basis for these considerations. The Handbook for National Quality Policy and Strategy provides guidance for the development of a national quality policy and strategy (WHO, 2018). It highlights the importance of defining national priorities, developing a local definition of quality, identifying relevant stakeholders, analysing the situation to identify care areas in need of improvement, assessing governance and organizational structure, and selecting quality improvement interventions (or strategies, according to the terminology of this book). In addition, it highlights the importance of improving the health information system to enable reliable measurement of selected quality indicators.

Indeed, the implementation of individual quality strategies is not enough to assure the provision of high-quality care in a country. Instead, a holistic approach – or an "overall strategy" – is required, encompassing a number of strategies that are aligned to achieve optimal outcomes of care. Ideally, the selection and implementation of different strategies should be focused on those aspects of the healthcare system that are in greatest need of improvement – also because evidence has shown that several of the strategies are most effective if focused on care areas or providers that are currently providing relatively poor care. Furthermore, regular re-evaluations of the impact and technical aspects of implemented strategies is of great importance to maintain and/or update good practice. The recommendation in most chapters in Part II is that policy-makers need to take a long-term perspective and that achieving quality improvements through implementation of any of the strategies will take many years. Government or system leadership is therefore key in providing direction and guidance, and understanding the specifics of different strategy options is instrumental in enabling relevant choices.

To make the individual strategies discussed in this book work in an optimal way, maintaining an overview is absolutely necessary, as well as being aware of conflicting standards, un-coordinated monitoring through a fragmented information infrastructure, bureaucratization, links between accountability mechanisms and improvement, and between learning mechanisms and the entrenchment of stakeholders in the healthcare system behind their own interests. Again, this extensive to-do list underlines the need for the development of a national quality strategy. To use a mechanical metaphor, each quality strategy can be considered a cogwheel and the task of a national quality strategy is to assure that all the cogwheels are connected and turning in the same direction resulting in the desired output and outcomes. If a more organic metaphor is used, the health system can be considered a human body with many different organisms and a delicate immune system. A national quality strategy tries to strengthen the immune system and make the organs and the body as a whole function well and be resilient against threats from outside.

References

Donabedian A (1966). Evaluating the quality of medical care. *Milbank Quarterly*, 44(3, Pt. 2):166–203.

Donabedian A (1980). The Definition of Quality and Approaches to Its Assessment. Vol 1. Explorations in Quality Assessment and Monitoring. Ann Arbor, Michigan: Health Administration Press.

Expert Group on Health Systems Performance Assessment (2016). So What? Strategies across Europe to assess quality of care. Available at: https://ec.europa.eu/health/sites/health/files/systems_performance_assessment/docs/sowhat_en.pdf, accessed 14 April 2019.

Juran JM, Godfrey A (1999). Juran's Quality Handbook. New York: McGraw-Hill.

Slawomirski L, Auraaen A, Klazinga N (2017). The economics of patient safety. Paris: Organization for Economic Development and Cooperation.

WHO (2007). Everybody's business: strengthening health systems to improve health outcomes: WHO's framework for action. Geneva: World Health Organization.

WHO (2018). Handbook for national quality policy and strategy – a practical approach for developing policy and strategy to improve quality of care. Geneva: World Health Organization.